Health Informatics

This series is directed to healthcare professionals leading the transformation of healthcare by using information and knowledge. For over 20 years, Health Informatics has offered a broad range of titles: some address specific professions such as nursing, medicine, and health administration; others cover special areas of practice such as trauma and radiology; still other books in the series focus on interdisciplinary issues, such as the computer based patient record, electronic health records, and networked healthcare systems. Editors and authors, eminent experts in their fields, offer their accounts of innovations in health informatics. Increasingly, these accounts go beyond hardware and software to address the role of information in influencing the transformation of healthcare delivery systems around the world. The series also increasingly focuses on the users of the information and systems: the organizational, behavioral, and societal changes that accompany the diffusion of information technology in health services environments.

Developments in healthcare delivery are constant; in recent years, bioinformatics has emerged as a new field in health informatics to support emerging and ongoing developments in molecular biology. At the same time, further evolution of the field of health informatics is reflected in the introduction of concepts at the macro or health systems delivery level with major national initiatives related to electronic health records (EHR), data standards, and public health informatics.

These changes will continue to shape health services in the twenty-first century. By making full and creative use of the technology to tame data and to transform information, Health Informatics will foster the development and use of new knowledge in healthcare.

More information about this series at http://www.springer.com/series/1114

William Hersh

Information Retrieval: A Biomedical and Health Perspective

Fourth Edition

Springer

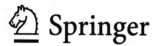

William Hersh
Oregon Health & Science University
Portland, OR
USA

ISSN 1431-1917 ISSN 2197-3741 (electronic)
Health Informatics
ISBN 978-3-030-47688-5 ISBN 978-3-030-47686-1 (eBook)
https://doi.org/10.1007/978-3-030-47686-1

This Springer imprint is published by the registered company Springer Nature Switzerland AG
The registered company address is: Gewerbestrasse 11, 6330 Cham, Switzerland

To Sally, Becca, Alyssa, and AJ

Preface

The main goal of this book is to provide an understanding of the theory, implementation, and evaluation of information retrieval (IR) systems in biomedicine and health. There is already a great deal of "how-to" information on searching for biomedical and health information (some listed in Chap. 1). Similarly, there are also a number of high-quality basic IR textbooks (also listed in Chap. 1). This volume is different from all of the above in that it covers basic IR as do the latter books, but with a distinct focus on the biomedical and health domain.

The first three editions of this book were published in 1996, 2003, and 2009. Although subsequent editions of books in many fields represent incremental updates, this edition is profoundly rewritten and is essentially a new book. The IR world has changed substantially since I wrote the first three editions of the book. At the time of the first edition, IR systems were available and not too difficult to access if you had the means and expertise. Also, in that edition, the Internet was a "special topic" in the very last chapter of the book. By the second edition, the World Wide Web had become a widespread platform for the use of information access and delivery, but had not achieved the nearly ubiquitous and saturated use it has now. At present, however, not only must health care professionals and biomedical researchers understand how to use IR systems to be effective in their work, but patients and consumers must also as well to attain optimal health care.

Similar to previous editions will be the maintenance of a Web site for errata and updates. The Website http://www.irbook.info/ will identify all errors in the book text as well as provide updates on important new findings in the field as they become available.

As in the first three editions, the approach is still to introduce all the necessary theory to allow coverage of the implementation and evaluation of IR systems in biomedicine and health. Any book on theoretical aspects must necessarily use technical jargon, and this book is no exception. Although jargon is minimized, it cannot be eliminated without retreating to a more superficial level of coverage. The reader's understanding of the jargon will vary based on their background, but anyone with some background in computers, libraries, health, and/or biomedicine should be able to understand most of the terms used. In any case, an attempt to define all jargon terms is made.

Another approach is to attempt wherever possible to classify topics, whether discussing types of information or models of evaluation. I have always found classification useful in providing an overview of complex topics. One problem, of course, is that everything does not fit into the neat and simple categories of the classification. This occurs repeatedly with IR, and the reader is forewarned.

This book had its origins in a tutorial taught at the former Symposium on Computer Applications in Medicine (SCAMC) meeting. The content continues to grow each year through my course taught to biomedical informatics students in the on-campus and disease-learning programs at OHSU. (Students often do not realize that next year's course content is based in part on the new and interesting things they teach me!) The book can be used in either a basic information science course or a biomedical and health informatics course. It should also provide a strong background for others interested in this topic, including those who design, implement, use, and evaluate IR systems.

Interest continues to grow in biomedical and health IR systems. I entered a fellowship in medical informatics at Harvard University in the late 1980s, during the initial era of medical artificial intelligence. I had assumed I would take up the banner of some aspect of that area, such as knowledge representation. But along the way I came across a reference from the field of "information retrieval." It looked interesting, so I looked at the references of that reference. It did not take long to figure out that this was where my real interests lay, and I spent many an afternoon in my fellowship tracing references in the Harvard University and Massachusetts Institute of Technology libraries. Even though I had not yet heard of the field of bibliometrics, I was personally validating all its principles. Like many in the field, I have been amazed to see IR become so "mainstream" with its routine use by almost everyone on the planet.

The book is divided into eight chapters. Chapter 1 provides basic definitions and models that will be used throughout the book. It also points to resources for the field and introduces evaluation of systems. Chapter 2 provides an overview of biomedical and health information, describing some of the issues in its production, dissemination, and use. Chapter 3 gives an overview of the great deal of content that is currently available. Chapters 4 and 5 cover the two fundamental intellectual tasks of IR, indexing and retrieval, with the predominant paradigms of each discussed in detail. Chapter 6 discusses the methods and challenges of larger information access. Chapter 7 focuses on evaluation research that has been done on state-of-the-art systems in the biomedical and health domain. Finally, Chapter 8 explores research about IR systems and their users, with an emphasis on applications in the biomedical and health domain. Within each chapter, the goal is to provide a comprehensive overview of the topic, with thorough citations of pertinent references. There is a preference for discussing biomedical and health implementations of principles, but where this is not possible, the original domain of implementation is discussed.

This book would not have been possible without the influence of various mentors, dating back to high school, who nurtured my interests in science generally and/or biomedical and health informatics specifically, and/or helped me achieve my academic and career goals. The most prominent include Mr. Robert Koonz (then of New Trier West High School, Northfield, IL), Dr. Darryl Sweeney (then of University of Illinois at Champaign-Urbana), Dr. Robert Greenes (then of Harvard Medical School), Dr. David Evans (then of Carnegie Mellon University), Dr. Mark Frisse (then of Washington University), Dr. J. Robert Beck (then of OHSU), Dr. David Hickam (then of OHSU), Dr. Brian Haynes (McMaster University), Dr. Lesley Hallick (then of OHSU), and Dr. Jerris Hedges (then of OHSU). I must also acknowledge the late Dr. Gerard Salton (Cornell University), whose writings initiated and sustained my interest in this field.

I would also like to note the contributions of institutions and people in the federal government who aided the development of my career and this book. While many Americans increasingly question the abilities of their government to do anything successfully, the NLM, under the former directorship of the late Dr. Donald A. B. Lindberg and the current directorship of Dr. Patricia Flatley Brennan, has led the growth and advancement of the field of biomedical and health informatics. The NLM's fellowship and research funding have given me the skills and experience to succeed in this field. I would also like to acknowledge the late Oregon Senator Mark O. Hatfield through his dedication to biomedical research funding that aided myself and many others.

Finally, this book also would not have been possible without the love and support of my family. All of my parents, Mom and Jon, Dad and Gloria, as well as my brother Jeff and sister-in-law Myra, supported the various interests I developed in life and the somewhat different career path I chose. I think that now as they have become Web users and searchers, they appreciate my interest in this area. And last, but most importantly, has been the contribution of my wife, Sally, and two children, Becca and Alyssa, whose unlimited love and support made this undertaking so enjoyable and rewarding.

March 2020
Portland, OR

William Hersh

Contents

Chapter 1
Foundations

The goal of this book is to present the field of *information retrieval* (IR), sometimes called *search*, with an emphasis on the biomedical and health domain. To many, "information retrieval" implies retrieving information of any type from a computer. However, to those working in the field, IR has a different, more specific meaning, which is the retrieval of information from databases that predominantly contain textual information. A field at the intersection of information science and computer science, IR concerns itself with the indexing and retrieval of information from heterogeneous and mostly textual information resources. The term was coined by Mooers in 1951, who advocated that it be applied to the "intellectual aspects" of description of information and systems for its searching [1].

The advancement of computer technology continues to alter the nature of IR. As recently as the 1970s, Lancaster stated that an IR system does not inform the user about a subject; it merely indicates the existence (or nonexistence) and whereabouts of documents related to an information request [2]. At that time, of course, computers had considerably less power and storage than today's personal computers, and there was no Internet connecting the world's computers and other information devices to each other. In the 1970s, computers and network systems were only sufficient to handle bibliographic databases, which contained just the title, source, and a few indexing terms for documents. Furthermore, the high cost of computer hardware and telecommunications usually made it prohibitively expensive for end users to directly access such systems, so they had to submit requests that were run in batches and returned hours to days later.

In the twenty-first century, however, the state of computers and IR systems is much different, leading to new perspectives on the nature of the field [3, 4]. End-user access to massive amounts of information in databases and on the World Wide Web is routine. A recent monograph traces the history of IR from early experiments in the 1960s through the advent of ubiquitous search systems in the 2000s [5].

Not only can IR databases contain the full text of resources, but they may also contain images, sounds, and even video sequences. Indeed, there is now the notion of the *digital library*, where journals and books are mostly provided in digital form

W. Hersh, *Information Retrieval: A Biomedical and Health Perspective*,
Health Informatics, https://doi.org/10.1007/978-3-030-47686-1_1

and library buildings are augmented by far-reaching computer networks [6, 7]. The scientific publishing enterprise has been transformed to increasingly *open science*, with access not only to research publications but also their underlying data [8]. New models for delivering knowledge have been proposed, such as the Mobilizing Computable Biomedical Knowledge initiative, whose manifesto calls for knowledge to be provided in "computable formats that can be shared and integrated into health information systems and applications" [9].

So transformative and ubiquitous has IR become that the name of the leading Web search engine, Google, has entered the vernacular in a variety of ways, including as a verb (i.e., using a search engine to look something up is called "Googling") [10]. The Google Trends[1] (formerly Zeitgeist) keeps a tally of the world's interests as measured by what humans collectively type into the Google search engine. In addition, some lament that the "Google generation," i.e., today's legions of technology-savvy young people, are not critical enough in their skills regarding seeking, synthesizing, and critically analyzing information [11].

One of the early motivations for IR systems was the ability to improve access to information. Noting that the work of early geneticist Gregor Mendel was undiscovered for nearly 30 years, Vannevar Bush called in the 1960s for science to create better means of accessing scientific information [12]. In current times, there is equal if not more concern with "information overload" and how to avoid missing important information. A well-known example occurred when a patient who died in a clinical trial in 2000 might have survived if information about the toxicity of the agent being studied from the 1950s (before the advent of MEDLINE) had been more readily accessible [13]. Indeed, a major challenge in IR is helping users find "what they don't know" [14].

Just how much information is out there? One analysis estimated the amount of digital data in the world to be 33 zettabytes in 2018, with a projection to grow to 175 zettabytes by 2025 [15]. (A zettabyte is 10^{21} bytes, or one billion terabytes.) Another report estimated the amount of computer network traffic to triple between 2017 and 2022 to 4.8 zettabytes per year, which would be about equal to all previous Internet traffic from 1984 to 2018 [16]. Another analysis noted that 3.8 million searches of Google are done every minute [17]. In the 2000s, Card published a figure comparing the exponential growth of information as it surpassed the estimate of the size of all documents created in human history (40,000 years), well above the estimated amount of information a human could learn in a year (see Fig. 1.1) [18]. A current estimate of the health information on a single human over their lifetime is over 1000 terabytes, with the major of information coming from social determinants of health and health behaviors, and only a tiny fraction representing clinical data (<1 terabyte) [19]. Of course, only a small part of this data is the kind of text and other information we might wish to retrieve using an IR system. Nonetheless, it was estimated in 2016 that Google had indexed 130 trillion Web pages in its search engine [20].

[1] https://trends.google.com

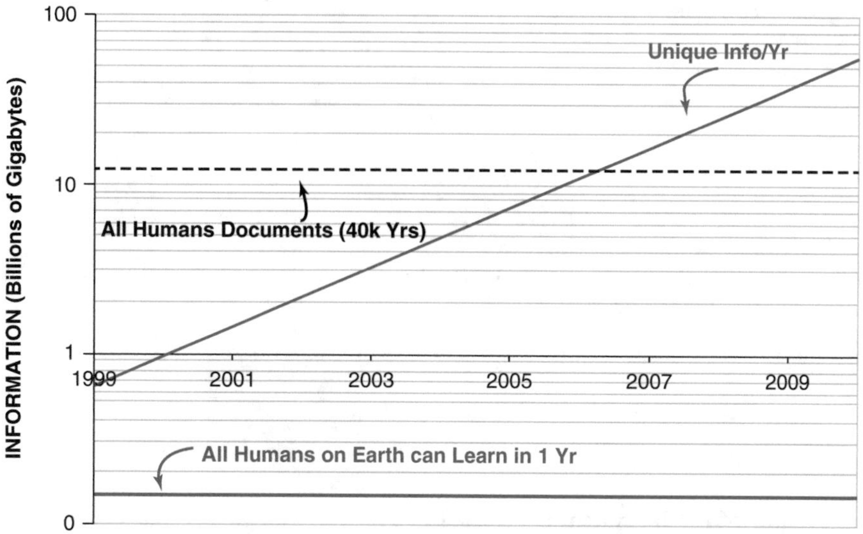

Fig. 1.1 Growth of information and comparison to all human documents and learning. (Courtesy of Stuart Card)

IR systems remain a unique type of computer application, and their use in all facets of life demands a better understanding of the principles underlying their operation. A workshop in 2018 brought together leading IR researchers to define key challenges in a number of broad areas for the field [21]:

- Conversational information seeking
- Fairness, accountability, confidentiality, and transparency in information retrieval
- IR for supporting knowledge goals and decision-making
- Evaluation
- Machine learning in information retrieval
- Generated information objects
- Efficiency challenges
- Personal information access

1.1 Basic Definitions

There are a number of terms commonly used in IR. An *IR system* consists of *content*, computer hardware to store and access that content, and computer software to process user input in order to retrieve it. Collections of content go by a variety of terms, including *database*, *collection*, or—in modern Web parlance—*site*. In conventional database terminology, the items in a database are called *records*. In IR, however, records are also called *documents*, and an IR database may be called a *document database*. In modern parlance, items in a Web-based collection may also be called *pages* and the collection of pages called a *Web site*.

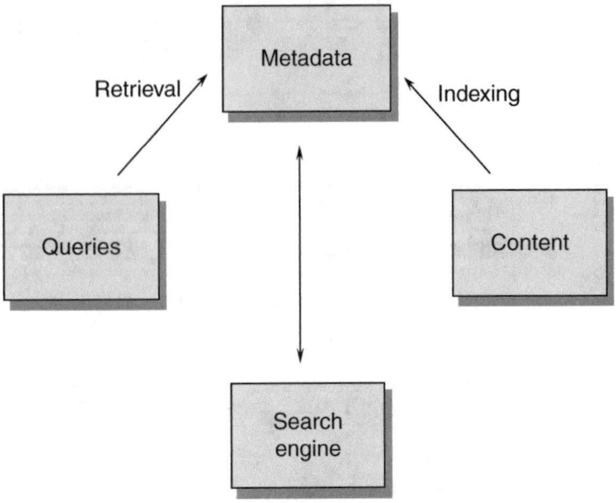

Fig. 1.2 Model of the IR system

A view of the IR system is depicted in Fig. 1.2. The goal of the system is to enable access by the user to content. Content consists of units of information, which may themselves be an article, a section of a book, or a page on a Web site. Content databases were easier to describe in the pre-Web era, as the boundaries of nonlinked databases and persistence of paper documents were, in general, more easy to delineate. The scope of Web content, however, varies widely: some sites organize information into long pages covering a great deal of matter, while others break it down into numerous short pages. The picture is further complicated by multimedia elements, which may be part of a page or may be found in their own separate file. In addition, Web pages may be composed of frames, each of which in turn may contain its own Web page of information. Furthermore, the content of Web pages may be generated dynamically and undergo constant change.

Users seek content by the input of queries to the system. Content is retrieved by matching *metadata*, which is meta-information about the information in the content collection, common to the user's query and the document [22]. As we will see in Chap. 4, metadata consists of both indexing *terms* and *attributes*. Indexing terms represent the subject of content, that is, what it is about. They vary from words that appear in the document to specialized terms assigned by professional indexers. Indexing attributes can likewise be diverse. They can, for example, consist of information about the type of a document or page (e.g., a journal article reporting a randomized controlled trial), its source (e.g., citation to its location in the *Journal of the American Medical Informatics Association* and/or its Web page address), or features in an image. A *search engine* is the software application that matches indexing terms and attributes from the query and document to return to the user.

There are two major intellectual or content-related processes in building and accessing IR systems: indexing and retrieval. *Indexing* is the process of assigning metadata to items in the database to facilitate and make efficient their retrieval. The term *indexing language*, sometimes used, refers to the sum of possible terms that can be used in the indexing of terms. There may be, and typically are, more than one set of indexing terms, hence indexing languages, for a collection.

In most bibliographic databases, for example, there are usually two indexing procedures and languages. The first indexing procedure is the assignment of indexing terms from a *controlled vocabulary* or *thesaurus* by human indexers. In this case, the indexing language is the controlled vocabulary itself, which contains a list of terms that describe the important concepts in a subject domain. The controlled vocabulary may also contain nonsubject attributes, such as the document publication type. The second indexing procedure is the extraction of all words that occur (as identified by a computer) in the entire database. Although one tends typically not to think of word extraction as indexing, the words in each document can be viewed as descriptors of the document content, and the sum of all words that occur in all the documents is an indexing language.

Retrieval is the process of interaction with the IR system to obtain documents. The user approaches the system with an *information need.* The user (or a specialized intermediary) formulates the information need into a *query*, which most often consists of terms from one or more of the indexing vocabularies, sometimes (if supported by the system) connected by the Boolean operators AND, OR, and NOT. The query may also contain specified metadata attributes. The search engine then matches the query and returns documents or pages to the user.

1.2 Scientific Disciplines Concerned with IR

The scientific disciplines historically most concerned with IR have been *library and information science* and *computer science*, although in recent years, many other disciplines have focused on search. *Information science* is a multidisciplinary field that studies the creation, use, and flow of information. Information scientists come from a wide variety of backgrounds, including information science itself, library science, computer science, systems science, decision science, and many professional fields. A broad attempt to define information science was recently undertaken by Zins, who assembled 57 leading scholars (including this author!) and carried them through an online Delphi process [23–26].

IR has strong relations to computer science as well. Croft has asserted that IR has always been a part of the overall computer science field and has a common heritage with database systems [27]. He also noted that the field grew and was validated by the success of Web search engines. Croft describes some known successes of the field:

- Search engines have become a significant means by which society accesses information.
- IR has long championed the "statistical" approach to using language, which has now been adopted by other areas of computer science, such as natural language processing.
- IR has focused on large-scale evaluation more extensively than other areas of computer science, which have come to adopt many of these techniques.

- IR has also focused on the importance of the user and interaction as part of its process.
- The global goals of information access and contextual retrieval are part of the vision of other grand research goals for computer science, as also noted by Gray [28].

The field of biomedical and health informatics (BMHI) has always had great interest in IR as well, though like computer science, IR is just a small part of the larger BMHI field. The National Library of Medicine (NLM), the leading funder of BMHI research and training in the United States, recently released an update of its strategic plan, *A Platform for Biomedical Discovery and Data-Powered Health*, which includes three overall goals, all of which are related to IR [29]:

- Accelerate discovery and advance health through data-driven research.
- Reach more people in more ways through enhanced dissemination and engagement.
- Build a workforce for data-driven research and health.

After 32 years of leadership from Donald A.B. Lindberg, MD, the National Library of Medicine named Patricia Flatley Brennan, RN, PhD as its fourth Director in 2016, who proceeded to outline her vision for the future of the NLM [30, 31].

Still, literature retrieval and analysis can be challenging for scientists and clinicians. Barnes and Gary have said, "Few areas of biological research call for a broader background in biology than the modern approach to genetics. This background is tested to the extreme in the selection of candidate genes for involvement with a disease process… Literature is the most powerful resource to support this process, but it is also the most complex and confounding data source to search" [32]. A leading neuroscientist, noting the advances in the Human Genome Project and related areas, advocated that biology should now be considered an "information science," with many advances likely to come from using data to form and test hypotheses [33]. Meanwhile, pharmaceutical (and likely other) companies fight for information and library talent [34]. One such talented individual quotes Harvard University Chemistry Professor Frank Westheimer, who once famously said, "Why spend a day in the library when you can learn the same thing by working in the laboratory for a month?" [35]. Likewise for clinicians, it has been asserted that "the skills needed to find potentially relevant studies quickly and reliably, to separate the wheat from the chaff, and to apply sound research findings to patient care have today become as essential as skills with a stethoscope" [36].

Another growing concern is *health information literacy*, whose need is increased in this era of proliferating online health information, which consists of the following skills as enumerated by the Medical Library Association (MLA)[2] [37]:

---

[2] http://www.mlanet.org/

- Recognize a health information need.
- Identify likely information sources and use them to retrieve relevant information.
- Assess the quality of the information and its applicability to a specific situation.
- Analyze, understand, and use the information to make good health decisions.

Health information literacy is especially a challenge for patients and consumers, as noted in a systematic review which found that low health literacy was associated with poorer health outcomes and poorer use of healthcare services [38]. This problem has led the US Institute of Medicine to hold several workshops on health literacy and numeracy, the most recent of which was in 2014 [39]. A growing population of concern for health-related content on the Web is aging baby boomers, who have the technology skills of those who are younger and are increasingly developing the health problems of those who are older [40]. Fiske et al. have proposed a new occupation of health information counselor to aid consumers in navigating all aspects of health information [41].

1.3 Models of IR

Another way to understand a field is to look at models of the processes that are studied. A model of the IR system has already been presented above. In this section, four models are discussed that depict the overall information world, the user's interaction with an IR system, factors that influence decision-making in healthcare, and knowledge acquisition and use.

1.3.1 The Information World

Figure 1.3 depicts the cyclic flow of information from its producers, into the IR system, and on to its users [42]. Starting from the creation of information, events occur in the world that lead to written observations in the form of books, periodicals, scientific journals, and so on. These are collected by database producers, who may create a bibliographic database of references to these sources or, as is happening with greater frequency, may create electronic versions of the full text. However a database is constructed, it is then organized into records and loaded into the IR system.

In the system, a file update program stores the data physically. Users, either directly or through trained intermediaries, query the database and retrieve content. Those users not only use the information but may also add value to it, some of which may make its way into new or other existing content. In addition, users also feed back observations to the database producers, who may correct errors or organize it better.

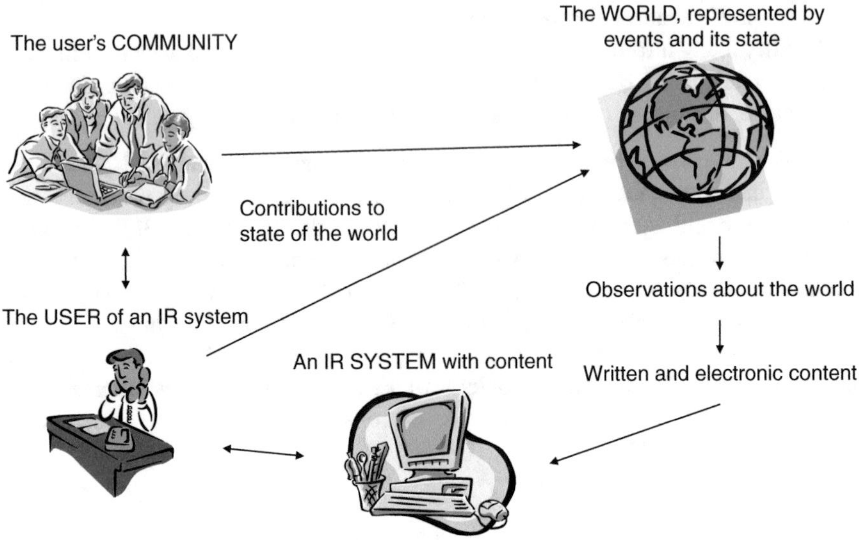

Fig. 1.3 Model of information flow in the world, adapted from [42]

Fig. 1.4 Model of the IR user, adapted from [43]

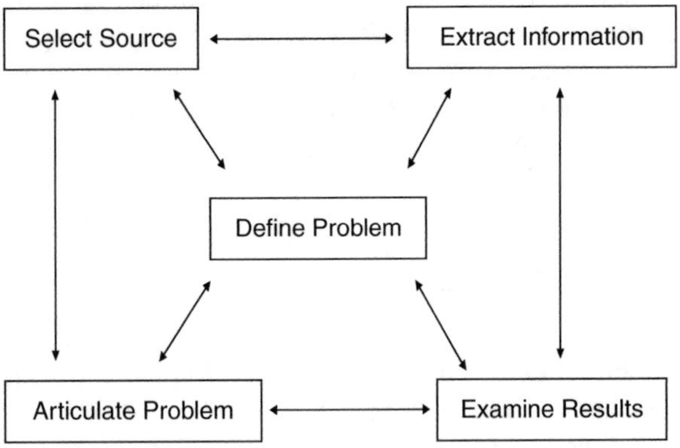

1.3.2 Users

Figure 1.4 shows the information-seeking functions of the user [43]. The central component is the user defining the problem (or information need). Once this has been done, the user selects the source for searching and articulates the problem (or formulates the query). The user then does the search, examines the results, and extracts information. Many of these tasks are interactive. Any step along the way, for example, may lead the user to redefine the problem. Perhaps some results obtained have provided new insight that changes the information need. Or examination of the results may lead the user to change the search strategy. Likewise, information extracted may cause the user to examine the rest of the searching results in a different manner.

A variety of other models of interaction between the user and IR system have been put forth. Marchionini looked beyond fact lookup to "exploratory search," where users also engage in learning and investigation [44]. Downey et al. developed a comprehensive model of user search activity that can be used to quantify various aspects of the process [45]. Another view of information seeking focusing on "strategies" and tactics" for searching, with a focus on the clinical domain, was put forth by Hung et al. [46].

1.3.3 Health Decision-Making

The ultimate goal of searching for health information is often to make a decision, such as whether to order a test or prescribe a treatment. The decision-maker may be a patient, his or her family, or a healthcare professional. A variety of factors go into making a health-related decision. The first of these categories is the scientific evidence, which answers the question of whether there has been objective-as-possible science to support a decision. An approach for finding and appraising this sort of information most effectively is called evidence-based medicine (EBM). As discussed in more detail in the next chapter, EBM provides a set of tools that enable individuals to more effectively find information and apply it to health decisions.

Evidence alone, however, is not sufficient for decisions. Both patients and clinicians may have personal, cultural, or other preferences that influence how evidence will be applied. The healthcare professional may also have limited training or experience to be able to apply evidence, such as a physician not trained as a surgeon or not trained to perform a specific treatment or procedure. There are other constraints on decision-making as well. There may be legal or other restrictions on what medical care can be provided. There may also be constraints of time (patient far away from the site at which a specific type of care can be provided) or financial resources (patient or entity responsible for paying for the care cannot afford it).

Figure 1.5, adapted from Mulrow et al., depicts the relationships among the factors that influence health decision-making [47]. The intersection of evidence and preferences provides the knowledge that can be used to make decisions. The intersection of evidence and constraints leads to guidelines. There is a growing interest in practice guidelines, with this specialized type of content discussed in Chap. 3. The ethical dimensions of healthcare lie at the intersection of preferences and constraints. Finally, the intersection of all three represents everything that is considered in a health decision.

1.3.4 Knowledge Acquisition and Use

Another model of information seeking and use is depicted in Fig. 1.6, with the process viewed as a funnel by which the user searches all of the scientific literature using IR systems to obtain a set of possibly relevant literature. In the current state of

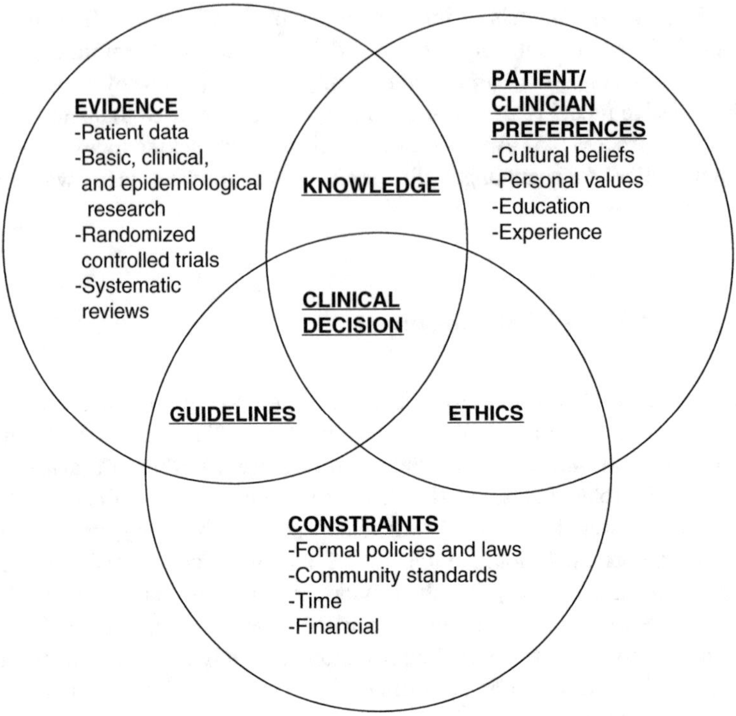

Fig. 1.5 Model of health decision-making, adapted from [47]

Fig. 1.6 Funnel of knowledge acquisition and use, showing the focus of the information retrieval field versus information extraction and text mining

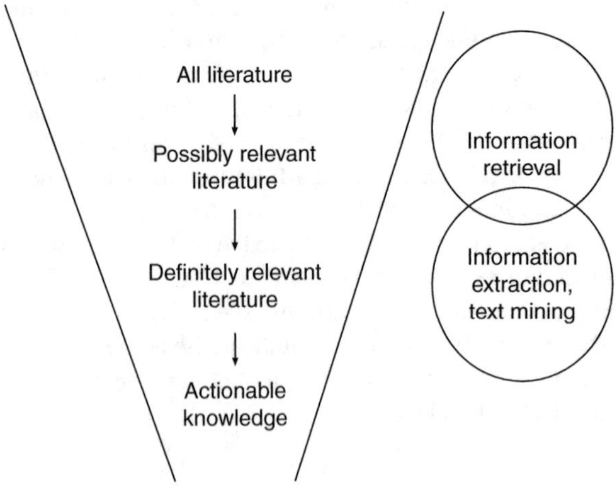

the art, he or she reviews this literature by hand, selecting which articles are definitely relevant and may become "actionable knowledge," i.e., part of his or her active store of knowledge. However, newer techniques from areas such as information extraction and text mining in the future may provide more automated assistance for determining what is relevant and converting it to actionable knowledge.

It is important to note that Fig. 1.6 also reminds us of the importance of IR systems for aiding processes like information extraction and text mining, which tend to apply more intensive processing to understand and create actionable knowledge as opposed to IR, which aims to deliver content to the user. Information extraction and text mining cannot, however, proceed effectively without good output from IR systems to feed their algorithms. We will cover these topics in the last chapter of the book.

1.4 IR Resources

It has already been noted that IR is a heterogeneous, multidisciplinary field. This section describes the field's organizations and publications. Because of the diversity of this field, the focus is on the organizations and publications most centrally committed to IR. Also included are those from the healthcare field that may not have IR as a central focus but do have an interest in it.

1.4.1 Organizations

A number of specialty organizations have interests that overlap with IR. The organization devoted specifically to information science is the *American Society for Information Science and Technology* (ASIST). The largest computer science organization devoted to IR is the *Special Interest Group in Information Retrieval* (SIGIR) of the *Association for Computing Machinery* (ACM). The library science field is closely related to information science, and there is much overlap in personnel, but its central issues are more related to the structure and functioning of libraries. The major library science organization is the *American Library Association* (ALA). Another organization more focused on technical libraries is the *Special Libraries Association* (SLA). There is also a professional group devoted specifically to document indexing, called the *American Society of Indexers* (ASI).

A number of health and biomedical information organizations have IR among their interests. The *American Medical Informatics Association* (AMIA) is devoted to all aspects of information technology in healthcare, biomedical research, and public health, including IR. The *Medical Library Association* (MLA) is concerned with the needs and issues of health science libraries, which of course include IR systems. Another organization that is not a professional society per se but is heavily involved in health-related IR is the *National Library of Medicine* (NLM), the US government agency that not only maintains many important medical databases but also funds research and training in medical informatics.

An additional group of organizations involved in IR are the companies that comprise the growing marketplace for search and retrieval products, which have by now become household names. In addition to the major Web search engines, whose names are household names (e.g., Google, Yahoo, and Microsoft), there are a variety of others that offer more specialized products, such as WebMD[3] in the biomedical domain.

1.4.2 Journals

There are a variety of scientific journals that are devoted fully or in part to IR research. Table 1.1 lists and divides these into general and biomedically oriented categories. Even general medical journals occasionally publish IR articles. Probably

Table 1.1 Journals noted for coverage of information retrieval

Journal	Web address
General information retrieval	
ACM Transactions on Information Systems (ACM TOIS)	https://tois.acm.org/
Journal of the American Society for Information Science and Technology (JASIST)	https://asistdl.onlinelibrary.wiley.com/journal/23301643
Information Processing and Management (IP&M)	https://www.journals.elsevier.com/information-processing-and-management
Information Research	http://informationr.net/ir/
Information Retrieval Journal (IRJ)	https://link.springer.com/journal/10791
Biomedical and health informatics (cover more than information retrieval)	
Applied Clinical Informatics (ACI)—also includes open-access *ACI Open*	https://www.thieme.com/books-main/clinical-informatics/product/4433-aci-applied-clinical-informatics
Journal of Biomedical Informatics (JBI)—also includes open-access *Journal of Biomedical Informatics: X*	https://www.journals.elsevier.com/journal-of-biomedical-informatics
Journal of the American Medical Informatics Association (JAMIA)—also includes open-access *JAMIA Open*	https://academic.oup.com/jamia/
Journal of Medical Internet Research (JMIR)—also includes family of area-specific journals	https://www.jmir.org/
Journal of the Medical Library Association (JMLA)	http://jmla.mlanet.org/ojs/jmla
Methods of Information in Medicine (MIM)	https://www.thieme-connect.com/products/ejournals/journal/10.1055/s-00035037

[3] http://www.webmd.com

the most notable of these is the *British Medical Journal* (BMJ), which not only publishes articles on the topic but has been a leader in innovating Web technology in electronic publishing of the journal.

1.4.3 Texts

There continue to be a variety of IR texts published. Since the last edition, a number of general IR textbooks have been published, including those by Baeza-Yates and Ribeiro-Neto [48], Buttcher et al. [49], Chowdhurry [50], Croft et al. [51], Manning et al. [52], Rubin [53], and Zhai and Massung [54]. Other books have focused on more specific topics such as:

- Crowdsourcing of health information [55]
- Evaluation [56, 57]
- Implementation of open-source search engines [58]
- Text mining [59–61]
- User interaction [62, 63]

Two publishers provide a series of 50–100-page monographs on a variety of IR topics:

- Morgan-Claypool, *Synthesis Lectures on Information Concepts, Retrieval, and Services.*[4]
- now publishers has created an additional series, *Foundations and Trends in Information Retrieval.*[5]

Some older "classic" texts in the field include Salton and McGill [64], which was written by the pioneer of "statistical" techniques in IR, and vanRijsbergen [65], whose text is maintained on the Web.[6] A text by Frakes described computer implementation of IR systems, providing source code in the C programming language [66].

1.4.4 Tools

When the first edition of this book was written, access to IR systems was expensive and, in many cases, required specialized software. Now, however, a plethora of search engines are just a mouse click away in anyone's Web browser. For those actually wanting to experiment implementing IR systems, there are several open-source search engines that are relatively easy to implement on basic personal computer

[4] https://www.morganclaypool.com/toc/icr/1/1

[5] https://www.nowpublishers.com/INR

[6] http://www.dcs.gla.ac.uk/Keith/Preface.html

systems (Windows, macOS, and Linux). Probably the most widely used open-source search engine is Lucene,[7] which was part of the original Apache open-source Web server platform. Two other widely used search engines are built on top of the Lucene code base:

- Solr[8] adds Web-based administration tools, including application programming interfaces (APIs) for other programming languages.
- Elasticsearch[9] adds commercial enterprise-level features.

A number of early research-oriented IR systems are no longer available, such as Salton's SMART [64], Harman's Prototype Indexing and Search Engine (PRISE) [67], and Robertson's Okapi [68]. However, two research search engines that are still supported include Terrier[10] and the Lemur Project,[11] of which the Indri search engine is part. A large number of academic IR researchers have converged on the use of Lucene as a foundation for research, using it as a platform to develop new approaches and evaluate them in a reproducible way[12] [69]. A code platform for experimentation has been developed in the Anserini system[13] [70], which also has available extensions for the Python programming language[14] and computational notebooks.[15]

1.5 The Internet and World Wide Web

This chapter has already alluded to the profound impact on IR of the Internet and World Wide Web. Indeed it is telling that in the first edition of this book, the Internet and the Web were described in the last chapter in the "special topics" section. In the second and third editions, they were introduced here in the first chapter and discussed widely throughout the rest of the book. But in this fourth edition, along with search in general, they have achieved near ubiquity in the lives of most knowledge professionals (including healthcare professionals and researchers) and assumed a major role in the lives of many who confront personal health issues. These technologies transformed IR from a task done by information professionals and a small number of other computer-savvy individuals to one done by people of all ages, levels of education, and geographic locations.

[7] http://lucene.apache.org/

[8] http://lucene.apache.org/solr/

[9] https://www.elastic.co/products/elasticsearch

[10] http://terrier.org/

[11] http://www.lemurproject.org/

[12] https://liarr2017.github.io/

[13] https://github.com/castorini/anserini

[14] https://github.com/castorini/pyserini

[15] https://github.com/castorini/anserini-notebooks

Few readers of this book are likely to need a description of the Internet and Web. However, it does help to define the key terms and point out some of their attributes relevant to IR. The Internet is the global computer network that connects computing devices of varying sizes and capacities using the communications protocol, TCP/IP. The Web is a software application that runs on the Internet, with servers making available pages coded in the Hypertext Markup Language (HTML) that are downloaded and displayed on client computers running a Web browser. In the hardware/software distinction of computers, the Internet can be viewed as the hardware and the Web as the software. But the Web is more than a simple computer application; essentially, it is a platform from which virtually any computer functions can be performed, including searching as well as database access and transactions.

1.5.1 Users

A number of analyses have the number of people who use the Internet and Web in different parts of the world. These statistics provide a picture of a world widely connected via computers and mobile devices, especially in but not limited to developed countries. There are several Web sites that track Internet use in different countries and languages:

- Internet World Statistics[16]—of 4.5 billion users worldwide (58% of world population), penetration in different regions is measured as follows from lowest to highest:
  - Africa—39.6%
  - Asia—54.2%
  - Middle East—67.90%
  - Latin America/Caribbean—68.9%
  - Oceania/Australia—68.4%
  - Europe—87.7%
  - North America—89.4%
- Pew Internet[17]—surveys focused on US Internet, mobile, and social media use.
  - Internet/broadband [71]

    90% of all Americans use the Internet, with higher use among lower age groups: 18–29, 100%; 30–49, 97%; 50–64, 88%; and over 65, 73%.

    Use of home broadband has plateaued at around 70%, probably due to those who use cellular connectivity to the Internet.
  - Mobile use [72]

    96% of Americans own a cell phone, with 81% owning a smart phone.

[16] https://www.internetworldstats.com/stats.htm

[17] https://www.pewinternet.org/

Smartphone usage is somewhat higher among those with more education and income, but a real differentiator is age: 18–29, 96%; 30–49, 92%; 50–64, 79%; and over 65, 53%.
74% of Americans own a desktop or laptop computer, while 52% own a tablet device.
- Social media use [73]
  Largest use of sites is YouTube, 73%; Facebook, 69%; Instagram, 37%; Pinterest, 28%; LinkedIn, 27%; Snapchat, 24%; Twitter, 22%; WhatsApp, 20%; and Reddit, 11%.
- A digital divide still exists between lower vs. higher income [74] and rural vs. urban setting [75], with the 10% of Americans not on the Internet likely to be poorer, older, and more rural [76].

Other organizations carry out various analyses of online information use. The Reuters Institute for the Study of Journalism measures the proportion of people who subscribe to online services, ranking the highest in Nordic countries (Norway, 34%; Sweden, 27%), with the United States much lower (16%, which rose after the 2016 election) [77]. Another site that reports on social media use is We Are Social.[18]

1.5.2 Usage

The statistics of the previous section show that use of the Internet and Web is ubiquitous, but for what do people use it? Even in the early days of the Web, Broder noted that while classic IR was driven by users seeking information, Web searching was often not just informational [78]. Instead, the user's intent might be navigational (e.g., finding a specific page) or transactional (e.g., purchase something, download a file, check the status of an account). He noted that navigational searches could be similar to what classic IR called a "known-item search," where the user aims to find a particular piece of content, such as an article or image. Broder also stated that "hub" pages (see Sect. 1.5.3) with lists of links that get to the target in one click may be acceptable to retrieve in a search. In transactional queries, the user needed not only to reach a site but also interact with it once he or she arrived there. He analyzed the frequency of these types of Web search by users of the AltaVista search engine and found the frequency for different types of interaction with search systems:

- Information tasks (39–48%)
- Navigational tasks (20–24%)
- Transactional tasks (30–36%)

Search engine use is very high among Internet users, if for no other reason that Web browsers redirect Uniform Resource Locators (URLs) to search engines when they are invalid. But it has become essentially ubiquitous for health-related

[18] https://wearesocial.com/us/

professionals. A 2012 survey conducted by Google and Manhattan Research described how much search is used by physicians [79]. Although the survey was conducted online and may not have been representative of all physicians, the authors claimed that those surveyed were representative of the age, gender, region, practice, and specialty setting of all physicians in the United States. The survey included 506 US physicians and found:

- Most had multiple devices: 99% with a desktop or laptop, 84% with a smartphone, and 54% with a tablet.
- They spent twice as much time using online resources as print resources.
- Even physicians aged 55+ were heavy users: 80% owned a smartphone, 84% used search engines daily, and 9 hours per week were spent online for professional purposes.
- Search engine use was a daily activity, with 84% using them daily, with an average of six searches per day and 94% using Google.
- When looking for clinical or treatment information, about a third clicked first on sponsored listings from a search.
- About 93% of physicians said they took action based on searching, everything from pursuing more information to sharing with a patient or colleague to changing treatment decisions.
- On smartphones, searching was preferred over mobile apps, with 48% of time spent with a search engine, 34% spent with mobile apps, and 18% spent going to specific Web sites in a browser or with a bookmark.
- They spent about 6 hours per week watching online video, with about half of that time spent for professional purposes.

Search is, of course, ubiquitous for most of the rest of the United States and almost all of the world. Pew Internet performed surveys about search in general and health in particular but discontinued regular updates around 2013. By 2012, 73% of all Americans (91% of all Internet users) were using search engines [80]. This study also presented data showing many search users were troubled by information collected about them, with 65% stating personalizing search in this manner was a "bad thing" [80]. Searching for health information was also a common use of searching. About 72% of US adult Internet users (59% of all US adults) reported looking for health information in the previous year [81]. About half the time, the searches were done on behalf of the health of someone else. A smaller but still nonetheless substantial percentage, 35% of all US adults, reported used the Internet to try to diagnose a medical condition they or someone else had. About 53% of "online diagnosers" talked with a clinician about what they found, and 41% had their condition confirmed by a clinician.

A previous analysis by Fox measured the most common types of searches done and the proportion having done them [82]:

- 66% for specific disease or medical condition
- 56% for certain medical treatment or procedure
- 44% for doctors or other health professionals
- 36% for hospitals or other medical facilities

- 33% for health insurance, including Medicare or Medicaid
- 29% for food safety or recalls
- 24% for drug safety or recalls
- 22% for environmental or health hazards

Fox also found that more than half of whites, women, adults providing unpaid care, or adults with higher income or some college education had searched for health information, while less than 50% of African-Americans, Latinos, adults with disability, adults over 65, or adults with high school education or less or lower income had done so.

Of course, one irony that few IR "old-timers" could ever have fathomed was the need, in the Web era, for the study of "adversarial IR," in other words, the development of techniques to *prevent* retrieval of certain content. One group of adversarial IR applications is the prevention of "spam" (i.e., unwanted) pages or emails [83, 84]. On the Web, this is called "link spam" [85]. There is now an annual conference devoted to research in this area. Singhal noted a continual tit-for-tat battle between those who developed search engines and those who tried to "game" them [86]. Indeed, a key modern business strategy is the attempt to drive traffic to one's Web site via search engines and other means, which is called *search engine optimization* (SEO). Many books and Web sites describe SEO, with the latter often provided by consulting firms that will help sites improve their rankings on the major search engines (e.g., Moz[19]). Even Google has a guide for SEO.[20]

A new form of adversarial IR came to the fore in the aftermath of the 2016 US elections, so-called fake news [87, 88]. The problem, however, is not limited to politics, and many other topics fall prey to methods that are exploited to proliferate incorrect information [89]. Analysis of false news has found it spreads more quickly than true news because it is more likely to be novel and elicit emotion from those who read it [90]. Social media "bots" play a role in amplifying false information, especially after it is first posted [91]. A case study of misinformation about vaccination found that bots and Russian trolls were responsible for amplifying scientifically incorrect anti-vaccine information [92]. These observations led to a call for developing better science toward combating the problem [93]. Some have noted that medicine is prone to these problems and needs solutions as well [94–96].

1.5.3 Hypertext and Linking

In both the paper and electronic information worlds, there are two ways of finding information: searching and browsing. In *searching*, information is sought by finding terms in an index that point to locations where material about that term may be. In books, for example, searching is done by looking up topics in the index in the back.

[19] https://moz.com/beginners-guide-to-seo

[20] https://support.google.com/webmasters/answer/7451184?hl=en

Searching in electronic resources is carried out by means of an IR system. *Browsing*, on the other hand, is done by delving into the text itself, navigating to areas that are presumed to hold the content that is sought. In books, browsing is usually started by consulting the table of contents, but the reader may also follow references within the text to other portions of the book. Electronic browsing in early computer systems was difficult if not impossible but has been made easier with the advent of *hypertext*, which is the electronic linking of nonlinear text.

The majority of the chapters of this book focus on searching as the means to find information. But computers also allow a unique form of information seeking that recognizes the nonlinearity of most text, especially scientific and technical reference information. Most paper-based resources allow some nonlinearity by referring to other portions of the text (e.g., "see Chap. X"). Computers allow these linkages to be made explicit.

The person most often credited with originating the notion of hypertext is Vannevar Bush, who proposed in 1945 that the scientist of the future would carry a device called a *memex* that linked all his or her information [97]. Another pioneer in the hypertext area was Ted Nelson, who implemented the first systems in the 1970s [98]. The popularity of hypertext did not take hold until the widespread proliferation of computers that used a graphical user interface (GUI) and a mouse pointing device. These systems allowed simple and easy-to-use hypertext interfaces to be built. Although not a true hypertext system, Apple Computer's HyperCard application, released in 1987, brought the concepts of hypertext to the mainstream. Another change brought by computers with GUIs was the ability to display nontextual information, such as images, sounds, video, and other media, often integrated with text. The term *hypermedia* is sometimes used to describe systems that employ hypertext combined with other nontextual information.

The Web brought Internet-based hypermedia to the mainstream, now exemplified by the World Wide Web platform. Kleinberg and Lawrence proposed a widely cited model for the Web, consisting of hubs and authorities [99]. *Hubs* are catalogs and resource lists of pages that point to *authorities*, which are the actual pages of content, on given topics. Another view of the Web divides it into the *visible* and *invisible* Web, as depicted in Fig. 1.7 [100]. The former contains all of the Web content that can be found by fixed or static URLs, while the latter contains content "hidden" behind password-protected sites or in databases [101]. In general, the visible Web is searched via general Web search engines. On the other hand, most of the commercial online databases to be described in later chapters reside on the invisible Web.

1.6 Evaluation

Another important topic to introduce early on concerns evaluation of IR systems, which is important for many reasons. Like any other technology, IR systems are expensive, if not to individuals then the institutions in which they work. And as with

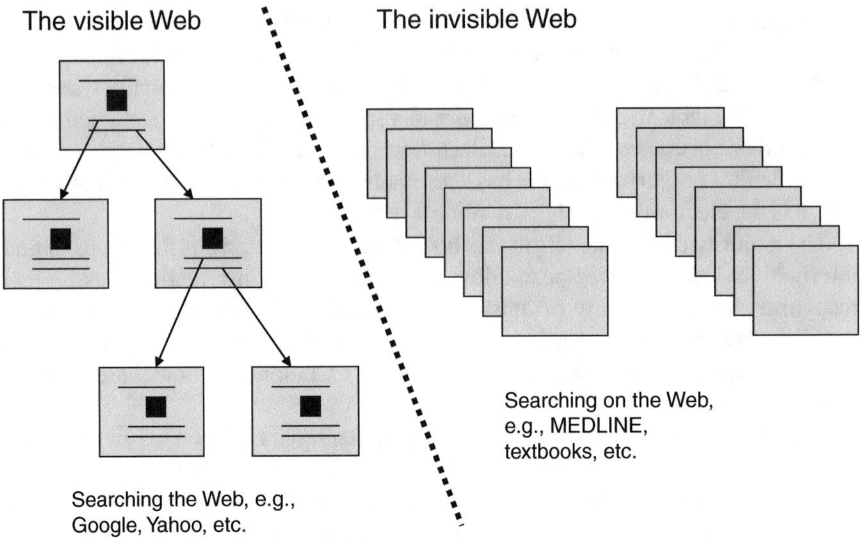

Fig. 1.7 Visible vs. invisible Web, adapted from [100]

many areas of computer use, there is a good deal of hype, marketing and otherwise, about the benefits of the technology. Thus the main reason to evaluate is to determine whether a system helps the users for whom it is intended. However, after this benefit has been demonstrated, it must also be shown that the system justifies its cost. And ultimately, the system's real-world results should indicate some measure of improvement on the tasks in which it is used. This notion has an analogy in the medical research world to outcomes research, where not only must an intervention demonstrate *efficacy* (benefit in controlled research) but also *effectiveness* (benefit in the real world outside the controlled research setting).

Evaluations of IR systems are often classified as macroevaluations or microevaluations. *Macroevaluations* look at the whole IR system and/or the user's interaction with it. This type of evaluation can take place in either a laboratory or a real-world setting. At times, however, one wishes to evaluate individual components of IR systems. Such evaluations are called *microevaluations*, and the motivations for doing them are to assess individual components of the system, to solve problems that arise with its use, and to determine how changes in the system might impact performance. They are typically performed in a laboratory or other controlled setting.

Another distinction often made when discussing IR evaluation is *system-oriented* versus *user-oriented*. System-oriented research focuses on evaluation of the system, either by part or as a whole, focusing on how well it performs a set of standardized tasks. The usual approach to system-oriented evaluation in IR is through the use of recall and precision. User-oriented evaluation, on the other hand, focuses on assessing the system in the hands of real users, who themselves may be in a simulated laboratory setting or real-world environment.

1.6.1 Classification of Evaluation

There are many classifications of evaluation or aspects therein that have been developed. One early and widely cited model was developed by Lancaster and Warner, who defined three levels of evaluation, as shown in Table 1.2 [102]. The first level is the evaluation of the effectiveness of the system and the user interacting with the system. (Health services researchers would actually state that efficacy and not effectiveness is being studied here, but Lancaster and Warner's own language shall be used.) At this level, the authors identify three general criteria for effectiveness: cost, time, and quality. While issues of cost and time are straightforward, those of quality are considerably more subjective. In fact, what constitutes quality in a retrieval system may be one of the most controversial questions in the IR field. This category also contains the relevance-based measures of recall and precision, which are the most frequently used evaluation measures in IR. The second level of retrieval evaluation in Lancaster and Warner's schema is *cost-effectiveness*. This level measures the unit costs of various aspects of the retrieval system, such as cost per relevant citation or cost per relevant document. The final level of evaluation in the schema is *cost-benefit*, which compares the costs of different approaches directly.

Fidel and Soergel developed a classification to catalog for researchers all the factors that need to be controlled in IR evaluations [103]. This classification can also, however, be used to review the components that should be studied (or at least considered) in effective IR evaluation. Its items include:

Table 1.2 Lancaster and Warner's classification of IR evaluation, adapted from [102]

I. Evaluation of effectiveness
A. Cost
1. Monetary cost to user (per search, document, or subscription)
2. Other, less tangible, cost considerations
a. Effort involved in learning how to use the system
b. Effort involved in actual use
c. Effort involved in retrieving documents
d. Form of output provided by system
B. Time
1. Time from submission of request to retrieval of references
2. Time from submission of request to retrieval of documents
3. Other time considerations, such as waiting to use system
C. Quality
1. Coverage of database
2. Completeness of output (recall)
3. Relevance of output (precision)
4. Novelty of output
5. Completeness and accuracy of data
II. Evaluation of cost-effectiveness
A. Unit cost per relevant citation retrieved
B. Unit cost per new (previously unknown) relevant citation retrieved
C. Unit cost per relevant document retrieved
III. Cost-benefit evaluation – value of systems balanced against costs of operating or using them

- Setting—where system used, e.g., library, clinic, laboratory, etc.
- User—type of searcher, e.g., researcher vs. clinician, or other attributes about him or her
- Request—type of information need, e.g., background, comprehensive, discussion, fact, update
- Database—content searched, e.g., type, cost, indexing
- System—retrieval system used, e.g., how accessed, cost, help provided, user interface
- Searcher—who did the search, e.g., intermediary vs. end user
- Process—how searches done experimentally, e.g., in batch process or an operational setting
- Outcome—results of search and their value to the user and his or her information need

While both Lancaster and Warner as well as Fidel and Soergel had "outcome" in their classifications, it may be desirable to expand what it means. In particular, there are (at least) six questions one can ask related to an IR resource (system or information collection) in a particular setting. These questions were developed for a systematic review assessing how well physicians use IR systems, but they could be applied to other users and settings [104].

1.6.1.1 Was the System Used?

An important question to ask about an IR resource is whether it was actually used by those for whom it was provided. Measurement of system or collection use can be gleaned from user questionnaires; preferably, however, it is done directly by system logging software. It is important to know how frequently people used a resource, since to be installed in the first place, someone had to have thought it would be beneficial to users. The non-use of a system or collection is a telling evaluation of its (non)value to users.

1.6.1.2 For What Was the System Used?

A related concern is knowing the tasks for which the system was being used. One might want to know what information collections were used (if there were more than one) and what types of questions were posed. In a clinical setting, there might be interest in what kind(s) of clinical problem led to use of which resource. Likewise, it may be important to know whether the system was used as a primary information resource or to obtain references for library lookup.

1.6.1.3 Were the Users Satisfied?

The next question to ask is whether users were satisfied with the IR system. User satisfaction is an important question both for administrators who make decisions to install and maintain systems and for researchers trying to determine the role of systems for users. It is also relatively straightforward to assess, with the use of instruments such as questionnaires, direct observation, and focus groups. A couple long-standing instruments for assessing computer software are the Questionnaire for User Interface Satisfaction (QUIS) [105] and the System Usability Scale (SUS) [106].

1.6.1.4 How Well Was the System Used?

Once it has been determined that systems were used and with satisfaction, the next issue is how effectively they were actually used. Whereas frequency of use and user satisfaction are relatively simple concepts, the notion of "how well" someone uses a system is more complex. Does one operate at the level of counting the number of relevant documents obtained, perhaps over a given time period? Or are larger issues assessed, such as whether use of the system results in better patient care outcomes? An example of the latter would be showing that the system had led a practitioner to make better decisions or had resulted in better patient outcomes. This issue will be addressed further shortly.

While many studies have focused on a wide variety of performance measures, the most widely used are still the relevance-based measures of recall and precision. These were first defined decades ago by Kent et al. [107] and achieved prominence by their use in the Cranfield studies of the 1960s [108]. Indeed, many consider them to be the "gold standard" of retrieval evaluation and call their use the "Cranfield paradigm." Yet as we see in this and other chapters, their use can lead to some serious problems, especially when they are the sole measurements in an evaluation. It is not that they are unimportant conceptually but rather that they are difficult to measure in operational settings and do not necessarily correlate with the success of using an IR system. In acknowledgment of their prevalence, however, we will cover them separately in Sect. 1.6.2.

1.6.1.5 What Factors Were Associated with Successful or Unsuccessful Use of the System?

Whether an IR system works well, or does not work well, there are likely explanations for the result. A variety of factors (e.g., demographic, cognitive, experiential) can be measured and correlated with the outcome of system use. Furthermore, if the system did not perform well, a researcher might wish to ask why. The assessment of system failure, called *failure analysis*, typically involves retrospectively determining the problems and ascertaining whether they were due to indexing, retrieval, user error, or some combination of these.

1.6.1.6 Did the System Have an Impact?

The final, and obviously most important question, is whether the system had an impact. In the case of clinical users, this might be measured by some type of improved healthcare delivery outcome, such as care of better quality or reduced cost. This item, which is addressed in the schemas of both Lancaster and Warner and Fidel and Soergel, takes on increased pertinence in healthcare, given the emphasis on quality of care and the desire to control costs. Of course, demonstrating that a computer system has an impact in actual patient outcome is difficult, because this effect is often indirect [109]. This is particularly true of IR systems, where not only is use for a given patient optional but also each new patient on whose behalf the system is used is likely to require a different kind of use. As such, there have been few studies of patient outcomes as related to IR systems. Such studies are easier to do for computer-based decision support systems, where the same function (e.g., recommended drug dose, alert for an abnormal laboratory test) is used for the same situation each time [110].

1.6.2 Relevance-Based Evaluation

Relevance-based measures are so prevalent in their usage and important conceptually that we will explore them further. Certainly a major goal of using an IR system is to find relevant documents. We measure how well systems do that through the measures of recall and precision. Furthermore, these two measures can be aggregated into a single measure using a number of different approaches, including the F measure, the recall-precision table, and mean average precision (MAP). For all of these measures, a system is assessed by calculating the average or mean across a set of topics in a given evaluation study.

1.6.2.1 Recall and Precision

Recall and precision quantify the number of relevant documents retrieved by the user from the database and in his or her search. Ignoring for a moment the subjective nature of relevance, we can see in Fig. 1.8 that for a given user query on a topic, there are relevant documents (Rel), retrieved documents (Ret), and retrieved documents that are also relevant (Retrel). Recall is the proportion of relevant documents retrieved from the database:

$$\text{Recall} = \frac{\text{Retrel}}{\text{Rel}} \tag{1.1}$$

In other words, recall answers the question, for a given search, what fraction of all the relevant documents have been obtained from the database?

One problem with Eq. (1.1) is that the denominator implies that the total number of relevant documents for a query is known. For all but the smallest of databases, however, it is unlikely, perhaps even impossible, for one to succeed in identifying all relevant documents in a database. Thus most studies use the measure of *relative*

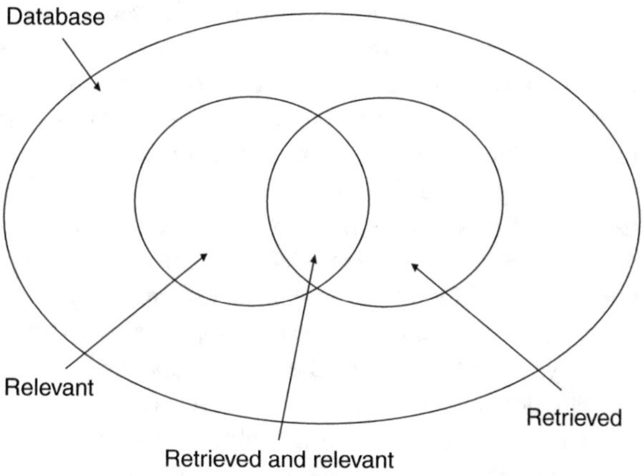

Fig. 1.8 Graphical depiction of the elements necessary to calculate recall and precision

Table 1.3 Table of retrieved and/or relevant documents for a query to calculate recall and precision

	Relevant	Not relevant	Total
Retrieved	30	70	100
Not retrieved	20	999,880	999,900
Total	50	999,950	1,000,000

recall, where the denominator is redefined to represent the number of relevant documents identified by multiple searches on the query topic.

Precision is the proportion of relevant documents retrieved in the search:

$$\text{Precision} = \frac{\text{Retrel}}{\text{Ret}} \tag{1.2}$$

This measure answers the question, for a search, what fraction of the retrieved documents are relevant?

A sample recall and precision matrix is shown in Table 1.3. The database contains a total of one million documents. For this particular query, there are 50 known relevant documents. The searcher has retrieved 100 documents, of which 30 are relevant to the query. The proportion of all relevant documents obtained, or recall, is 30/50, or 60%. The fraction of relevant documents from the set retrieved is 30/100, or 30%.

Table 1.3 is very similar to the matrix used to calculate the diagnostic test performance measures of sensitivity and specificity. In fact, if "relevance" is changed to "presence of disease" and "number retrieved" is changed to "number with positive test result," then recall is identical to sensitivity, while precision is the same as positive predictive value. (Specificity would be a much less useful number in IR research, since the numbers of both relevant and retrieved articles for a given query tend to be small. With large databases, therefore, specificity would almost always approach 100%.)

It is known in medical testing that there is a trade-off between sensitivity and specificity. That is, if the threshold is changed for a positive test, it will change not only the proportion of people correctly diagnosed but also the proportion incorrectly diagnosed. If the threshold for diagnosis is lowered, then the test will usually identify more true positive cases of the disease (and thus raise sensitivity) but also will identify more false-positive instances. The relationship between sensitivity (recall) and positive predictive value (precision) is not quite so direct, but it usually occurs in IR systems. The trade-off can be demonstrated qualitatively by comparing searchers of different types, such as researchers and clinicians. A researcher would more likely want to retrieve everything on a given topic. This searcher (or an intermediary) would thus make the query statement broad to be able to retrieve as many relevant documents as possible. As a result, however, this searcher would also tend to retrieve a high number of nonrelevant documents as well. Conversely, a clinician searching for a small number of good articles on a topic is much less concerned with complete recall. He or she would be more likely to phrase the search narrowly, aiming to obtain just a few relevant documents, without having to wade through a large number of nonrelevant ones.

Another medical measurement analogy from recall and precision has been defined by Bachmann et al. [111]: the number needed to read (NNR), which is the inverse of precision, i.e., 1/precision. The NNR defines the total number of articles that must be read to find each relevant one. This analogy can actually be carried back to the medical measurement realm, with the inverse of the positive predictive value (equivalent of precision) representing the number needed to test.

1.6.2.2 F Measure

Another measure commonly used to combine recall and precision is the F measure [65]. This measure is the harmonic mean of recall and precision and uses a parameter α that gives added value to recall as it increases. When $\alpha = 1$, the measure is called F1, and it represents the harmonic mean of recall and precision. For a search situation where precision was important, one would set α to a lower level, i.e., less than one.

$$F = \frac{(1+\alpha) * R * P}{(\alpha * P) + R} \tag{1.3}$$

1.6.2.3 Ranked Systems

Many IR systems use relevance ranking, whereby the output is sorted by means of measures that attempt to rank the importance of documents, usually based on factors related to frequency of occurrence of terms in both the query and the document. In general, systems that feature Boolean searching do not have relevance ranking, while those featuring natural language searching tend to incorporate it. Systems that use relevance ranking tend to have larger but sorted retrieval outputs, and users can decide how far down to look. Since the more relevant documents tend to be ranked higher, this approach gives users a chance to determine whether they want lower recall and higher precision (just look at the top of the list) or higher recall and lower precision (keep looking further down the list).

One problem that arises when one is comparing systems that use ranking versus those that do not is that nonranking systems, typically using Boolean searching, tend to retrieve a fixed set of documents and as a result have fixed points of recall and precision. Systems with relevance ranking, on the other hand, have different values of recall and precision depending on the size of the retrieval set the system (or the user) has chosen to show. For this reason, many evaluators of systems featuring relevance ranking will create a recall-precision table (or graph) that identifies precision at various levels of recall. The original approach to this was defined by Salton, who pioneered both relevance ranking and this method of evaluating such systems [64].

To generate a recall-precision table for a single query, one first must determine the intervals of recall that will be used. A typical approach is to use intervals of 0.1 (or 10%), with a total of 11 intervals from a recall of 0.0 to 1.0. The table is built by determining the highest level of overall precision at any point in the output for a given interval of recall. Thus, for the recall interval 0.0, one would use the highest level of precision at which the recall is anywhere greater than or equal to zero and less than 0.1. Since the ranked output list is scanned from the top, the number of relevant documents is always increasing. Thus, each time a new relevant document in the list is identified, it must first be determined whether it is in the current interval or the next one (representing higher recall). For the appropriate interval, the new overall precision is compared with the existing value. If it is higher, then the existing value is replaced.

When there are fewer relevant documents than there are intervals (e.g., 10 intervals but fewer documents), one must interpolate back from the higher interval. For example, if there are only two relevant documents, then the first relevant one would fall at a recall level of 0.5 and would require interpolation of the current overall precision value back to the preceding levels of recall (i.e., 0.4, 0.3, 0.2, 0.1, and 0.0). Conversely, when there are more relevant documents than intervals, one must compare each level of precision within the recall interval to all the others to determine the highest one.

An example should make this clearer. Table 1.4 contains the ranked output from a query of 20 documents retrieved, and 7 are known to be relevant. Table 1.5 is a recall-precision table for the documents listed in Table 1.4 with recall intervals of 0.1. Note that there are fewer relevant documents than intervals, so interpolation is needed.

The first document in Table 1.4 is relevant. Because there are seven relevant documents, the recall is 1/7 or 0.14. The overall precision at this point is 1/1 or 1.0, and its value is entered into the table for the recall level of 0.1. Since there are fewer than ten relevant documents, there will be separate precision for the recall level of

Table 1.4 Example ranked output of 20 documents with 7 known to be relevant

Rank	Relevance[a]	Recall and precision[b]
1	Rel	R = 1/7, P = 1/1
2	NRel	
3	Rel	R = 2/7, P = 2/3
4	NRel	
5	Rel	R = 3/7, P = 3/5
6	Rel	R = 4/7, P = 4/6
7	Nrel	
8	NRel	
9	Rel	R = 5/7, P = 5/9
10	NRel	
11	NRel	
12	NRel	
13	NRel	
14	Rel	R = 6/7, P = 6/14
15	NRel	
16	NRel	
17	NRel	
18	NRel	
19	NRel	
20	Rel	R = 7/7, P = 7/20

[a]Rel, relevant document; Nrel, nonrelevant one

[b]Each time a relevant document is encountered, recall (R) and precision (P) are calculated to be entered into the recall-precision table (see Table 1.5)

Table 1.5 Recall-precision table resulting from the data in Table 1.4

Recall	Precision
0.0	1.00
0.1	1.00
0.2	0.67
0.3	0.60
0.4	0.60
0.5	0.67
0.6	0.56
0.7	0.56
0.8	0.43
0.9	0.35
1.0	0.35

0.0, so the value from the recall level of 0.1 is interpolated back to the 0.0 level. The second document is not relevant, but the third document is. The overall level of recall is now 2/7 or 0.28, so the new level of precision, 2/3 or 0.67, is entered into the recall level of 0.2 in Table 1.5. The following document is not relevant, but the fifth document is, moving the overall recall level up to 3/7 or 0.42. The new precision is 3/5 or 0.60, and it is entered into Table 1.5 at the recall level of 0.4. Notice that there was no value to enter into the recall level of 0.3, so the value at the 0.4 level is interpolated back to the 0.3 level. The rest of the results are shown in Table 1.5.

For a whole set of queries, the values at each recall level are averaged. In general, the values for precision over a set of queries will fall with increasing level of recall. To compare different systems, or changes made in a single system, three or more of the precision levels are typically averaged. When the recall interval is 0.1, one might average all 11 intervals or just average a few of them, such as 0.2, 0.5, and 0.8.

An approach that has been used more frequently in recent times has been the MAP, which is similar to precision at points of recall but does not use fixed recall intervals or interpolation [112, 113]. MAP is calculated from the mean of average precision (AP) for each topic. AP represents the average of precision at each point a relevant document is retrieved or, for relevant documents not retrieved, a value of 0. As such, it is a recall-oriented measure (despite having "precision" in its name), since it measures retrieval across the entire set of relevant documents for a topic.

Here is how AP would be calculated for the ranked output of Table 1.4:

$$\text{AP} = \frac{\frac{1}{1}+\frac{2}{3}+\frac{3}{5}+\frac{4}{6}+\frac{5}{9}+\frac{6}{14}+\frac{7}{20}}{7} = \frac{4.27}{7} = 0.61 \quad (1.4)$$

If the retrieved documents in positions 14 and 20 in the output were not relevant, and those other relevant documents had not been retrieved at all, then AP would be calculated as follows:

$$\text{AP} = \frac{\frac{1}{1}+\frac{2}{3}+\frac{3}{5}+\frac{4}{6}+\frac{5}{9}+\frac{0}{0}+\frac{0}{0}}{7} = \frac{3.49}{7} = 0.50 \quad (1.5)$$

Another approach to aggregating recall and precision with ranked output has been proposed by Jarvelin and Kekalainen [114], who have put forth two measures related to the value to the degree of relevance and rank of the document in the output list. The measure to add value based on relevance is called cumulative gain (CG). A cumulative score is kept, with additional score added based on the degree of relevance of the document:

$$\text{CG}(i) = \text{CG}(i-1) + G(i) \quad (1.6)$$

where i is the document's rank in the output list (e.g., the top-ranking document has $i = 1$) and $G(i)$ is the relevance value. The measure based on document rank is called the discounted cumulative gain (DCG):

$$\mathrm{DCG}(i) = \mathrm{DGC}(i-1) + \frac{G(i)}{\log(i)} \tag{1.7}$$

When $i = 1$, CG(1) is set to 1 if there is no relevant document and DCG(1) is set to 1 to avoid dividing by zero. The authors advocate that CG be plotted versus DCG, with the performance of systems assessed based on the value of CG relative to DCG.

As test collections get larger (to reflect the growing size of real-world collections), there is a need for better methods to select documents to get the best sampling for relevance judgments. There is also a need for new performance measures that optimize use of incomplete judgments. An early approach was to employ the B-Pref measure [115]. Yilmaz et al. developed some measures, most notably inferred average precision (infAP) and inferred normalized discounted cumulative gain (infNDCG), which "infer" mean average precision and normalized discounted cumulative gain by making use of random sampling for judgments [116].

For all of the above measures, a system is evaluated by taking the mean or average of a given measure over a set of topics. For a recall-precision table, the average precision at each point of recall is calculated, while for AP, the MAP across all topics is calculated. We will explore these measures and their usage further in Chaps. 7 and 8, along with actual evaluation results of systems. We will also explore some of their limitations.

1.6.3 Challenge Evaluations

The field of computer science has a long history of *challenge evaluations*, where developers of different systems compare their efficacy with some sort of standardized task and/or data collection. The IR field is no exception. The largest and best-known IR challenge evaluation is the Text REtrieval Conference (TREC),[21] organized by the US National Institute for Standards and Technology (NIST) [117]. Challenge evaluations are usually based on test collections, which have three basic components:

- Documents—used very generically here, documents can be articles, Web pages, bibliographic records, images, or any other item that is a unit of retrieval.
- Topics—statements of information need, ideally derived from real-world situations. It should be noted that the statements themselves are usually described as topics whereas the search statements entered into actual systems are typically called queries.
- Relevance judgments—judgments of relevance of documents to the topics. This is typically done via the pooling method where a certain number of top-ranking

[21] https://trec.nist.gov/

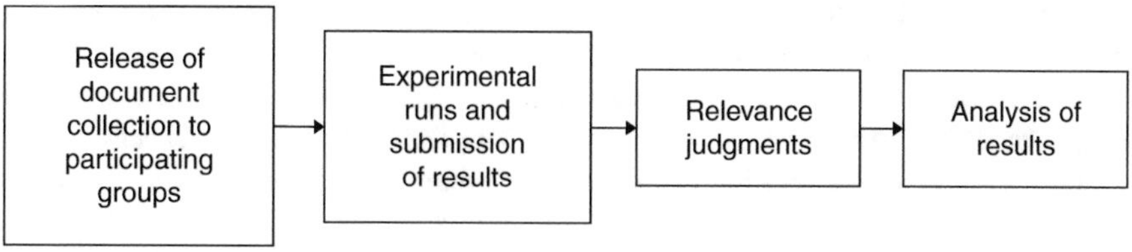

Fig. 1.9 Annual cycle of most TREC tracks and tasks

documents from each system participating in the challenge evaluation are included in a pool for relevance judging for each topic.

1.6.3.1 Text REtrieval Conference (TREC)

Started in 1992, TREC has provided a series of challenge evaluations and a forum for presentation of their results. TREC is organized as an annual event at which the tasks are specified and queries and documents are provided to participants. Figure 1.9 shows the usual steps in the annual cycle for each task organized in TREC. The original TRECs were numbered, e.g., TREC-1 (in 1992), TREC-2 (in 1993), etc. until TREC-9 (in 2000). Thereafter, each year's TREC was named with the year, e.g., TREC 2001.

One of the motivations for starting TREC was the observation that much IR evaluation research (prior to the early 1990s) was done on small test collections that were not representative of real-world databases. Furthermore, some companies had developed their own large databases for evaluation but were unwilling to share them with other researchers. TREC was therefore designed to serve as a means to increase communication among academic, industrial, and governmental IR researchers. Although the results were presented in a way that allowed comparison of different systems, conference organizers advocated that the forum not be a "competition" but instead a means to share ideas and techniques for successful IR. In fact, participants are required to sign an agreement not to use results of the conference in advertisements and other public materials [117].

The original TREC featured two common tasks for all participants. An *ad hoc retrieval task* simulated an IR system, where a static set of documents was searched using new topics, similar to the way a user might search a database or Web search engine with an information need for the first time. A *routing task*, on the other hand, simulated a standing query against an oncoming new stream of documents, similar to a topic expert's attempt to extract new information about his or her area of interest. The original tasks used newswire and government documents, with queries created by US government information analysts. System performance was measured by a variety of measures similar to those described previously. Relevance judgments were performed by the same information analysts who create the queries [112].

By the third TREC (TREC-3), interest was developing in other IR areas besides ad hoc tasks and routing. At that time, the conference began to introduce *tracks* geared to specific interests, each of which developed one or more tasks in each annual cycle. A more detailed overview of the various tracks is presented in Chap. 8. TREC celebrated its 25th anniversary in 2016.[22] The Webcast of the 25th anniversary conference features a talk by this author, *The TREC Bio/Medical Tracks*, which describes the various tracks in the biomedical domain at TREC over the years (starting around the 50-minute mark of Part 3 of the video).

1.6.3.2 TREC Biomedical Tracks

TREC has, for the most part, focused on general searching tasks over content such as newswire, government, and Web documents. There have, however, been so-called "domain-specific" tracks, a number of which have been focused in biomedicine and health. The methods and results of these tracks are described in more detail in Chap. 8 but are listed here:

- TREC Genomics Track [118]—retrieval of journal abstracts and articles focused on questions about genomics and related areas
- Medical Records Track [119]—searching de-identified electronic health record (EHR) documents to identify patients who might be eligible for a clinical study or trial
- Clinical Decision Support Track [120]—retrieval of full-text journal articles that might answer clinical questions about diagnosis, tests, and treatments
- Precision Medicine Track [121]—searching journal abstracts and clinical trials descriptions for genetic variants associated with different types of cancer

1.6.3.3 Other Aspects of TREC

The TREC experiments have led to research about evaluation itself. Voorhees, for example, has assessed the impact of different relevance judgments on results in the TREC ad hoc task [112]. In the TREC-6 ad hoc task, over 13,000 documents among the 50 queries had duplicate judgments. Substituting one set of judgments for the other was found to cause minor changes in the MAP for different systems but not their order relative to other systems. In other words, different judgments changed the MAP number but not the relative performance among different systems. Zobel has demonstrated that the number of relevant documents in the ad hoc track is likely underestimated; hence recall may be overstated [122].

TREC has also had its share of critics. Those who have argued that system assessments based solely on topical relevance assessments and not employing real users are implicitly criticizing the TREC model [123–125]. Blair noted the problems in calculating recall that have been put forth by others and further argued that the TREC ad hoc experiments overemphasized the importance of recall in the

[22] https://trec.nist.gov/celebration/25thcelebration.html

operational searching environment [126]. He did not, however, acknowledge the TREC Interactive Track, which addressed some of his concerns [127].

Some TREC tracks were so successful that they spawned their own separate organizational structures. The first of these was the Cross-Language Track, which spawned two TREC-like initiatives:

- Cross-Language Evaluation Forum, later named the Conference and Labs of the Evaluation Forum (CLEF)[23]—Focused on European languages, CLEF features a number of tracks that mimic those in TREC, such as ad hoc and Web searching [128]. CLEF has also included an image retrieval task, ImageCLEF,[24] which itself includes a medical image retrieval task [56].
- NTCIR[25]—Focused on East Asian languages (predominantly Japanese and Chinese), this forum also provides a full spectrum of IR tasks, including retrieval, question-answering, Web searching, and text summarization.

Another track that spawned its own initiative was the Video Track, which has evolved into the separate TRECVID.[26] The TREC Question-Answering Track inspired work at IBM on Watson [129, 130].

1.6.3.4 Beyond TREC

There is growing interest in retrieval (and challenge evaluations) using highly personal data, such as email, confidential documents, and patient records. This makes the standard approach to challenge evaluations difficult, in particular distributing the data of the test collections. One approach to solving this problem is the notion of Evaluation as a Service (EaaS), where the data is stored in a highly secure site and IR researchers send their experimental systems to the data. Of course, a limitation of this approach is that the researchers just get results, and not the actual data retrieved, for analysis.

Other biomedical challenge evaluations have been developed as well:

- BioCreative (Critical Assessment of Information Extraction in Biology)[27]—focused on tasks for annotators of biological literature.
- n2c2 (formerly i2b2)[28]—long-standing yearly challenge focused on natural language processing (NLP) and information extraction, covering the following tasks:
  - 2006—De-identification and smoking status
  - 2008—Obesity
  - 2009—Medications

[23] http://www.clef-initiative.eu/

[24] https://www.imageclef.org/

[25] http://research.nii.ac.jp/ntcir/index-en.html

[26] https://trecvid.nist.gov/

[27] https://biocreative.bioinformatics.udel.edu/

[28] https://n2c2.dbmi.hms.harvard.edu/

  - 2010—Relations
  - 2011—Coreferences
  - 2012—Temporal relations
  - 2014—De-identification and heart disease
  - 2016—Research domain criteria (RDoC) for psychiatry
  - 2018—Cohort selection for clinical trials and adverse drug events and medication extraction in EHRs
- ImageCLEFmed—in addition to ad hoc medical image retrieval, the tasks included modality classification (e.g., identify magnetic resonance imaging [MRI] or plain film X-ray images) and identification of similar cases based on a given image (e.g., with description and an image of a patient with pneumonia, find other cases of pneumonia). In the early ImageCLEF medical tasks, the "documents" of the test collection were comprised of images and their annotations [131, 132].
- CLEF eHealth[29]—focused on three domains:
  - Information extraction (IE)
  - Information management
  - Information retrieval (IR)—tasks including:
    - Patient-centered IR
    - Cross-language IR
    - Total-recall task to identify studies for inclusion in systematic reviews
- bioCADDIE—retrieval of metadata for research datasets [133, 134].

Other collections made available for research have included query logs. Such logs from major Web engines have provided a snapshot of the information people are looking for (or at least type into search engines). This research lets us know, for example, that most users enter very short queries and rarely look at results beyond the first page of ten results [135, 136]. America On-Line created a stir in 2006 when it released, with great fanfare, a collection of 20,000 user queries from its system. After it was quickly discovered that the queries contained some personally identifiable information, the dataset was withdrawn and never posted again [137].

References

1. Mooers C. Zatocoding applied to mechanical organisation of knowledge. Am Doc. 1951;2:20–32.
2. Lancaster F. Information retrieval systems: characteristics, testing, and evaluation. New York: Wiley; 1978.
3. Tunkelang D. Beyond algorithms: optimizing the search experience. O'Reilly 2015.
4. Zobel J. What we talk about when we talk about information retrieval. SIGIR Forum. 2017:18–26.

[29] http://clef-ehealth.org/

5. Harman D. Information retrieval: the early years. Foundations and trends in information retrieval, vol. 5. Hanover, MA: Now Publishers; 2019.
6. Lesk M. Understanding digital libraries. 2nd ed. San Francisco, CA: Morgan Kaufmann; 2005.
7. Banerjee K, Reese T. Building digital libraries, 2nd edn. Amazon Digital Services; 2018.
8. Anonymous. Open science by design – realizing a vision for 21st century research. Washington, DC: National Academies Press; 2018.
9. Anonymous. Mobilizing Computable Biomedical Knowledge (CBK): A Manifesto 2018 October 7, 2018.
10. Heffernan V. Just Google it: a short history of a newfound verb. WIRED. 2017 Nvoember 15, 2017.
11. Anonymous. Information behaviour of the researcher of the future. London, England: Centre for Information Behaviour and the Evaluation of Research 2008 January 16, 2008.
12. Bush V. Science is not enough. New York: Morrow; 1967.
13. McLellan F. 1966 and all that – when is a literature search done? Lancet. 2001;358:646.
14. Belkin N. Helping people find what they don't know. Commun ACM. 2000;43:58–61.
15. Reinsel D, Gantz J, Rydning J. The digitization of the world – from edge to core. Framingham, MA: International Data Corporation 2018 Contract No.: IDC White Paper – #US44413318.
16. Cooney M. Cisco predicts nearly 5 zettabytes of IP traffic per year by 2022. Network World. 2018 November 28, 2018.
17. Desjardins J. What happens in an internet minute in 2019? Visual capitalist 2019.
18. Card S. Information foraging theory. Palo Alto, CA: Palo Alto Research Center 2003 January, 2003.
19. Singhal S, Carlton S. The era of exponential improvement in healthcare? McKinsey on Healthcare: McKinsey & Company; 2018.
20. Schwartz B. Google's search knows about over 130 trillion pages. Search Engine Land. 2016;
21. Culpepper J, Diaz F, Smucker M. Research frontiers in information retrieval: report from the third strategic workshop on information retrieval in Lorne (SWIRL 2018). SIGIR Forum. 2018:34–90.
22. Riley J. Understanding metadata: what is metadata, and what is it for? Baltimore, MD: National Information Standards Organization 2017 January 1, 2017.
23. Zins C. Conceptual approaches for defining "data", "information", and "knowledge". J Am Soc Inf Sci Technol. 2007;58:479–93.
24. Zins C. Conceptions of information science. J Am Soc Inf Sci Technol. 2007;58:335–50.
25. Zins C. Classification schemes of information science: 28 scholars map the field. J Am Soc Inf Sci Technol. 2007;58:645–72.
26. Zins C. Knowledge map of information science. J Am Soc Inf Sci Technol. 2007;58:526–35.
27. Croft W editor. Salton award lecture – information retrieval and computer science: an evolving relationship. Proceedings of the 26th Annual International ACM SIGIR Conference on Research and Development in Information Retrieval; 2003; Toronto, Canada: ACM Press.
28. Gray J. What next? A dozen information technology research goals. J ACM. 2003;50:41–57.
29. Anonymous. A platform for biomedical discovery and data-powered health – National Library of Medicine strategic plan 2017–2027. Bethesda, MD: National Library of Medicine 2017 December, 2017.
30. Brennan P. Crafting the third century of the National Library of Medicine. J Am Med Inform Assoc. 2016;23:858.
31. Brennan P. The National Library of Medicine: accelerating discovery, delivering information, improving health. Ann Intern Med. 2016;165:808–9.
32. Barnes M, Gary R. Bioinformatics for geneticists. West Sussex: Wiley; 2003.
33. Insel T, Volkow N, Li T, Battey J, Landis S. Neuroscience networks: data-sharing in an information age. PLoS Biol. 2003;1:E17.
34. Davies K. Search and deploy. Bio-IT World. 2006 October 16, 2006.
35. Corey E, Frank H. Westheimer, major figure in 20th century chemistry, dies at 95. Harvard Gazette. 2007 April;19:2007.

36. Glasziou P, Burls A, Gilbert R. Evidence based medicine and the medical curriculum. Br Med J. 2008;337:a1253.
37. Schardt C. Health information literacy meets evidence-based practice. J Med Libr Assoc. 2011;99:1–2.
38. Berkman N, Sheridan S, Donahue K, Halpern D, Crotty K. Low health literacy and health outcomes: an updated systematic review. Ann Intern Med. 2011;155:97–107.
39. French M. Health literacy and numeracy: workshop summary (2014). Washington, DC: National Academies Press; 2014.
40. LeRouge C, VanSlyke C, Seale D, Wright K. Baby boomers' adoption of consumer health technologies: survey on readiness and barriers. J Med Internet Res. 2014;16(9):e200.
41. Fiske A, Buyx A, Prainsack B. Health information counselors: a new profession for the age of big data. Acad Med. 2019;1:37–41.
42. Meadow C, Boyce B, Kraft D, Barry C. Text information retrieval systems. 3rd ed. San Diego, CA: Academic Press; 2007.
43. Marchionini G. Interfaces for end-user information seeking. J Am Soc Inf Sci. 1992;43:156–63.
44. Marchionini G. Exploratory search: from finding to understanding. Commun ACM. 2006;41(4):41–6.
45. Downey D, Dumais S, Horvitz E, editors. Models of searching and browsing: languages, studies, and applications. International Joint Conference on Artificial Intelligence 2007; 2007; Hyderabad, India.
46. Hung P, Johnson S, Kaufman D, Mendonça E. A multi-level model of information seeking in the clinical domain. J Biomed Inform. 2008;41:357–70.
47. Mulrow C, Cook D, Davidoff F. Systematic reviews: critical links in the great chain of evidence. Ann Intern Med. 1997;126:389–91.
48. Baeza-Yates R, Ribeiro-Neto B. Modern information retrieval: the concepts and technology behind search. 2nd ed. Reading, MA: Addison-Wesley; 2011.
49. Buttcher S, Clarke C, Cormack G. Information retrieval: implementing and evaluating search engines. Cambridge, MA: MIT Press; 2010.
50. Chowdhurry G. Introduction to modern information retrieval. 3rd ed. New York, NY: Neal-Schuman Publishers; 2010.
51. Croft W, Metzler D, Strohman T. Search engines: information retrieval in practice. Boston, MA: Addison-Wesley; 2009.
52. Manning C, Raghavan P, Schutze H. Introduction to information retrieval. Cambridge: Cambridge University Press; 2008.
53. Rubin R. Foundations of library and information science. 4th ed. New York, NY: Neal-Schuman Publishers; 2016.
54. Zhai C, Massung S. Text data management and analysis: a practical introduction to information retrieval and text mining. Association for Computing Machinery: New York, NY; 2016.
55. Yom-Tov E. Crowdsourced health: how what you do on the internet will improve medicine. Cambridge, MA: MIT Press; 2016.
56. Müller H, Clough P, Deselaers T, Caputo B, editors. Image CLEF: experimental evaluation in visual information retrieval. Heidelberg: Springer; 2010.
57. Sakai T. Laboratory experiments in information retrieval – sample sizes, effect sizes, and statistical power. Springer: Singapore; 2018.
58. Turnbull D, Berryman J. Relevant search: with applications for solr and Elasticsearch. Greenwich, CT: Manning Publications; 2016.
59. Aggarwal C, Zhai C, editors. Mining text data. New York, NY: Springer; 2012.
60. Shatkay H, Craven M. Mining the biomedical literature. Cambridge, MA: MIT Press; 2012.
61. Cohen K, Demner-Fushman D. Biomedical natural language processing. Amsterdam: John Benjamins Publishing; 2014.
62. Hearst M. Search user interfaces. Cambridge: Cambridge University Press; 2009.
63. White R. Interactions with search systems. Cambridge: Cambridge University Press; 2016.

64. Salton G, McGill M. Introduction to modern information retrieval. New York: McGraw-Hill; 1983.
65. van Rijsbergen C. Information retrieval. London: Butterworth; 1979.
66. Frakes W, Baeza-Yates R, editors. Information retrieval: data structures and algorithms. Englewood Cliffs, NJ: Prentice-Hall; 1992.
67. Harman D, Candela G. Retrieving records from a gigabyte of text on a minicomputer using statistical ranking. J Am Soc Inf Sci. 1990;41(8):581–9.
68. Robertson S, Zaragoza H. The probabilistic relevance framework: BM25 and beyond. Foundations and trends in information retrieval. Delft: Now Publishers; 2009.
69. Lin J, Crane M, Trotman A, Callan J, Chattopadhyaya I, Foley J et al., editors. Toward reproducible baselines: the open-source IR reproducibility challenge. European Conference on Information Retrieval; 2016.
70. Yang P, Fang H, Lin J. Anserini: reproducible ranking baselines using Lucene. J Data Inf Qual. 2016;10(4):16.
71. Anonymous. Internet/broadband fact sheet. Washington, DC: Pew Research Center 2019 June 12, 2019.
72. Anonymous. Mobile fact sheet. Washington, DC: Pew Research Center 2019 June 12, 2019.
73. Anonymous. Social media fact sheet. Washington, DC: Pew Research Center 2019 June 12, 2019.
74. Anderson M, Kumar M. Digital divide persists even as lower-income Americans make gains in tech adoption. Washington, DC: Pew Research Center 2019 May 7, 2019.
75. Perrin A. Digital gap between rural and nonrural America persists. Washington, DC: Pew Research Center 2019 May 31, 2019.
76. Anderson M, Perrin A, Jiang J, Kumar M. 10% of Americans don't use the internet. Who are they? Washington, DC: Pew Research Center 2019 April 22, 2019.
77. Newman N, Fletcher R, Kalogeropoulos A, Nielsen R. Digital News Report 2019. Oxford: Reuters Institute for the Study of Journalism; 2019.
78. Broder A. A taxonomy of Web search. SIGIR Forum. 2002;36(2):3–10.
79. Anonymous. From screen to script: The Doctor's digital path to treatment. New York, NY: Manhattan Research; Google 2012.
80. Purcell K, Brenner J, Rainie L. Search engine use 2012. Washington, DC: Pew Internet & American Life Project 2012 March 9, 2012.
81. Fox S, Duggan M. Health online 2013. Washington, DC: Pew Internet & American Life Project 2013 January 15, 2013.
82. Fox S. Health topics. Washington, DC: Pew Internet & American Life Project 2011 February 1, 2011.
83. Metaxas P, DeStefano J, editors. Web spam, propaganda and trust. First international workshop on adversarial information retrieval on the Web; 2005; Chiba, Japan.
84. Cormack G, Lyman T. Online supervised spam filter evaluation. ACM Transactions on Information Systems. 2007;25(3):Article 11.
85. Noruzi A. Link spam and search engines. Webology. 2006;3(1).
86. Singhal A. Challenges in running a commercial web search engine. Mountain View, CA: Google 2004.
87. Holan A. 2016 Lie of the year: fake news. St. Petersburg, FL: Politifact 2016 December 13, 2016.
88. Guess A, Nyhan B, Reifler J. Selective exposure to misinformation: evidence from the consumption of fake news during the 2016 U.S. presidential campaign: European Research Council 2018 January 9, 2018.
89. Kavanagh J, Rich M. Truth decay – an initial exploration of the diminishing role of facts and analysis in American public life. Santa Monica, CA: RAND Corporation; 2018.
90. Vosoughi S, Roy D, Aral S. The spread of true and false news online. Science. 2018;359: 1146–51.

91. Shao C, Ciampaglia G, Varol O, Yang K, Flammini A, Menczer F. The spread of low-credibility content by social bots. Nat Commun. 2018;9:4787.
92. Broniatowski D, Jamison A, Qi S, AlKulaib L, Chen T, Benton A, et al. Weaponized health communication: Twitter bots and Russian trolls amplify the vaccine debate. Am J Public Health. 2018;108:1378–84.
93. Lazer D, Baum M, Benkler Y, Berinsky A, Greenhill K, Menczer F, et al. The science of fake news. Science. 2018;359:1094–6.
94. Wenzel R. Medical education in the era of alternative facts. N Engl J Med. 2017;377:607–9.
95. Chou W, Oh A, Klein W. Addressing health-related misinformation on social media. J Am Med Assoc. 2018;320:2417–8.
96. Merchant R, Asch D. Protecting the value of medical science in the age of social media and "fake news". J Am Med Assoc. 2018;320:2415–6.
97. Bush V. As we may think. Atl Mon. 1945;176:101–8.
98. Nelson T. Computer Lib. 2nd ed. Redmond, WA: Microsoft Press; 1987.
99. Kleinberg J, Lawrence S. The structure of the Web. Science. 2001;294:1849–50.
100. Sherman C, Price G. The invisible web: uncovering information sources search engines can't see. Chicago: Independent Publishers Group; 2001.
101. Anonymous. Invisible web: what it is, why it exists, how to find it, and its inherent ambiguity: University of California Berkeley Library2002 July 1, 2002.
102. Lancaster F, Warner A. Information retrieval today. Arlington, VA: Information Resources Press; 1993.
103. Fidel R, Soergel D. Factors affecting online bibliographic retrieval: a conceptual framework for research. J Am Soc Inf Sci. 1983;34:163–80.
104. Hersh W, Hickam D. How well do physicians use electronic information retrieval systems? A framework for investigation and review of the literature. J Am Med Assoc. 1998;280:1347–52.
105. Chin J, Diehl V, Norman K, editors. Development of an instrument measuring user satisfaction of the human-computer interface. Proceedings of CHI '88 – Human Factors in Computing Systems; 1988; New York: ACM Press.
106. Brooke J. SUS: a retrospective. J Usability Stud. 2013;8(2):29–40.
107. Kent A, Berry M, Leuhrs F, Perry J. Machine literature searching VIII: operational criteria for designing information retrieval systems. Am Doc. 1955;6:93–101.
108. Cleverdon C, Keen E. Factors determining the performance of indexing systems (Vol. 1: Design, Vol. 2: Results). Aslib Cranfield Research Project: Cranfield; 1966.
109. Friedman C, Wyatt J. Evaluation of biomedical and health information resources. In: Shortliffe E, Cimino J, editors. Biomedical informatics: computer applications in health care and biomedicine. 4th ed. London: Springer; 2014. p. 355–87.
110. Garg A, Adhikari N, McDonald H, Rosas-Arellano M, Devereaux P, Beyene J, et al. Effects of computerized clinical decision support systems on practitioner performance and patient outcomes: a systematic review. J Am Med Assoc. 2005;293:1223–38.
111. Bachmann L, Coray R, Estermann P, TerRiet G. Identifying diagnostic studies in MEDLINE: reducing the number needed to read. J Am Med Inform Assoc. 2002;9:653–8.
112. Voorhees E, editor. Variations in relevance judgments and the measurement of retrieval effectiveness. Proceedings of the 21st Annual International ACM SIGIR Conference on Research and Development in Information Retrieval; 1998; Melbourne, Australia: ACM Press.
113. Buckley C, Voorhees E. Retrieval system evaluation. In: Voorhees E, Harman D, editors. TREC: Experiment and Evaluation in Information Retrieval. Cambridge, MA: MIT Press; 2005. p. 53–75.
114. Jarvelin K, Kekalainen J, editors. IR evaluation methods for retrieving highly relevant documents. Proceedings of the 23rd Annual International ACM SIGIR Conference on Research and Development in Information Retrieval; 2000; Athens, Greece: ACM Press.

115. Buckley C, Voorhees E, editors. Retrieval evaluation with incomplete information. Proceedings of the 27th Annual International ACM SIGIR Conference on Research and Development in Information Retrieval; 2004; Sheffield, England: ACM Press.
116. Yilmaz E, Kanoulas E, Aslam J, editors. A simple and efficient sampling method for estimating AP and NDCG. Proceedings of the 31st Annual International ACM SIGIR Conference on Research and Development in Information Retrieval; 2008; Singapore.
117. Voorhees E, Harman D, editors. TREC: Experiment and Evaluation in Information Retrieval. Cambridge, MA: MIT Press; 2005.
118. Hersh W, Voorhees E. TREC genomics special issue overview. Inf Retr. 2009;12:1–15.
119. Voorhees E, editor. The TREC Medical Records Track. Proceedings of the International Conference on Bioinformatics, Computational Biology and Biomedical Informatics; 2013; Washington, DC.
120. Roberts K, Simpson M, Demner-Fushman D, Voorhees E, Hersh W. State-of-the-art in biomedical literature retrieval for clinical cases: a survey of the TREC 2014 CDS track. Inf Retriev J. 2016;19:113–48.
121. Roberts K, Demner-Fushman D, Voorhees E, Hersh W, Bedrick S, editors. Overview of the TREC 2017 Precision Medicine Track. The Twenty-Sixth Text REtrieval Conference (TREC 2017) Proceedings; 2017; Gaithersburg, MD.
122. Zobel J, editor. How reliable are the results of large-scale information retrieval experiments? Proceedings of the 21st Annual International ACM SIGIR Conference on Research and Development in Information Retrieval; 1998; Melbourne, Australia: ACM Press.
123. Swanson D. Information retrieval as a trial-and-error process. Libr Q. 1977;47:128–48.
124. Harter S. Psychological relevance and information science. J Am Soc Inf Sci. 1992;43:602–15.
125. Hersh W. Relevance and retrieval evaluation: perspectives from medicine. J Am Soc Inf Sci. 1994;45:201–6.
126. Blair D. Some thoughts on the reported results of TREC. Inf Process Manag. 2002;38:445–51.
127. Hersh W. Interactivity at the Text Retrieval Conference (TREC). Inf Process Manag. 2001;37:365–6.
128. Ferro N, Peters C, editors. Information retrieval evaluation in a changing world – lessons learned from 20 Years of CLEF. Cham: Springer; 2019.
129. Ferrucci D, Brown E, Chu-Carroll J, Fan J, Gondek D, Kalyanpur A, et al. Building Watson: an overview of the DeepQA Project. AI Mag. 2010;31(3):59–79.
130. Ferrucci D, Levas A, Bagchi S, Gondek D, Mueller E. Watson: beyond Jeopardy! Artificial Intelligence. 2012;199–200:93–105.
131. Hersh W, Müller H, Jensen J, Yang J, Gorman P, Ruch P. Advancing biomedical image retrieval: development and analysis of a test collection. J Am Med Inform Assoc. 2006;13:488–96.
132. Hersh W, Müller H, Kalpathy-Cramer J. The ImageCLEFmed medical image retrieval task test collection. J Digit Imaging. 2009;22:648–55.
133. Cohen T, Roberts K, Gururaj A, Chen X, Pournejati S, Hersh W et al. A publicly available benchmark for biomedical dataset retrieval: the reference standard for the 2016 bioCADDIE Dataset Retrieval Challenge. Database. 2017;27:bax061.
134. Roberts K, Gururaj A, Chen X, Pournejati S, Hersh W, Demner-Fushman D et al. Information retrieval for biomedical datasets: the 2016 bioCADDIE Dataset Retrieval Challenge. Database. 2017;2017:bax068.
135. Jansen B, Spink A, Bateman J, Saracevic T. Real life information retrieval: a study of user queries on the Web. SIGIR Forum. 1998;32:5–17.
136. Spink A, Jansen B, Wolfram D, Saracevic T. From e-sex to e-commerce: Web search changes. Computer. 2002;35:107–9.
137. Hafner K. Researchers Yearn to Use AOL Logs, but They Hesitate. New York Times. 2006 August 23, 2006.

Chapter 2
Information

Chapter 1 defined the basic terminology of information retrieval (IR) and presented some models of the use of IR systems. Before proceeding with the details of IR systems, however, it is worthwhile to step back and consider the more fundamental aspects of information, especially as it is used in the biomedical and health domain. In this chapter, the topic of information itself will be explored by looking at what it consists of and how it is produced and used. Consideration of this topic allows a better understanding of the roles as well as the limitations of IR systems.

2.1 What Is Information?

The notion of *information* is viewed differently by different people. Dictionary.com offers a number of different definitions of the word that include the following (mostly quoted)[1]:

- Knowledge communicated or received concerning a particular fact or circumstance
- Knowledge gained through study, communication, research, instruction, etc.
- An office, station, service, or employee whose function is to provide information to the public
- Law
  - An official criminal charge presented, usually by the prosecuting officers of the state, without the interposition of a grand jury
  - A criminal charge, made by a public official under oath before a magistrate, of an offense punishable summarily
  - The document containing the depositions of witnesses against one accused of a crime

[1] https://www.dictionary.com/browse/information

W. Hersh, *Information Retrieval: A Biomedical and Health Perspective*,
Health Informatics, https://doi.org/10.1007/978-3-030-47686-1_2

- (In information theory) An indication of the number of possible choices of messages, expressible as the value of some monotonic function of the number of choices, usually the logarithm to the base 2
- Computers
  - Important or useful facts obtained as output from a computer by means of processing input data with a program.
  - Data at any stage of processing (input, output, storage, transmission, etc.)

Others have attempted to define information by comparing it on a spectrum containing data, information, and knowledge [1]. *Data* consist of the observations and measurements made about the world. *Information*, on the other hand, is data brought together in aggregate to demonstrate facts. *Knowledge* is what is learned from the data and information and what can be applied in new situations to understand the world. Some add the notion of *wisdom* to this hierarchy, pointing to human appreciation and perspective of underlying knowledge, information, and data [2].

Whatever the definition of information, its importance cannot be overemphasized. This is truly the information age, where information (or access to it) is an indispensable resource, as important as human or capital resources. Most corporations have a chief information officer (CIO) who wields great power and responsibility. Some of best-known very wealthy Americans (e.g., Bill Gates, Paul Allen, Michael Bloomberg, and Mark Zuckerberg) made their fortunes in the information industry. Information is important not only to managers but to workers as well, particularly those who are professionals. Most healthcare and other knowledge-based professionals spend a significant proportion of their time acquiring, managing, and utilizing information.

2.2 Theories of Information

One way of understanding a complex concept like information is to develop theories about it. In particular, one can develop models for the generation, transmission, and use of information. This section will explore some of the different theories of information, which provide different ways to view information. More details in all the theoretical aspects of information can be found in books by Losee [3] and Stone [4].

The scientists generally credited with the origin of information theory are Claude Shannon and Warren Weaver [5]. Shannon was an engineer, most concerned with the transmission of information over telephone lines. His theory, therefore, viewed information as a signal transmitting across a channel. His major concerns were with coding and decoding the information as well as minimizing transmission noise. Weaver, on the other hand, was more focused on the meaning of information and how that meaning was communicated.

Figure 2.1 depicts Shannon and Weaver's model of communication. In information communication, the goal is to transfer information from the source to the destination. For the information to be transmitted, it must be encoded and sent by the

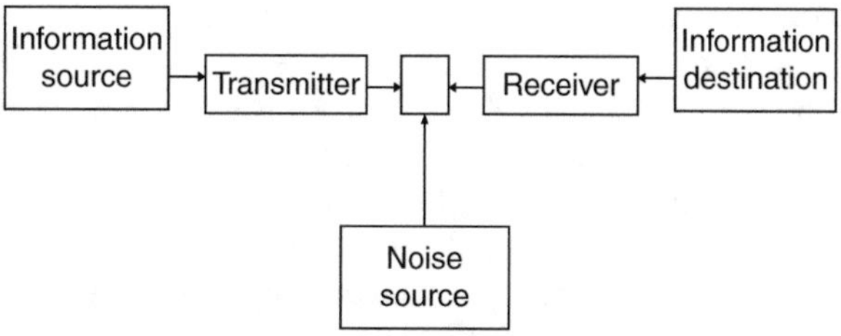

Fig. 2.1 Shannon and Weaver's model of communication, adapted from [5]

transmitter to a channel, which is the medium that transmits the message to the destination. Before arriving, however, it must be captured and decoded by the receiver. In electronic means of communication, the signal is composed of either waves (i.e., the analog signals of telephone or radio waves) or binary bits (i.e., in a digital computer).

From the standpoint of the sender, the goal is to deliver information as efficiently as possible. Therefore, information is a measure of *uncertainty* or *entropy*. Shannon actually defines this quantitatively. The simplest form of this expression is:

$$I = \log_2\left(\frac{1}{p}\right) = -\log_2(p) \tag{2.1}$$

where p is the probability of a message occurring. If base two is used for the logarithm, then information can be measured in terms of bits. An alternative view is that the quantity of information is measured by q, the logarithm of the number of different forms that a message can possibly take. In this case, the measurement of information is expressed as:

$$I = \log_2(q) \tag{2.2}$$

Obviously, messages of greater length have a higher number of possible forms.

As an example of the measure of information, consider the transfer of a single letter. If each letter has an equal probability of occurring, then the chance of any one letter occurring is 1/26. The information contained in one of these letters, therefore, is—$\log_2(1/26) = 4.7$ bits. This can be alternatively expressed as having 26 different forms, with the information contained in a letter as $\log_2(26) = 4.7$ bits. Similarly, the information in a coin flip is—$\log_2(1/2) = \log_2(2) = 1$ bit. Therefore, there is more information in a single letter than a coin flip. These examples indicate that the more likely a message is to occur, the less information it contains. Shannon's measure is clearly valuable in the myriad of engineering problems in transmitting messages across electronic media.

The quantification of information can provide other insights. For example, consider deoxyribose nucleic acid (DNA), the blueprint of life. Human DNA contains about three billion base pairs, each of which can have one of four possible "letters" (A, C, G, T), giving a total size of about 750 megabytes [6]. If nothing else, this demonstrates the efficiency of tiny living cells as storage mechanisms, even as computer storage has decreased in size through hard disks, optical disks, and now flash memory. None of these computer memory devices can store so much information in such a small volume of space. Also of note, from an information size standpoint, is that the amount of information in human DNA could actually be viewed as higher (e.g., the 200 gigabytes of overlapping reads coming from a modern gene sequencer) or lower (e.g., the uncertain role of "noncoding" DNA or the relatively small amount of variation from the "reference" genome, estimated to be about 0.1% and represented in about 125 megabytes).

Weaver, as mentioned above, was more concerned with the transmission of meaning [5]. He noted that Shannon's view of communication was only one of three levels of the communication problem and that the other two levels also must be considered in the communication of information. These levels were:

1. Technical—issues of engineering, such as how to efficiently encode information and move it across a channel with a minimum of noise
2. Semantic—issues of conveying meaning, such as whether the destination understands what the source is communicating
3. Effectiveness—issues of whether information has the desired effect at the destination level. A well-engineered communication system may have good semantic representation, but if it does not provide proper behavioral outcomes at other end, then the system is not effective.

Others attempted to refine and extend Shannon and Weaver's model. Bar Hillel and Carnap attempted to add a layer of semantics to the measurement of information [7]. They noted that information does not consist just of isolated bits; it actually contains objects with relationships (or predicates) between them. These objects and relationships can be encoded in logical forms, and therefore, information can be defined as the set of all statements that can be logically excluded from a message. In other words, information increases as statements become more precise. Belis and Guiasi worked at Weaver's effectiveness level by adding values of utility of messages for both the sender and receiver [8]. Certainly a message over a paramedic's radio that a patient in cardiac arrest is on the way to the emergency department has a great deal more utility for sender and receiver than one announcing that someone with a fractured wrist is coming. Belis and Guiasi added factors based on utilities of these types to Shannon's original equations.

Whereas information science is concerned with these theoretical notions of information and communication, most work has a more practical basis. In particular, information scientists are most concerned with written communication, which plays an important role in the dissemination of historical events as well as scholarly ideas. Information scientists focus on written information, from both archival and retrieval perspectives. Written information has been viewed not only from theoretical perspectives, such as the measuring of the "productivity" of scientists, but also from practical standpoints, such as deciding what books and journals to put in libraries and, more recently, how to build and disseminate IR systems.

2.3 Properties of Scientific Information

As just noted, information scientists study many facets of information but are usually most concerned with the written form. In the course of this work, they have identified many properties of information. Since the focus of information science is also usually based on scholarly and scientific information, most of these properties turn out to be quite pertinent to health information. This section will explore the growth, obsolescence, fragmentation, and linkage of scientific information.

2.3.1 Growth

Scientific information has been growing at an exponential level for several centuries and shows no signs of abating. The most widely cited description of this came from Price, who found that from the first known scientific journals in the 1600s, the doubling time of the scientific literature was about 15 years [9]. Pao noted that Price's model predicted an accumulation of 2.3 million scientific papers by 1977 (based on an initial paper in 1660) [10], which was very close to the 2.2 million documents that were indexed by members of the National Federation of Abstracting and Indexing Services in that year [11]. A couple decades later, based on the estimated Price doubling time, the number of all scientific papers published by 2006 should have been about 50 million, which was verified by Jinha by other means [12]. By 2009, it was estimated that there were 25,400 journals in science, technology, and medicine, publishing 1.5 million articles annually and increasing at a rate of 3.5% [13].

There is also plenty of evidence for growth of the scientific literature in biomedicine and health. In 2010, it was estimated that 75 clinical trials and 11 systematic reviews were being published per day [14]. Another measure of growth comes from the MEDLINE PubMed Production Statistics of the National Library of Medicine (NLM).[2] According to data from US Fiscal Year 2019, a total of 956,390 new records were added from 5243 journals to MEDLINE, bringing the total number of records to over 26 million. Inspection of the data back to 2013 shows an annual growth rate of around 5%. Durack [15] and Madlon-Kay [16] followed the weight growth of the (no longer produced) *Index Medicus* books of the medical literature index, noting that they also followed Price's doubling time. They lamented practically that this might exceed the shelving space of libraries, though did not foresee the transition to electronic publication of science, which has actually reduced the shelf space needs of most libraries.

There is a consensus that scientific information continues to grow exponentially, although it has become harder to measure with its growth beyond the confines of traditionally published journals that could be tracked through publications like the

[2] https://www.nlm.nih.gov/bsd/medline_pubmed_production_stats.html

Science Citation Index (Clarivate Analytics; see Chap. 3). Science is increasingly published in additional venues, such as conference proceedings, open archives, and Web sites [17, 18].

There are other aspects of the scientific literature that have been growing in recent times. One of these is the growth in the number of authors per paper. There continues to be an increase in the number of papers with more than 50, 100, and even 1000 authors [19]. Clearly that many people cannot have contributed to the writing of such papers, but they likely did participate in the research, so authorship is one method to acknowledge that. With the growth of numbers of authors, one concern is the order. There is a tradition of course for the first author to be the leader of the overall scientific effort and for the last author to be the "senior" author. In between, however, the roles are unclear. One growing trend is to list all authors alphabetically, although one study shows that this benefits those whose names occur early in the alphabet and are more likely to be seen [20]. Related to this are a small number of "hyperprolific" authors, those who publish a paper every 5 days in a given year [21]. Many of these authors come from physics, the field with the largest number of papers with the largest number of authors. There is no evidence of misconduct for these authors, but their achievements raise questions about what is required to achieve authorship of scientific publications.

2.3.2 Obsolescence

Despite its exponential growth in size, another property of scientific information is that it becomes obsolete, sometimes rather quickly. Newer literature not only reports on more recent experiments but is also more likely to provide a more up-to-date list of citations to recent work. Furthermore, new experimental findings often cause underlying views of a topic change over time. As new results are obtained, older experiments may be viewed in a different light.

A classic example of how views change over time because of new experimental results was seen with the view of the role of serum cholesterol in the heart disease [22]. When the link between serum cholesterol and coronary artery disease was first discovered, there was no evidence that lowering the cholesterol level was beneficial. But as experimental studies began to demonstrate that benefits could occur, then the earlier beliefs were displaced (though such assertions remained in the literature in the form of outdated papers). Even more recently, however, it has become clear that not everyone benefits from lowering serum cholesterol. In particular, for primary prevention of heart disease, many individuals must be treated to obtain benefit in a relatively few, and those likely to benefit are difficult to predict [23].

Some phenomena, such as medical diseases, change over time. For example, the presentation of many infectious diseases has changed drastically since the beginning of the antibiotic era, while the incidence of coronary artery disease continues to decline. Even phenomena from chemistry and physics, which themselves do not change, are seen in a different light when new methods of measuring and detecting them are developed.

These changes over time indicate that more recent literature is clearly advantageous and that some information becomes obsolete. The actual rate of information obsolescence varies by field. Price found that half of all references cited in chemistry papers were less than 8 years old, while half of those in physics papers were less than 5 years old [9]. This type of observation is not just theoretical; it has practical implications for those designing libraries and IR systems. For the former, there are issues of shelves to build and librarians to hire, while for the latter, there are issues of how much data to store and maintain.

Fortunately, knowledge itself becomes obsolete less quickly than citations. A famous early study demonstrated the "truth survival" of conclusions in the domain of liver cirrhosis and hepatitis [24]. The goal of the study was to determine whether information generated by the best evidence-based means had a longer survival when obtained in studies of higher methodological quality. The authors identified 474 conclusions in the published literature from 1945 to 1999 and found that 285 (60%) were still true in 2000, 91 (19%) were obsolete, and 98 (21%) were false. The half-life of truth in this domain was 45 years (in stark contrast to the half-life figures for citations presented above for chemistry and physics). The survival of conclusions was not higher in studies of better methodological quality than those of lesser quality and that the 20-year survival of conclusions derived from systematic reviews (a type of summarization of the literature described in Sect. 2.5.4) was lower (57%) than those from nonrandomized studies (87%) or randomized controlled trials (RCTs) (85%).

Another study of information obsolescence assessed only systematic reviews, determining how quickly "signals" for their updating became known [25]. These signals could be quantitative or qualitative. The former were defined as changes in statistical significance or 50% or more relative change in effect magnitude of one of the primary outcomes or of any mortality measure. The latter were defined as "substantial" changes with new information about harms or concerns about previously described findings. Based on this approach applied to 100 systematic reviews, the authors discovered a signal for updating 57% of all reviews, with a median duration of "survival-free" signal for updating of 5.5 years. The signal for updating occurred within 2 years for 23% of systematic reviews and by the publication date for 7% of them. A more recent study of systematic reviews found that some have significant delay between their completion and publication, leading to the possibility that new evidence has been published that might influence the results of the review [26].

Of course, just because literature is old does not mean it is obsolete. When a healthy volunteer died after being given the compound hexamethonium in a 2001 clinical trial, it was noted that this compound's toxicity had been documented in earlier literature [27]. Since the pertinent literature had been published before the advent of MEDLINE in 1966, it was not included in the MEDLINE database. This case led to the call for more systematic searching of older literature by researchers.

Related to information obsolescence is the long lead time for the dissemination of information. A common dictum in healthcare is that textbooks are out of date the moment they are published. As it turns out, they may be out of date before the authors even sit down to write them. Antman et al. showed that the information of experts as disseminated in the medical textbooks, review articles, and practice recommendations they produce often lagged far behind the edge of accumulated knowledge [28]. As a result, important advances go unmentioned and/or ineffective treatments are still advocated. Extending the analysis of Antman et al., Balas and Boren estimated that the average medical treatment advance takes 17 years to go from original discovery to clinical trials and into routine clinical practice [29].

2.3.3 Fragmentation

Ziman noted another property of the scientific literature, namely, that a single paper typically reports only on one experiment that is just small part of overall picture [30]. Ziman observed that the scientific literature is mainly written for scientists to communicate with their peers and thus presumes a basic understanding of the concepts in the field. Ziman also maintained that the literature is not only fragmented but also derivative, in that it relies heavily on past work and is edited, which provides a quality control mechanism.

Part of the reason for the fragmentation of the scientific literature is that scientists desire to "seed" their work in many different journals, where it may be seen by a larger diversity of readers. In addition, the academic promotion and tenure process encourages scientists in academic settings to "publish or perish." A common quip among academicians is to slice results into "least publishable units" (or "minimal publishable units") so that the maximum number of publications can be obtained for a body of work [31]. The extent to which this is done is not clear, but to the extent that the practice exists, more fragmentation of the scientific literature is a result. Another study found that the more publications that result from a project, the more likely those publications will be cited in total, especially when the articles are long [32].

Another aspect of fragmentation has been the tendency of science to segregate into fields, which further specialize as they grow in size [33]. Fortunately, the globally connected Internet buffers this somewhat, leading to easier access to information across fields, as demonstrated by the increased amount of citations across fields [34].

2.3.4 Linkage and Citations

Another property of scientific information is linkage, which occurs via the citation. The study of citations in scientific writing is a field unto itself called *bibliometrics* [35, 36]. This field is important in a number of ways, such as measuring the importance of individual contributions in science, indicating the likely places to find information on a given topic, and, as is known to Google users and we will discuss in Chap. 5, offering potential ways to enhance IR systems (i.e., the Google PageRank algorithm).

The bibliography is an important part of a scientific paper. It provides background information, showing the work that has come before and indicating what research has motivated the current work. It also shows that the author is aware of others working in the field. Authors also use citations to substantiate claims. Thus, a scientific paper on a new treatment for a disease will usually cite papers describing the disease, its human toll, and the success of existing therapies. An author arguing for a certain experimental approach or a new type of therapy, for example, may cite evidence from basic science or other work to provide rationale for the novel approach.

Citations can be viewed as a network or as a directed acyclic graph. Although reasons for citation can often be obtuse (i.e., a medical paper may cite a statistical paper for a description of an uncommon method being used), networks can give a general indication of subject relationship. One of the early workers in bibliometrics was Garfield, who originated the *Science Citation Index* (described above), a publication that now lists all citations of scientific papers from about 8500 journals in about 150 disciplines [37].

Being cited is important for scientists. Academic promotion and tenure committees look at, among other things, how widely cited an individual's work is, as do those who review the work of candidates for grant funding. In a study of several different fields, Price found that in certain fields, half of all citations formed a core of a small number of papers representing authors and publications with major influence on a given subject [38]. Some advocate using citation patterns to judge the quality of the work of scientists, but others have warned against it [39, 40]. One recent study found that quality and impact of papers were not associated well with their being cited, with citation rates actually underestimating the impact of highly impactful papers [41].

What factors are associated with increased likelihood of a paper being cited? One important factor in the modern era is the paper's easy electronic availability. Lawrence was the first to find that computer science papers freely available on the Web had a higher likelihood of being cited than those that were not [42]. Antelman verified this for four other fields: philosophy, political science, mathematics, and electrical engineering [43]. Likewise, Eysenbach found that for articles published in *Proceedings of the National Academy of Sciences*, which offers both open access (a more open approach to publishing described in Sects. 2.6.1 and 6.4.3) and non-open access publishing to authors, those published under the former approach were 2–3 times more likely to be cited [44]. Of course, these articles were not "randomized," so there may have been confounders leading to the different citation rate. It has also been found sharing research data in biomedicine is also associated with a higher rate of citation [45].

Others, however, have questioned whether open-access publishing and other forms of making articles freely available may not lead to increased citation. In reviewing more recent studies on this question, Craig et al. noted other possible explanations for their higher citation impact, such as selection bias, where more prominent authors are likely to post their articles online, and early-view bias, where the earlier availability of articles leads to more citations [46]. In other words, more widespread availability of articles may lead to quicker citation of articles, especially of those by more prominent researchers.

What other factors lead to higher rates of citations? A pair of studies has looked at Norwegian scientists, most of whom publish in international journals and are cited by international authors. The first study looked compared highly cited with "ordinary" cited papers [47]. It found that while most papers were regular articles (81%), review articles (12%) were overrepresented relative to their regular rate of appearance. Highly cited papers followed the usual pattern of initial rise and then decline of citation frequency over time. They received citations from many different journals and from both close and remote fields, which was also true of ordinary papers, although their high rate of citation made them appear in higher absolute numbers in different journals and fields. The second study found that in general, the rate of citation of papers correlated well with scientists' perceived importance of the research [48]. However, due to individual variance, it was difficult to apply this at the single-paper level.

The nature of linkage has been changing in the modern era of electronic publishing. Since 1990, the number of highly cited papers coming from highly cited journals has been diminishing [49]. Also in recent years, the number of highly cited papers in "non-elite" journals has increased, perhaps reflecting a democratizing effect of the ease of access of journals in electronic form [50]. However, there are still a number of "landmark" publications (about 1000 papers published between 1980–1990, 0.02% of all published papers) that achieved high impact quickly and sustained a high rate of citation [51].

Other research also provides more insights into citations. Letchford et al. found that papers with shorter titles [52] and with shorter abstracts containing more frequently used words [53] were more likely to be cited. Greenberg noted, however, that while citations can indicate authority of papers, they can also lead to unfounded authority of claims [54]. Trinquart et al. found in papers on one topic, the controversy of the role of reducing salt intake, that papers tended to be polarized in their citations, with more citations supporting the conclusions of a given paper [55]. Vucetic et al. found that in computer science doctoral programs, there is strong correlation with subjective rank of the program (as measured by *US News & World Report*) and faculty article citations [56]. Piwowar et al. found that articles published under the open access model (described in Chap. 6) were 18% more likely to be cited than those that were not freely available [57]. Larivière et al. noted that there is a higher propensity for scientists to cite researchers in their own country, which could skew citations indexes in favor of larger countries, especially a scientifically emergent China [58].

Sometimes cited papers take on lives of their own, receiving repeated citations that are unwarranted. For example, Leung et al. reported on a letter published in the *New England Journal of Medicine* (NEJM) [59] in 1980 [60] that asserted that opioid addiction was rare. The paper was an opinion piece and not a scientific investigation. Leung et al. identified 608 citations of the publication, noting a large increase after the introduction of OxyContin (a long-acting formulation of oxycodone) in 1995. Of the articles that referenced the 1980 letter, 439 (72.2%) cited it as evidence that addiction was rare in patients treated with opioids. Some authors were found to misrepresent the conclusions of the original letter, and the recent epidemic of opioid addiction has shown that addiction is not rare.

A similar example has been described by Koberlein, describing an experiment that supposedly proved Einstein's determination of the nonexistence of the "ether" in space was wrong [61]. The experiment was referenced in a letter in the esteemed journal, *Nature* [62], and Koberlein was able to find an experiment in a journal called *Speculations in Science and Technology* that indeed reported the experiment, although there are other explanations for its results [63].

Another challenge is that sometimes papers that do not even exist get cited and then those papers are cited subsequently by other papers. This was shown in "the most influential paper Gerard Salton never wrote," a paper from the IR pioneer that was cited repeatedly (fortunately never by this author!) [64].

As mentioned, the field of bibliometrics is concerned with measuring the individual contributions in science as well as the distribution of publications on topics. This field has also generated two well-known laws that deal with author productivity and subject dispersion in journals, Lotka's law and Bradford's law, respectively. It has also developed the impact factor, which attempts to measure the importance of journals, and various measures of individual scientist impact, such as the h-index. Alternatives to citations as measures of impact have also been explored, such as altmetrics.

2.3.4.1 Author Productivity: Lotka's Law

Most readers who work in scientific fields know that there is a small core of authors who produce a large number of publications. A mathematical relationship describing this has been described by Lotka and verified experimentally by Pao [65]. *Lotka's law* states if x is the number of publications by a scientist in a field and y is the number of authors who produce x publications each, then:

$$x^n * y = C \tag{2.3}$$

where C is a constant. For scientific fields, the value for n is usually near 2.0. Thus in scientific fields, the square of the number of papers published by a given author is inversely proportional to the number of authors who produce that number of papers.

Lotka's law is also known as the *inverse square law of scientific productivity* [65]. If the number of single paper authors is 100, then the number of authors producing two papers is $100/2^2 = 25$, and the number of authors producing three papers is $100/3^2 = 11$, etc. In general, 10% of the authors in a field produce half the literature in a field, while 75% produce less than 25% of the literature. Of course, the amount of publishing by an author does not measure their impact, which will be described below.

2.3.4.2 Subject Dispersion: Bradford's Law

Bradford observed [66] and others verified [67, 68] a phenomenon that occurs when the journals with articles on a topic are arranged by how many articles on that topic each publication contains. The journals tend to divide into a nucleus of a small number of journals followed by zones containing n, n^2, n^3, etc. journals with approximately the same number of articles. This observation is known as *Bradford's law of scattering*. Its implication is that as a scientific field grows, its literature becomes increasingly scattered and difficult to organize. But Bradford's law also indicates that most articles on a given topic are found in a core of journals. This fact is of importance to libraries, which must balance the goal of comprehensiveness with space and monetary constraints. Bradford's law has been found to apply to other phenomena in IR, such distribution of query topics to a database [69].

This phenomenon has been demonstrated in a number of areas in the medical literature, such as in the area of the acquired immunodeficiency syndrome (AIDS) [70]. In 1982, shortly after the disease was identified, only 14 journals had literature on AIDS. By 1987, this had grown to over 1200. The authors plotted the cumulative percent of journal titles versus journal articles for AIDS (Fig. 2.2) and found a Bradford distribution, with the first third of articles in 15 journals, the second third in 123 journals (=15 * 8.2), and the final third in 1023 journals ($\approx$15 * 8.2^2).

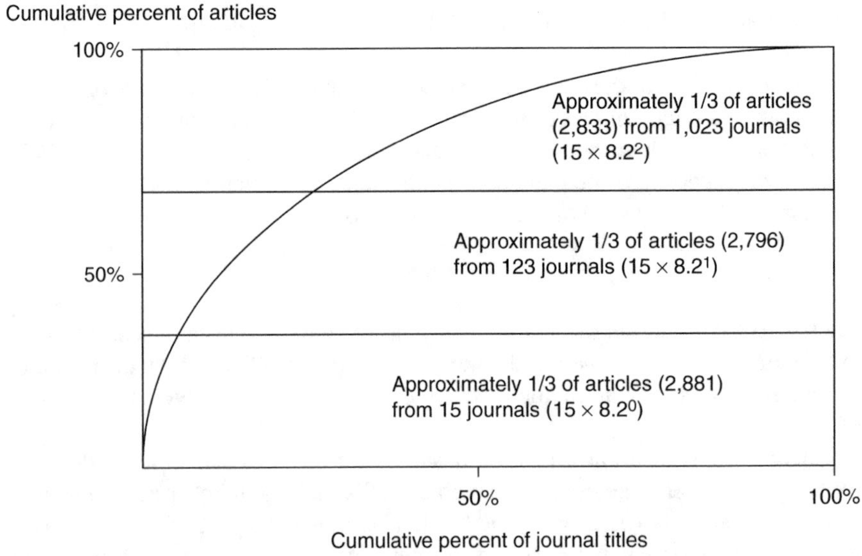

Fig. 2.2 The Bradford distribution for articles on AIDS, adapted from [70]

Other data support the notion of scattering. Wilczynski et al. found in the area of nephrology that 2779 articles cited in systematic reviews were concentrated in 466 journals and that 90% of the titles were in a set of 217 [71]. For systematic reviews of the Cochrane Collaboration in two respiratory diseases, Bradford's law was found to hold for RCTs included in the reviews but was not useful in predicting the long tail of how many journals should be searched to find trials [72]. In the field of neurosurgery, Bradford's law was found to hold in the main field and all of its subspecialties [73].

One implication of both Lotka's law and Bradford's law is that scientists and journals that are already successful in writing and attracting articles are likely to continue to be so in the future. In Sect. 2.5.2 on peer review, aspects of the scientific publishing process that indicate why successful scientists in a field continue their good fortune are explored.

2.3.4.3 Journal Importance: Impact Factor

Linkage information can also be used to measure the importance of journals, based on the *impact factor* (IF), which was introduced by Garfield [74]. The assumption underlying the IF is that the quantity of citations of a journal's papers is associated with that journal's importance. As with other linkage measures, IF can be used to make decisions about the journals to which a library should subscribe.

IF is usually measured with a formula that is the ratio of the number of citations in a given time period to the number of articles published. The formula also has a variant that adjusts for self-citations within a journal. The IF for current year citations of articles published over the last 2 years would thus be:

$$\text{IF} = \frac{\text{Citations in current year to articles published in prior two years}}{\text{Number of articles published in prior two years}} \tag{2.4}$$

Table 2.1 shows the most recent IF for the top journals in general medicine, medical informatics, and information systems.

Table 2.1 Impact factors of journals from selected fields for 2018, adapted from *Journal Citation Reports* (Clarivate Analytics)

Rank	Full journal title	Journal impact factor
General medical		
1	*New England Journal of Medicine*	70.67
2	*Lancet*	59.102
3	*JAMA—Journal of the American Medical Association*	51.273
4	*Nature Reviews Disease Primers*	32.274
5	*BMJ – British Medical Journal*	27.604
6	*JAMA Internal Medicine*	20.768
7	*Annals of Internal Medicine*	19.315

(continued)

Table 2.1 (continued)

Rank	Full journal title	Journal impact factor
8	*PLOS Medicine*	11.048
9	*Journal of Cachexia, Sarcopenia and Muscle*	10.754
10	*BMC Medicine*	8.285
11	*Cochrane Database of Systematic Reviews*	7.755
12	*Mayo Clinic Proceedings*	7.091
13	*Canadian Medical Association Journal*	6.938
14	*Journal of Internal Medicine*	6.051
15	*Journal of Clinical Medicine*	5.688
Medical informatics		
1	*Journal of Medical Internet Research*	4.945
2	*JMIR mHealth and uHealth*	4.301
3	*Journal of the American Medical Informatics Association*	4.292
4	*IEEE Journal of Biomedical and Health Informatics*	4.217
5	*Artificial Intelligence in Medicine*	3.574
6	*Computer Methods and Programs in Biomedicine*	3.424
7	*JMIR Serious Games*	3.351
8	*JMIR Medical Informatics*	3.188
9	*Journal of Biomedical Informatics*	2.95
10	*Medical Decision Making*	2.793
11	*International Journal of Medical Informatics*	2.731
12	*Journal of Medical Systems*	2.415
13	*Statistical Methods in Medical Research*	2.388
14	*Health Informatics Journal*	2.297
15	*BMC Medical Informatics and Decision Making*	2.067
Information science		
1	*International Journal of Information Management*	5.063
2	*Journal of Computer-Mediated Communication*	4.896
3	*Journal of Knowledge Management*	4.604
4	*MIS Quarterly*	4.373
5	*Government Information Quarterly*	4.311
6	*Journal of the American Medical Informatics Association*	4.292
7	*Information & Management*	4.12
8	*Journal of Strategic Information Systems*	4
9	*Information Processing and Management*	3.892
10	*Journal of Informetrics*	3.879
11	*Telematics and Informatics*	3.714
12	*International Journal of Geographical Information Science*	3.545
13	*Information Systems Journal*	3.286
14	*Journal of Information Technology*	3.125
15	*Journal of the Association for Information Systems*	3.103

Not everyone agrees that IF is the best determinant of journal quality. West pointed out that the importance of scientific articles is influenced by other factors, such as the nature of the underlying research; variations in the number of references different publications include; journal editorial policies that limit the number of references per article; different sized readerships, which may lead to differences related to audience size; scientists' conformity in often citing papers that are currently cited; authors' tendencies to cite their own work; and referees' tendencies to recommend inclusion of references to their work [75]. A number of authors have criticized IF over the years, noting that journals place too much emphasis on it and find ways to "game" it [76, 77].

However, a number of studies have found positive association between IF and other measures of journal quality. Lee et al. noted that IF and other measures of journal quality (e.g., citation rate, acceptance rate, listing in MEDLINE, circulation) were associated with higher methodological quality of a given publication [78]. Saha et al. asked 113 physicians who were predominantly practitioners and 151 physicians who were graduates of advanced training programs in clinical and health services research to rate the quality of nine general medical journals [79]. The correlation of IF with physicians' ratings of journal quality was high overall and somewhat higher for the group of researchers than the practitioners. McKibbon et al. also found an association between IF and the quantity of high-quality (i.e., evidence-based) studies published by medical journals [80].The inventor of the IF, Garfield, defended the measure in a *Journal of the American Medical Association* (*JAMA*) commentary [81]. He noted the value of quantitative measurement of a journal's importance for decision-making concerning the value of journals as well as decisions for library subscriptions. He did, however, warn against its use for evaluating the contributions of individual scientists. Dong et al. also recently reviewed the IF and provided a list of how the measure can be biased, including [82]:

- Incomplete journal coverage by the Science Citation Index (SCI), with an over-representation of English-language journals
- Different citation patterns across research fields and subject areas
- Differences among journals that increase IF but have nothing to do with quality, such as citations to "non-citable" items (i.e., items not counted in the IF denominator), availability of the abstract and/or full text online, and presence of longer articles.
- Inaccuracy of data
- IF calculated for whole journals whereas citations are to single articles
- Journals manipulating IF, such as by requesting authors to cite papers in their journal

They noted that while IF was effective in measuring the quality of a journal, it had little value in assessing individual articles, whether for their scientific contribution or how evidence-based they were.

Another category of criticism of IF consists of what some consider its misapplication to measuring the value of the work of individual scientists. Many commentators have noted that IF is really a measure that should be applied to journals and not individual scientists [83, 84]. In an analysis of literature of the role of `beta-amyloid` in `Alzheimer's disease`, Greenberg found that articles discounting the connection were less likely to be cited, resulting in "unfounded authority" and a "citation bias" in this area of science [54]. This was posited to harm science, giving researchers the incentive to publish sooner and more frequently than might be warranted by their work [85]. Another concern is that papers being commented upon, often because other researchers criticize the methods and/or disagree with the conclusions, have higher rates of citations than non-commented papers, potentially giving higher citation to papers whose methods or conclusions may be suspect [86]. As this study notes, similar to show business, any publicity is good publicity. Another analysis focusing on post-publication review finds that IF and number of citations are poor measures of scientific merit [87]. Ioannidis et al. surveyed highly cited scientists and found that their most cited work is not necessarily their best work [40]. (This is true for this author, as his top-cited paper ever is one published in 1994 describing his first test collection; see discussion on Google Scholar profiles below for details.) All of these concerns have led to a statement, the *San Francisco Declaration on Research Assessment*, originated by the American Society for Cell Biology, calling for journal-based metrics, most prominently IF, to not be used to evaluate the output of individual scientists.[3]

Just as scientific literature is linked, so is information on the Web. Indeed, Ingwersen proposed a Web impact factor (WIF), which is defined as the proportion of pages that link to a site from some defined area of the Web, such as a site or a group sites devoted to a specific topic [88]. It is defined mathematically as follows:

$$\text{WIF} = \frac{\text{number of pages linking to a site}}{\text{total number of pages in site}} \tag{2.5}$$

The value of the WIF in assessing the impact of research output has been limited due to use of the Web for activities other than publishing research [89]. Thelwall elaborated the different types of links among academic Web sites, also attempted to categorize links between academic Web sites, finding four general categories of links [90]:

- General navigation—allowing browsing to nonspecific information
- Ownership – allowing navigation to co-owners or co-authors of a project
- Social—recognition that the site being linked to is important in the social context of a field
- Gratuitous—links acknowledging institutions or other entities

[3] https://sfdora.org/

2.3.4.4 Author Impact

If the IF of published papers should not be used to judge the impact of individual scientists, what measure should be used? The measure that has gained the most prominence is the *h-index*, which is a measure of the number of papers of a scientist that have >h citations [91]. The h-index gives value to the most highly cited papers by a scientist. The h-index has been popularized by its prominent use by Google Scholar, which allows researchers to create a profile page that lists their publications and their citations (captured by Google crawling), such as the one for this author[4] or his daughter.[5] By default, the Google Scholar profile sorts papers by their number of citations, which may not represent what authors consider to be their best or most important work. For example, the most highly cited paper for this author is a 1994 paper describing an IR test collection that has been widely used, which he would not consider to be his most valuable research work [92]. Another tool for calculating h-index is the software package *Publish or Perish*,[6] which uses a number of citation sources (including Google Scholar) to calculate a wide range of measures for a scientist, with tools to control for author names, in particular authors from different fields who have the same names.

There are some challenges to the different citation packages on the Internet that use automated methods to calculate metrics like h-index. Kulkarni et al., for example, found that three sources of citations—Web of Science, Scopus, and Google Scholar—varied "quantitatively and qualitatively" in their citation counts for articles published in three journals, *JAMA*, *Lancet*, and *NEJM* [93]. Different sites also use different approaches for calculating h-index. Because the Google Scholar h-index calculation includes a variety of resources on the Web beyond just academic papers, it tends to be higher than when calculated just for published papers, as is done by Elsevier Scopus. For example, the current Google Scholar h-index for this author at the time of this writing is 71, compared to an h-index of 42 at the same time calculated by Elsevier Scopus.[7]

Another challenge for the Google Scholar h-index is that it does not always correctly disambiguate author names (such as William H. Hersh of Queens College[8]). It has also been shown that uploads of false papers that are found and included by Google Scholar can manipulate its metrics [94].

A number of other measures have been proposed to measure scientific impact. One proposed variant of the h-index is the *g-index*, which measures the number of papers of a scientist that have >g citations, on average [95]. The g-index correlates with the total number of citations for an author, whereas the h-index is correlated with the most citations from the most highly cited papers. For fields like

[4] https://scholar.google.com/citations?user=xFn_7nUAAAAJ

[5] https://scholar.google.com/citations?user=Ed5VVnUAAAAJ

[6] https://harzing.com/resources/publish-or-perish

[7] https://ohsu.pure.elsevier.com/en/persons/william-bill-hersh

[8] https://scholar.google.com/citations?hl=en&user=DCt8udIAAAAJ

informatics, where scientific output also includes tools and databases, Callahan et al. have proposed the U-index to account for these other contributions [96]. One more effort to catalog citations of scientists comes from Ioannidis et al., who both include and exclude self-citation [97].

Another measure whose use has been advocated by the US National Institutes of Health (NIH) is the *relative citation ratio* (RCR) [98]. The RCR uses the co-citation network of the paper to normalize the number of citations it has received for a given field. In other words, it adjusts citations relative to a discipline and allows comparison of peers within it. As such, a paper will have an RCR >1.0 if it is more cited relative to other papers in its discipline. The NIH has developed a dataset of citations for biomedical researchers and a Web site that calculates RCR for individual researchers[9] [99]. One analysis found that while amount and length of grant funding were associated with RCR, there was a diminishing of returns for funding over time [100].

An additional well-known project of bibliographic linkage is the Erdös Number Project. This project is, according to its Web site,[10] part of the "folklore of mathematicians," who measure their distance in co-authorship from the prolific Hungarian mathematician, Paul Erdös. Erdös published over 1400 scientific papers and had over 500 co-author collaborators. The mathematical community has built a collaboration graph for its community with approximately 337,000 authors of 1.6 million authored items in the *Math Review* database. Erdös is at the center of that graph. An "Erdös number" is thus the smallest number of co-authorship links between an individual and Erdös. Therefore, someone who co-authored with Erdös has an Erdös number of 1. Anyone who co-authored with any one of those co-authors has an Erdös number of 2. This author has an Erdös Number of 4, thanks to his former postdoc Andrew Turpin,[11] who was a graduate student of Alistair Moffat,[12] who has one of the lowest Erdös numbers (2) in the IR community.

A more tongue-in-cheek citation measure is the "Kardashian Index," which measures the discrepancy between a scientist's social media profile (from their Twitter handle) and publication record (from Google Scholar) based on a comparison of numbers of citations and Twitter followers [101]. The index can be calculated from a Web site that has users enter their Twitter handle and Google Scholar ID, with index of 5 indicating one is a "science Kardashian."[13] As of this writing, this author's Kardashian Index is 2.6, indicating his social media presence is not out of proportion to his scientific citation profile.

[9] https://icite.od.nih.gov/

[10] https://oakland.edu/enp/

[11] https://people.eng.unimelb.edu.au/aturpin/

[12] https://cis.unimelb.edu.au/people/staff.php?person_ID=13222

[13] http://theinformationalturn.net/kardashian-index/

2.3.4.5 Co-citation Analysis

Another type of analysis done in bibliometrics is *co-citation analysis*, which measures the number of times that pairs of authors are cited together by another paper. Co-citation analysis can help show authors whose work is similar in scope. Andrews performed such an analysis for the field of medical informatics, with a particular focus on members of the American College of Medical Informatics, a body of elected fellows who have made significant and sustained contributions to the field [102]. This analysis showed that the work of this author at the time was closest to that of Keith Campbell, Betsy Humphreys, Mark Tuttle, and Christopher Chute. In addition, he was found to be the 21st most highly cited individual in this group of leaders of the field.

Another analysis of publication and citation in the medical informatics field was recently carried out by Eggers et al. [103]. They analyzed 10 years of publications and citations in 22 journals in the field. In addition to measuring numbers of publications, they calculated an "authority score," based on frequency of citation by other highly frequent publishers. This author ranked tenth in the list of authority scores. They also mapped closeness of authors, which converged into five topic areas of the field. This analysis placed this author close to Homer Warner, Steve Johnson, Arthur Elstein, and Patricia Brennan, which seems less logical than Andrews' analysis.

Related to co-citation analysis is the recognition of the importance of research collaboration, especially with the emergence of "team science" and the large teams that take part in large, cutting-edge research projects. Indeed, a motivation of the NIH Roadmap initiative is to encourage collaboration of multidisciplinary teams of scientists to accelerate research findings into benefit for human health [104]. Co-citation analysis has also been proposed as a means to identify fields ripe for cross-disciplinary ideas [105].

2.3.4.6 Alternatives to Citations

Can the impact of science be determined by measures other than citations? One approach that has been adopted is article-level metrics, or altmetrics [106]. Lin et al. defined an ontology of article-level metrics that includes five categories and provides examples how each can be measured both for scholars and the public [107]. This has been developed into an altmetrics score that gives relative weight to different types of "mentions" about a publication, from appearing in the major news media to social media, Wikipedia, online course syllabi, and other Web platforms, as enumerated in Table 2.2.[14] These mentions carry varying weight and are used to calculate a real-time altmetrics score that journals and others can display on their Web sites. The altmetrics score was first adopted by the *Public Library of Science* (PLoS) family of journals [108], but many others now provide it, such as *JAMA* and

[14] http://altmetrics.org/

Table 2.2 Elements of the altmetrics measure for article citation (adapted from[a])

Source	Weight
News	8
Blog	5
Policy document (per source)	3
Patent	3
Wikipedia	3
Twitter (tweets and retweets)	1
Peer review (Publons, Pubpeer)	1
Weibo (not trackable since 2015, but historical data kept)	1
Google+ (not trackable since 2019, but historical data kept)	1
F1000	1
Syllabi (Open Syllabus)	1
LinkedIn (not trackable since 2014, but historical data kept)	0.5
Facebook (only a curated list of public pages)	0.25
Reddit	0.25
Pinterest (not trackable since 2013, but historical data kept)	0.25
Q&A (Stack Overflow)	0.25
YouTube	0.25
Number of Mendeley readers	0
Number of dimensions and Web of science citations	0

[a]https://www.altmetric.com/about-our-data/our-sources/

British Medical Journal (BMJ) [109]. One concern for altmetrics is that the highest values tend to show focus on minor and/or uncertain issues rather than major health issues [110].

2.3.5 Propagation

A final property of information is propagation. Interest in this area has been revived with the growth of the Internet and Web, which provide a vast new medium for information spread. The notion of the propagation of information can be traced back to Dawkins, whose book laid out the ideas of *memes*, which are information patterns that are held in a person's memory but can be copied to another [111]. The field that studies the replication and evolution of memes is called *memetics*. There are many Web sites devoted to memetics.[15]

Dawkins gave examples of memes as "tunes, ideas, [and] catch-phrases," which propagate from "brain to brain." Memes have been likened to genes but may be more appropriately compared to viruses, which cannot replicate themselves but take over a cell's DNA to cause it to make millions of copies of itself. According to

[15] http://pespmc1.vub.ac.be/MEMES.html

Dawkins, memes can affect the mind like a parasite, causing an individual to change his or her behavior and/or pass the idea on to others. Memes are selected or, in genetic terms, have fitness by a variety of properties such as novelty, coherence, and self-reinforcement. If they do not have the capability to survive, then they may die out. The Internet is a medium for the wide spread of memes. The frequent forwarding of emails and the use of social media sites are common means for memes to propagate. One consequence of such easy spread of information is the propagation of misinformation, including that related to science [112].

2.4 Classification of Health Information

Now that some basic theories and properties of information have been described, attention can be turned to the type of information that is the focus of most of this book, textual health information. It is useful to classify it, since not only are varying types used differently but alternative procedures are applied to its organization and retrieval.

Table 2.3 lists a classification of textual health information. *Patient-specific* information applies to individual patients. Its purpose is to tell healthcare providers, administrators, and researchers about the health and disease of a patient. This information comprises the patient's medical record. Patient-specific data can be either *structured*, as in a laboratory value or vital sign measurement, or in the form of *free (narrative) text*. Of course, many notes and reports in the medical record contain both structured and narrative text, such as the history and physical report, which contains the vital signs and laboratory values. For the most part, this book does not address patient-specific information although Chap. 8 discusses the processing of clinical narrative text. As will be seen, the goals and procedures in the processing of such text are often different from other types of medical text.

The second major category of health information is *knowledge-based* information. This is information that has been derived and organized from observational or experimental research. In the case of clinical research, this information provides clinicians, administrators, and researchers with knowledge derived from experiments and observations, which can then be applied to individual patients. This information is most commonly provided in books and journals but can take a wide variety of other forms, including computerized media. Some patient-specific information

Table 2.3 A classification of textual health information

1. Patient-specific information
   a. Structured—lab results, vital signs
   b. Narrative—history and physical, progress note, radiology report
2. Knowledge-based information
   a. Primary—original research (in journals, books, reports, etc.)
   b. Secondary—summaries of research (in review articles, books, practice guidelines, etc.)

does make it into knowledge-based information sources, but with a different purpose. For example, a case report in a medical journal does not assist the patient being reported on but rather serves as a vehicle for sharing the knowledge gained from the case with other practitioners.

Knowledge-based information can be subdivided into two categories. *Primary* knowledge-based information (also called primary literature) is original research that appears in journals, books, reports, and other sources. This type of information reports the initial discovery of health knowledge, usually with original data. Revisiting the earlier serum cholesterol and heart disease example, an instance of primary literature could include a discovery of the pathophysiological process by which cholesterol is implicated in heart disease, a clinical trial showing a certain therapy to be of benefit in lowering it, a cost-benefit analysis that shows which portion of the population is likely to best benefit from treatment, or a systematic review that uses meta-analysis to combine all the original studies evaluating one or more therapies.

Secondary knowledge-based information consists of the writing that reviews, condenses, and/or synthesizes the primary literature. The most common examples of this type of literature are books, monographs, and review articles in journals and other publications. Secondary literature also includes opinion-based writing such as editorials and position or policy papers. It also encompasses clinical practice guidelines, systematic reviews, and health information on Web pages. In addition, it includes the plethora of pocket-sized manuals that are a staple for practitioners in many professional fields. As will be seen later, secondary literature is the most common type of literature used by physicians.

Another approach to classifying knowledge-based information comes from Haynes [113], taking the perspective of evidence-based medicine (EBM) [114, 115]. As depicted in Fig. 2.3, Haynes defines a hierarchy of evidence, dubbed the 4S model. At the base are the original *studies* forming the foundation of knowledge. These studies are in turn aggregated into *syntheses*, often called *systematic reviews* or *evidence reports*, which systematically identify and synthesize all the evidence

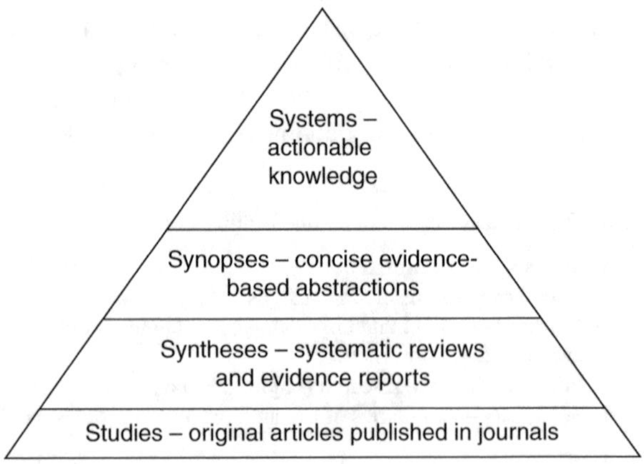

Fig. 2.3 The "4S model" of hierarchy of evidence, adapted from [113]

on a given topic. Where appropriate in systematic reviews, meta-analysis is performed, in which the results of multiple appropriately homogenous studies are combined to achieve an aggregate result, which usually also has larger statistical power. Systematic reviews are distinct from *narrative reviews*, which just provide a general overview of a topic that is usually broader but less exhaustive in coverage. A further distillation of knowledge occurs with *synopses*, which provide a summary (ideally derived from an evidence-based synthesis) on a topic. The ultimate level of the hierarchy is *systems*, which consist of actionable knowledge structured in a way that can be used by information systems, such as a clinical decision support module of an electronic health record. Haynes and colleagues subsequently expanded this 4S model into 5S [116] and 6S [117] versions, adding summaries explicit for each level, but the original is simplest and provides an overview of the types of information formats in which is scientific information is provided and published.

Although the scope of EBM is beyond this book, it is well-described in other references [114, 115]. But the process of EBM requires IR throughout, so an overview of EBM provides some perspective about the use of IR with it. The process of EBM involves three general steps:

- Phrasing a clinical question that is pertinent and answerable
- Identifying evidence (studies in articles) that address the question
- Critically appraising the evidence to determine whether it applies to the patient

There are two general types of clinical question: background questions and foreground questions [118]. *Background* questions ask for general knowledge about a disorder, whereas foreground questions ask for knowledge about managing patients with a disorder. Background questions are generally best answered with textbooks and classical review articles, whereas foreground questions are answered using EBM techniques. Background questions contain two essential components: a question root with a verb (e.g., what, when, how) and a disorder or aspect of a disorder. Examples of background questions include `What causes pneumonia?` and `When do complications of diabetes usually occur?`

Foreground questions have four essential components, based on the PICO mnemonic: the patient and/or problem, the intervention, the comparison intervention (if applicable), and the clinical outcome(s). Some expand the mnemonic with two additional letters, PICOTS, adding the time duration of treatment or follow-up and the setting (e.g., inpatient, outpatient, etc.) [119]. There are four major categories of foreground questions:

- Therapy (or intervention)—benefit of treatment or prevention
- Diagnosis—test diagnosing disease
- Harm—etiology of disease
- Prognosis—outcome of disease course

EBM has evolved since its inception. The original approach to EBM focused on clinicians finding original studies in the primary literature and applying critical appraisal, a challenging and time-consuming task for most. This led to a next generation of EBM that focused on the use of syntheses and synopses, where the literature searching, critical appraisal, and extraction of statistics operations were performed ahead of time [120]. Others argued we should put more emphasis on teaching information management (seeking) than the techniques of EBM [121], and we will see many examples of evidence-based information resources now available in Chap. 3.

2.5 Production of Biomedical and Health Information

Since the main focus of this book is on indexing and retrieval of knowledge-based information, the remainder of this chapter will focus on that type of information (except for Chap. 8, where patient-specific information is discussed, but only in the context of processing the text-based variety). This section covers the production of biomedical health information, from the original studies and their peer review for publication to their summarization in the secondary literature for clinicians and consumers.

2.5.1 Generation of Scientific Information

How is scientific information generated? Figure 2.4 depicts the "life cycle" of scientific information. The process begins with scientists themselves, who make and record observations, whether in the laboratory or in the real world. These observations are then written up and submitted for publication in the primary literature, where they undergo peer review. If the paper passes the test of peer review, it is published, usually in a scientific journal. If the paper does not pass muster in peer review, the author usually revises it and resubmits it to the same or a different

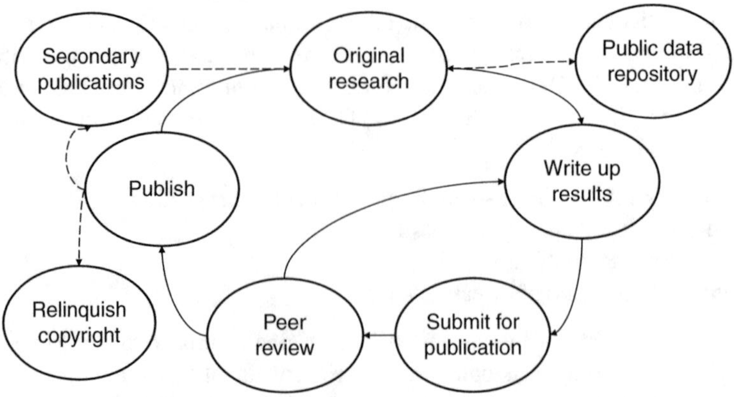

Fig. 2.4 The "life cycle" of scientific information

journal. Other steps that may occur if the paper is published is that the author may be required to relinquish the copyright, usually to the publisher of the journal, and/or the information in the paper may make its way into secondary publications, such as a textbook or clinical practice guideline. In addition, there is growing encouragement, sometimes requirement (especially in the genomic sciences) for underlying data to be published. Finally, research results typically generate new questions and motivate new research that may then follow a new cycle through this process.

One of the most widely cited descriptions of the scientific process is Thomas Kuhn's *The Structure of Scientific Revolutions* [122]. Kuhn noted that science proceeds in evolutions and revolutions. In the evolutionary phase of a science, there is a stable, accepted paradigm. In fact, Kuhn argued, a field cannot be a science until there is such a paradigm that lends itself to common interpretation and agreement on certain facts. A science evolves as experiments and other observations are performed and interpreted under the accepted paradigm. This science is advanced by publication in peer-reviewed journals. In the revolutionary phase, however, evidence in conflict with the accepted paradigm mounts until it overwhelmingly goes against the paradigm, overturning it. The classic example of this described by Kuhn came from the work of Copernicus, who contributed little actual data to astronomy but showed how the astronomical observations of others fit so much better under a new paradigm in which the planets revolved around the sun rather than around the earth. A more recent example comes from cancer research, where existing notions of the "hallmarks" of cancer are overturned piece by piece, leading to significant changes in our understanding of the disease and its treatment [123].

Just about all research undergoes *peer review* by scientist colleagues, whom decide whether the paper describing the research is worthy of publication. The goal of this process is to ensure that the appropriate experimental methods were used, that the findings represent a new and informative contribution to the field, and that the conclusions are justified by the results. Of course, what is acceptable for publication varies with the scope of the journal. Journals covering basic biomedical science (e.g., *Cell*) tend to publish papers focusing on laboratory-based research that is likely to focus on mechanisms of diseases and treatments, whereas clinical journals (e.g., *JAMA*) tend to publish reports of large clinical trials and other studies pertinent to providing clinical care. Specialized journals are more likely to publish preliminary or exploratory studies. Bourne provided some simple rules to those aspiring to achieve scientific publication in the field of computational biology, but these easily apply to other fields and still pertinent in recent times [124].

Peer-reviewed journals are not the only vehicle for publication of original science. Other forums for publication include the following:

- Conference proceedings – usually peer-reviewed, publishing either full papers or just abstracts
- Technical reports—may be peer-reviewed, frequently providing more detail than journal papers
- Books—may be peer-reviewed.

In general, however, non-journal primary literature does not carry the scientific esteem accorded to journal literature. These varying sources of non-journal primary literature are sometimes called "grey literature," and their identification can be important, as they may impact the results of systematic reviews and meta-analyses. In particular, they are less likely to show a treatment effect and thus may lead to exaggeration of meta-analysis results when not included [125].

It has been posited for a long time that the scientific method is the best method humans have devised for discerning the truth about their world [30]. While a number of limitations with the peer review process and the scientific literature itself will be seen in ensuing sections, the present author agrees that there is no better method for understanding and manipulating the phenomena of the world than the scientific method. Flaws in science are usually due more to flaws in scientists and the experiments they devise than to the scientific method itself, although some note systemic flaws as well [126].

To bring more standardization to the biomedical and health publishing process, the editors of the major medical journals formed a committee (International Committee of Medical Journal Editors, ICMJE[16]) to establish policy, such as providing general recommendations on the submission of manuscripts to journals. They defined the so-called Vancouver format for publication style, which journals will agree to accept upon submission even if their own formats vary and will require editing later. Equally important, however, they defined a number of additional requirements and other statements for biomedical publishing [127]:

- Redundant or duplicate publication occurs when there is substantial overlap with an item already published. One form of redundant publication that is generally acceptable is the publication of a paper whose preliminary report was presented as a poster or abstract at a scientific meeting. Acceptable instances of secondary publication of a paper include publication in a different language or in a journal aimed at different readers. In general, editors of the original journals must consent to such publication, and the prior appearance of the material should be acknowledged in the secondary paper.
- Authorship should be given only to those who make substantial contribution to study conception or design and data acquisition, analysis, or interpretation; drafting of the article or revising it critically for important intellectual content; and giving final approval for publication.
- A peer-reviewed journal is one that has most of its articles reviewed by experts who are not part of the editorial staff.
- While journal owners have the right to hire and fire editors, the latter must have complete freedom to exercise their editorial judgment.
- All conflicts of interest from authors, reviewers, and editors must be disclosed. Financial support from a commercial source is not a reason for disqualification from publishing, but it must be properly attributed.

[16] http://www.icmje.org/

- Advertising must be kept distinguishable from editorial content and must not be allowed to influence it.
- Competing manuscripts based on the same study should generally be discouraged, and this requires careful intervention by editors to determine an appropriate course of action.

The ICMJE has also published guidelines concerning conflicts of interest and authorship [128], planned for update in 2020 [129], as well a statement on data sharing [130], both of which are described below. They recently published a statement, *Recommendations for the Conduct, Reporting, Editing, and Publication of Scholarly Work in Medical Journals.*[17]

Scientific information would not be generated at all were it not for research funding. The process to determine research funding is also done via peer review. The largest grantor of biomedical research funding in the world is the NIH, which maintains a site containing a wealth of data about its grant review and funding process.[18] Some highlights from this site include:

- The NIH budget for the most recent US fiscal year was $36 billion.
- About 80% of the funding goes to extramural researchers outside the NIH, with remaining funding administration as well as intramural researchers.
- In recent years, the NIH received about 54,000 grant proposals and awarded about 11,000 grants for a success rate of about 20%, which varies across institutes and research initiatives.
- About 30,000 scientists participate in NIH peer review.
- The process supports about 126,000 graduate (mostly PhD) students and 43,000 postdocs, many of whom carry out parts of the funded research.

There are some additional concerns about the generation of knowledge. One is that some knowledge is never obtained because it is "forbidden" to be studied [131]. Knowledge may be forbidden because it can only be obtained through unethical means, e.g., human experiments conducted by Nazi scientists. But other research is prohibited by what Kempner et al. call "informal constraints." This may involve fear from results being attacked by political groups across the spectrum, from religious groups to animal rights activists. Clearly there must be some ethical constraints on the conduct of science, but not merely if they offend the political agenda of a particular group.

A new wrinkle on this problem has emerged with efforts to undermine government science in the United States. Until recently, for example, research on gun safety has not been allowed to be funded by US government agencies [132]. One recent analysis identified over 300 instances of government Web sites having scientific information on politically controversial topics modified or removed [133]. This has been particularly notable for government Web sites on climate change [134]. Another concern is the potential subverting of open data reuse policies for political

[17] http://www.icmje.org/recommendations/

[18] https://report.nih.gov/nihdatabook/

agendas. For example, the US Environmental Protection Agency recently adopted a "transparency rule" that allowed it to exclude data that was not freely shared [135]. As a number of large environmental science studies have personally identifying information, excluding them from consideration in environmental regulations means ignoring large amounts of research that could impact policy. Several university associations wrote letters objecting to this policy [136].

Another concern about the production of biomedical literature is that the clinical trials carried out do not meet the needs of "decision-makers," in particular, those who develop policy, practice guidelines, and so forth. This has given rise to the development of pragmatic clinical trials [137, 138]. The characteristics of these trials include the selection of clinically relevant interventions for comparison, diverse populations of study participants, recruitment from heterogeneous practice settings, and data collection from a broad range of clinical outcomes.

There are a number of other characteristics of the scientific process. One is that it is based on *trust*, i.e., all who participate should have a disinterested pursuit of the truth. Smith advocates that scientists especially should have extraordinary honesty, since their methods and results are mostly taken without direct verification [139]. Conflicts of interest that undermine science will be explored further below, but some have called for more financial independence for research and the education of researchers [140]. Other have noted, however, that much more must be done to maintain trust in scientific research, including addressing systematically some of the flaws that will be described later in this chapter [126]. Jamieson et al. propose a number of approaches for authors and journals that would lead to more effective signals of trustworthiness. These include article badging, checklists, a more extensive withdrawal ontology, identity verification, better forward linking, and greater transparency [141].

Objective scientific research also shows us that new is not necessarily better. This was borne out in an analysis that assessed 10 years of articles in NEJM that concerned a medical practice and tested a new practice [142]. The study found that 77% of the times, the new practice was beneficial, but the remainder of the times it was not. By the same token, studies of established practices found that, over half the time, the practice was no better or worse, so actually reversing the established practice, or it was inconclusive. Another analysis looked at four cohorts of randomized control trials in the Cochrane Database of Systematic Reviews and found that slightly more than half of new treatments were superior to established ones [143]. Further analyses like these have identified many more "reversals" of earlier research [144, 145]. Indeed, this points to another characteristic of science, which is that when it works properly, it is *self-correcting*.

Science has also undergone profound change, especially with the emergence of new information technologies and the global Internet. There has been essentially a complete change of publishing medium from paper to electronic. This is certainly noticeable over the editions of this book, where original IR systems were used to be directed to paper copies of articles and books to now the entire process being electronic, from finding the content to accessing and using it. This has impacted all of the sections to follow, from peer review to primary and secondary literature.

2.5.2 *Peer Review*

Although peer review had its origins centuries ago, it did not achieve its present form until the twentieth century [146]. As noted earlier, the goal of peer review is to serve as a quality filter to the scientific literature. Theoretically, only research based on sound scientific methodology will be published. In reality, of course, the picture is more complicated. Awareness that what constitutes acceptable research may vary based on the quality or scope of the journal has led to the realization by some that the peer review process does not so much determine whether a paper will be published as where it will be published.

Most journals have a two-phase review process. The manuscript is usually reviewed initially by the editor or an associate editor to determine whether it fits the scope of the journal and whether there are any obvious flaws in the work. If the manuscript passes this process, it is sent out for formal peer review. Most of the high-profile journals have low acceptance rates, e.g., the <10% in *Nature*[19] and 4–10% (depending on paper type) for *JAMA*.[20] Among smaller journals, the rate of acceptance has always varied widely, in one older analysis from 13 to 91% [147].

The peer review process serves other purposes besides assessing the quality of science. For example, review of papers by peers also leads to improvement in the reporting of results and conclusions. Purcell et al. found that peer review identified five types of problem with papers: too much information, too little information, inaccurate information, misplaced information, and structural problems [148]. These can be corrected during the editorial process. Even if the paper is not accepted, peer review can be beneficial to authors who are likely to implement suggested changes before submitting their material to a different journal [149].

2.5.2.1 Is Peer Review Effective?

Has peer review been shown to improve the quality of publications or, better yet, the advancement of human health or scientific knowledge? One early systematic review found that all studies to date had focused on surrogate and intermediate measures and none compared peer review with other methods [150]. Twenty-one studies of the process were found and led to a variety of conclusions (number supporting each conclusion in parentheses):

- Concealing identities of peer reviewers or authors does not appear to affect quality of reviews (9).
- Checklists and other attempts at standardizing the process do not appear to help (2).
- Training of referees does not improve the quality of reviews (2).

[19] https://www.nature.com/nature/for-authors/editorial-criteria-and-processes

[20] https://jamanetwork.com/journals/jama/pages/for-authors

- Electronic media do not improve quality (2).
- Peer review does not detect bias against unconventional drugs (1).
- The process may improve readability and general quality of papers (2).

Other studies have highlighted problems with the peer review process. A famous study from the 1980s generated a great deal of controversy. Two psychologists took 12 psychology articles that were already published in prestigious psychology journals and resubmitted them with different author names and slight rewording of titles [151]. These articles were eventually disseminated to 38 reviewers, only 3 (8%) of whom detected that the article was a resubmission. For the remaining 9 articles, 16 of 18 reviewers recommended against acceptance, and all but one of the articles were rejected for publication. The most common reason for rejection of these previously accepted papers was "serious methodologic flaw." While there was some criticism of their methods, this study showed that the prestige of the authors influenced the peer review process.

Other early studies raised additional concerns. Ingelfinger, a former editor of NEJM, noted that for nearly 500 consecutive papers submitted to that journal, the concordance between the 2 reviewers for each article was only slightly better than chance [152]. Among the problems he cited in the peer review process were reviewers wrongly assumed to be knowledgeable on a particular topic based on their stature in the field as a whole, reviewers not skilled in detecting poor writing that obscured the quality of an underlying message, and reviewer bias toward or against others in the individual's field. Another early study showed that in secondary review of accepted manuscripts, although there was high concordance among reviewers for accepting or rejecting the paper, there was a wide divergence in the identification of problems deemed to warrant further revision [153].

A more recent study of peer review gave reviewers papers of identical methods but positive vs. neutral results and found a higher rate of recommending publication for positive (97.3%) over neutral (80.0%) papers [154]. Siler et al. assessed over 1000 articles submitted to three elite medical journals, of which about 800 articles were eventually published [155]. While there was an association between peer review scores and subsequent citations, the top 14 cited articles had been rejected by these elite journals. An analysis from a highly selective computer science conference compared "single-blind" (reviewers were aware of names and affiliations of paper authors) versus "double-blind" (names and affiliations hidden) reviewing, finding the former were more likely to recommend acceptance of papers from famous authors, top universities, and top companies [156]. Nicholson has noted that at least eight Nobel Prize for science winners had papers describing some of their work rejected [157], which happened again in 2019 [158].

Another group of concerns have emanated from the growth of open-access publishing, which will be discussed in Chap. 6. These journals, which typically have an "author pays" model, have financial incentive to accept articles. While some of these journals have achieved high prestige, such as *BioMed Central* (BMC) and PLoS, some of them serve as money-making vehicles for those who publish them [159]. Journals with scientific-sounding names but minimal if any peer review have been dubbed "predatory journals" [160]. This problem is not limited to publishing in journals. There are also a growing number of for-profit conferences that invite legitimate researchers, some of whom are attracted by the opportunity to present their work [161].

Results like these have led to commentary about the peer review process. Some have posited that the peer review system tends to serve to keep control of science in the hands of those who already have it [162]. Other have noted the so-called "winner's curse," with positive research results more likely to be accepted and published, leading to distortion of the larger picture of all scientific results [163]. This may lead to a "decline effect" of scientific results to the most dramatically positive findings being published first and foremost [164]. One major critic of peer review has been Richard Smith, the former editor of BMJ who has called peer review "an empty gun" [165]. Smith proposed a variety of steps for radically altering publishing of scientific results, essentially requiring publication of protocols and results with data, after which studies meeting a certain screen would be published with a unique identifier [166]. Reviewers would then assess the studies, and authors could use that feedback to improve their work, in an auditable way. This would make it easy to publish but also allow a great deal more transparency of the results and their meaning.

The peer review process of grant proposals has also been studied. One early analysis noted a number of problems, which also occur with journal peer review [167]:

- For scientific pioneers, there are often few peers who are knowledgeable enough to adequately review their work.
- For all scientists, the closest peer is a competitor, who may not be appropriate as a reviewer.
- While reviewers have the opportunity to criticize every aspect of the submitter's work, there is little if any chance for rebuttal.
- Reviewers are anonymous, hence are shielded from their own deficiencies and/or bias.

More recently, an assessment of more than 130,000 research project (R01) grants funded by the NIH from1980 to 2008 and found that better peer review scores were consistently associated with better research outcomes [168]. A one-standard deviation worse peer review score among awarded grants was associated with 15% fewer citations, 7% fewer publications, 19% fewer high-impact publications, and 14% fewer follow-on patents. Re-analysis of this data found, however, that for scientists with highly scoring proposals, i.e., those likely to receive funding, the correlation disappeared [169]. A study by Pier et al. found low agreement among reviewers evaluating the same NIH grant applications [170]. Of encouragement to young scientists, Wang et al. found that scientists who had early "near misses" with grant funding were likely to either achieve long-term success or disappear from the literature, with the former doing better than those with early "near wins" [171]. All of these results led Smaldino et al. to advocate for funding decisions based on "modified lotteries," which would allocate funding randomly among proposals that pass a baseline for methodological rigor [172]. They believe this would reduce the rate of false discoveries, especially when paired with other improvements that increase the publication of negative results and improve the quality of peer review.

Many researchers would no doubt agree with the information scientist Tefko Saracevic, who has said (personal communication) that the peer review process determines more where an article is published than whether it is published. Perhaps another lesson can be learned from observations about professional basketball, which is that those who are already successful tend to continue achieving success. In the book, *The Jordan Rules* [173], an analysis of NBA referees found a tendency to give this superstar (and probably others) the benefit of the doubt in foul calls.

2.5.2.2 How Can Peer Review Be Improved?

There is a fairly substantial body of disparate literature on what works in peer review and how it can be improved. One simple suggestion for improving peer review has been the separation of improving writing from judgment of scientific merit [174]. A variety of other studies have looked at who makes good reviewers, how they are best helped, and where the process falls down. Bourne and Korngreen provided simple rules for individuals being good reviewers [175].

Some research has attempted to identify the characteristics of good peer reviewers. The only consistent factor associated with high-quality reviewing has been younger age, in particular advanced enough to know the field but not too senior so as to be too busy or cynical. One researcher found that the best reviews came from faculty of junior academic status [176], while another showed the best reviews came from younger faculty working at top academic institutions or who were known to the editors [177]. Nylenna et al. found that younger referees with more experience refereeing had a better chance at detecting flaws in problematic papers [178]. Black et al. also showed that younger reviewers and those who had training in epidemiology or statistics produced better reviews, though their study found in general that reviewer characteristics could explain only 8% of the variation in review quality [179]. Callaham et al. found that subjective ratings of reviewers correlated with the ability to detect flaws in manuscripts [180].

One common practice in peer review, especially outside medicine, is to ask authors for suggested reviewers. Does this make a difference? One analysis of 329 manuscripts from 10 leading journals found that the quality of the reviews was judged similar but that author-suggested reviewers tended to make more favorable recommendations concerning publication [181]. Similar findings were found in another analysis [182]. However, this process has been shown in some instances to lead to fraud, as those submitting papers conspire to list colleagues or even non-scientists as suggested peer reviewers [183, 184].

A related problem is that most editors of peer-reviewed journals are not trained in editorial practices, tending to come from the ranks of accomplished academicians and clinicians. Most of these individuals are likely to have had prior experience with publishing and/or peer reviewing, however. While the editors of the major journals devote full-time effort to editing, editors of specialty journals usually devote part-time effort. Most specialist clinical medical journals tend to be edited by practicing clinicians who are self-taught, part-time editors [185]. Moher et al. have proposed a set of core competencies for scientific journal editors that included having a broad knowledge of the field covered by the journal, communication skills, understanding of publication ethics and research integrity, and a mastery of editorial principles and practices [186].

Some have noted that the modern Internet and Web provide the possibility for more open and transparent peer review. A growing number of journals have experimented with publishing peer reviews and have adopted the process as policy [187, 188]. Two large private biomedical researchers—UK Wellcome Trust and the Howard Hughes Medical Institute—along with ASAPbio, a nonprofit organization that encourages innovation in life sciences publishing, have published a statement calling for publication of peer reviews in the sciences [189].

2.5.3 *Primary Literature*

As already noted, the primary literature consists of reports of original research. Key features of primary literature are that it reports on new discoveries and observations, describes earlier work to acknowledge it and place the new findings in the proper perspective, and draws only conclusions that can be justified by the results.

2.5.3.1 Characteristics of the Primary Literature

Historically, a key feature of most primary literature is that it has not been published elsewhere, especially in non-peer-reviewed forums. Indeed, most journals adhere to the "Ingelfinger rule," which states that a manuscript will be accepted for publication only if it has not been published elsewhere [190]. Exceptions are made for articles that have been presented at scientific meetings, situations in which early publication would have a major impact on public health, and cases in which findings have been released for government deliberations [191].

Where do scientists choose to publish? In a study of where the highest-quality (i.e., most evidence-based) studies were published, McKibbon et al. noted they were mostly clustered in a relatively small number of high-profile clinical journals [80]. A study of submission patterns among different journals found a pattern of researchers aiming for high-impact general journals initially and, if articles were not accepted, aiming for more focused journals in their own fields [192]. While biomedicine remains firmly wedded to the notion of journal articles being the primary vehicle for dissemination of science, other fields such as computer science consider the critical metric of success as having a paper published in highly selective (i.e., those with low acceptance rates, on the order of 10–20%) conferences. This is clearly exemplified by data showing that papers from those conferences have higher rates of subsequent citation, comparable to major journals in the field, although some have concern that the tight timeline of publishing of conference papers does not provide for the back and forth between authors and peer reviewers seen in journals [193]. This has led some to call for a policy of "publish now, judge later," as the large numbers of papers that must be rejected (often 80%) means that peer reviewers will look for obvious flaws and not delve into more nuanced ones. Some of these flaws could potentially be corrected, but the additional short time cycle to publication also prevents papers from being improved along the process. Biomedical scientists most value journal readership, while they believe their peers most value prestige and related metrics such as IF when submitting their work for publication [194].

Like many aspects of science in the Internet and Web era, the Ingelfinger rule has been challenged in a number of ways. Most prominent among them is the growth of scientific preprints [195]. Some fields, such as physics and computer science, have embraced preprints for several decades. The rationale for preprints is that they distribute science earlier, but under the recognition that such publications have not been fully peer-reviewed. The main site for posting preprints in computer science, math, physics, and other fields been has been ArXiv.[21] The use of preprints in biomedicine and health is more recent. The first biology preprint server was bioRxiv,[22] and it has been followed by medRxiv[23] and psyRxiv.[24] Some have advocated that preprints become a universal part of science, with results of research published upon completion of the work and then the longer peer review process proceeding from there [196].

Abdill and Blekhman analyzed all 37,648 preprints uploaded to bioRxiv in its first 5 years through 2018 [197]. The rate of preprints being posted increased to over 2100 per month by the end of 2018. About two-thirds of bioRxiv preprints posted in 2016 or earlier were later published in peer-reviewed journals, with the majority published less than 6 months after being posted. Preprints with more downloads were more likely to be published in journals with a higher impact factor.

Not everyone agrees that preprints are good for biomedical research. Maslove raises several concerns, such as biomedical research being different from fields like physics, where the larger public may see and take action on papers they find that have not been subject to peer review [198]. As posted papers are given official identifiers (Digital Object Identifiers– DOI), they may take on the look of more officially reviewed papers. Sheldon expresses concern they may promote confusion, especially among journalists who may not be able to adequately explain their meaning to their readers [199]. However, Oakden-Rayner et al. advocate their value in providing more open peer review, which may improve reproducibility of the work [200].

[21] https://arxiv.org/

[22] https://www.biorxiv.org/

[23] https://www.medrxiv.org/

[24] https://psyarxiv.com/

One alternative to preprints might be the use of *registered reports*, where if the methods are approved proactively, the results are automatically accepted [201]. The purported advantage to this approach is to guarantee publication acceptance of quality science regardless of the results.

Another major change facilitated by technology is the publication of data. While some disciplines have required publishing of data for several decades (e.g., genomics and physics), such publishing is relatively new to most fields, including clinical medicine. However, there is value to it, as shown in one 1 of 37 re-analyses of RCT data found that 13 (35%) led to interpretation of results different from the original paper, with a majority identifying a larger group of patients who might benefit from treatment [202].

However, there are also concerns with publication of clinical data, especially that from RCTs [203]. One obvious concern is privacy, as there is always the potential to reidentify individuals who took part in trials. Surveys of participants in clinical trials have found that most are willing to allow reuse of their data with appropriate privacy safeguards [204, 205]. The former found that 93% of patients would be willing to have their data shared with academics and 82% with industry researchers, while the latter found a willingness of other research stakeholders, including researchers themselves, to allow sharing of data.

Another concern is whether the data will be used responsibly. Mello et al. laid out principles for responsible reuse of RCT data [206]. Many journals have developed policies around availability of data from the papers they publish, although adherence to such policies was found to be incomplete in a majority of papers from high IF journals [207]. This study also found that journals lacking data availability policies had no publicly available data.

The momentum for sharing biomedical and health data gained steam with a controversy resulting from the publication of an editorial in NEJM suggesting those who do secondary analysis of such data might be "research parasites" [208]. This sets off a fury of debate across the spectrum, from those who argued that primary researchers labored hard to devise experiments and collect their data, thus having claim to control over it, to those who argued that since most research is government-funded, the taxpayers deserve to have access to that data [209]. Some of those in the latter group celebrated the adoption of the "research parasite" moniker [210]. This led to calls for dialogue between researchers who produce the data and those who want to reuse it [211].

Many groups and initiatives have advocated for the potential value of wider reuse of data from clinical research. The cancer genomics community has long seen the value of a data commons to facilitate sharing among researchers [212]. Recent US federal research initiatives, such as the AllOfUs (formerly Precision Medicine) Initiative [213] and the 21st Century Cures Act [214], envision an important role for large repositories of data to accompany patients in cutting-edge research. There are a number of large-scale efforts in clinical data collection that are beginning to accumulate substantial amounts of data, such as the National Patient-Centered Clinical

Research Network (PCORNet[25]) [215] and the Observational Health Data Sciences and Informatics (OHDSI[26]) [216] initiatives.

As with many contentious debates, there are valid points on both sides. The case for requiring publication of data is strong. As most research is taxpayer-funded, it only seems fair that those who paid are entitled to all the data for which they paid. Likewise, all of the subjects were real people who potentially took risks to participate in the research, and their data should be used for discovery of knowledge to the fullest extent possible. And finally, new discoveries may emerge from re-analysis of data. This was actually the case that prompted the Longo "research parasites" editorial, which was praising the "right way" to do secondary analysis, including working with the original researchers. The paper that the editorial described had discovered that the lack of expression of a gene (CDX2) was associated with benefit from adjuvant chemotherapy [217].

Some researchers, however, have pushed back. They argue that those who carry out the work of designing, implementing, and evaluating experiments certainly have some exclusive rights to the data generated by their work. Some also question whether the cost is a good expenditure of limited research dollars, especially since the demand for such datasets may be modest and the benefit is not clear. One group of 282 researchers in 33 countries, the International Consortium of Investigators for Fairness in Trial Data Sharing, noted that there are risks, such as misleading or inaccurate analyses as well as efforts aimed at discrediting or undermining the original research [218]. They also expressed concern about the costs, given that there are over 27,000 RCTs performed each year. As such, this group called for an embargo on reuse of data for 2 years plus another half-year for each year of the length of the RCT. Even those who support data sharing point out the requirement for proper curation, wide availability to all researchers, and appropriate credit to and involvement of those who originally obtained the data [219].

There are also some practical challenges to more widespread dissemination of RCT data for reuse. A number of pharmaceutical companies have begun making such data available over the last few years. Their experience has shown that the costs are not insignificant (estimated to be about $30,000–$50,000 per RCT) and a scientific review process is essential [220]. Another analysis found that the time to reanalyze datasets can be long, and so far the number of publications has been few [221]. An additional study found that identifiable datasets were only explicitly visible from 12% of all clinical research funded by the National Institutes of Health in 2011 [222]. This meant that from 2011 alone, there are possibly more than 200,000 datasets that could be made publicly available, indicating some type of prioritization might be required.

There are also a number of informatics-related issues to be addressed. These not only include adherence to standards and interoperability [223] but also attention to workflows, integration with other data, such as that from electronic health records

[25] https://pcornet.org/

[26] https://www.ohdsi.org/

(EHRs), and consumer/patient engagement [224]. In a study of 120 recent publications that used data from the US National Inpatient Sample, the majority of users did not adhere to required practices [225].

One incentive for data sharing would be for those who produce data to get academic credit for such data authorship [226]. A system in which researchers are regularly recognized for generating data that become useful to other researchers could transform how academic institutions evaluate faculty members' contributions to science, although there would be a need for identifiers to connect data to researchers and track its use [227]. Certainly, the trialists who generate the data must be given incentives when their data is reused [228].

The ICMJE now requires data sharing statements for clinical trials [130]. As described in more detail in Chap. 6, the CrossRef standard allows linking of clinical trials publications with their data [229]. There are a number of venues for sharing research data. The Open Science Framework (OSF)[27] aims to streamline the entire open science process. The Dryad Digital Repository[28] is a nonprofit membership association that makes data underlying scientific publications discoverable, freely reusable, and citable. Dryad is used by about 100 journals, including several informatics journals, such as *Journal of the American Medical Informatics Association* (JAMIA), *JAMIA Open*, *Journal of Biomedical Informatics*, *Bioinformatics*, and a number of BMC journals. As an example, a recent *JAMIA Open* paper of this author has its data stored in the Dryad repository [230].

How widespread is data sharing? One of the most proactive journals has been the PLoS family of journals. An analysis of data availability statements from 47,593 papers published in PLoS ONE from March, 2014 (when the policy went into effect), to May, 2016, found that while compliance with the policy increased over time, only 20% of statements indicate that data are deposited in a repository, which PLoS policy stated was the preferred method [231]. More commonly, authors stated that their data were in the paper itself or in its supplemental information.

What has been the impact of data sharing? Naudet et al. analyzed data from RCTs published in two journals with strong data sharing policies, BMJ and *PLoS Medicine* [232]. They identified 37 RCTs that met eligibility criteria for data publishing. Only 17 (46%) met the criteria for adequate publishing of their data, with 14 able to be fully reproduced for all of their primary outcomes. Two of the remaining three had errors identified but reached the same conclusions of the original papers, and another had insufficient information in the Methods section to allow reproducing. Barriers found to accessing data included contacting corresponding authors, lack of resources in preparing the datasets, and meaningful heterogeneity in data sharing practices. Another study from Tannenbaum et al. surveyed authors of studies in journals with proactive data sharing policies (BMJ, *Annals of Internal Medicine*, and *PLoS Medicine*) found that many authors had received requests for data sharing and had been willing to do so [233]. Barriers to data sharing included

[27] https://osf.io/

[28] https://datadryad.org/stash/

a lack of preparation and an unwillingness to share when requests conflicted with the investigators' own research interests.

There is definitely great potential for reuse of RCT and other clinical research data to advanced research and ultimately health and clinical care for the population. However, it must be done in ways that represent an appropriate use of resources and result in data that truly advances research, clinical care, and ultimately individual health.

2.5.3.2 Methodological Issues in Primary Literature

Problems in the methodology used in clinical studies have been a problem for decades. An early analysis by Fletcher and Fletcher lamented that weak methods were quite prevalent in the biomedical literature, such as studies using nonrandomized designs or very small sample sizes [234]. Even now, studies of case series or case reports, with no experimental or observational control, sometimes still get published. While such studies can have value in generating hypotheses for further research, their appearance in the literature (and literature databases, such as MEDLINE) gives them an aura of value that may not be warranted.

It has also been found that lower-quality studies are more likely to be later "overturned" [235]. This is probably due to their relatively small sample sizes that prevent complete knowledge of all effects, especially relatively uncommon adverse ones. Ioannidis has further generalized this observation to assert that "most published research findings are false" [236]. He makes this claim based on the observations that most studies and the effects they discover are small and that the proper range of hypotheses is not tested. He also expresses concern about research groups "vigorously chasing" statistical significance such that research findings may just be a result of "prevailing bias."

There are also a number of practical issues in the conduct of biomedical research that raise concerns. Some studies are stopped early because a strong and statistically significant treatment effect has occurred [237]. These studies are usually published in the major five medical journals and funded by industry. However, despite this happening more commonly, they often fail to fully document their reasons for stopping early. Mueller et al. reviewed the ethical issues in this setting and advocate continuing recruitment and monitoring of patients randomized to the favorable group to minimize the risk of overestimate of its benefit [238]. An additional problem with peer review is that once the process is completed, and the paper published, there are many obstacles to correcting errors later discovered [239].

Another common problem in methodology is inappropriate use of statistics. One early analysis found that nearly half of all studies in medical journals utilized statistics incorrectly, with the most common error being the inappropriate use of the *t*-test in comparing more than two groups of means [240]. A related issue was inadequate statistical power, where an inadequate sample size may fail to discern a statistically significant difference that may actually exist. Moher et al. found that many published clinical trials do not have a large enough sample size to be able to detect clinically meaningful relative differences [241], while Halpern et al. deemed the continued performing and reporting of underpowered clinical trials as an ethical dilemma [242].

Another issue is discrepancy between reported p-values and confidence intervals and recalculations of them by other researchers. Georgescu and Wren assessed reported and recalculated values for several thousand papers [243]. They found that discrepancies were less frequent in percent-ratio calculations (2.7%) than in ratio-CI and p-value calculations (5.6–7.5%), and smaller discrepancies were more frequent than large ones. Systematic discrepancies (i.e., multiple incorrect calculations of the same type) were higher for more complex tasks (14.3%) than simple ones (6.7%). Discrepancy rates decreased with increasing IF.

A related problem is the reporting of statistically nonsignificant results of primary outcomes in RCTs, with 1 analysis of 72 such reports finding "spin" in the titles (18%), abstracts (58%), and main text (50%) [244]. This phenomenon has also been found in about 30% of studies of diagnostic imaging accuracy [245]. Another study looked at studies with nonsignificant primary endpoints that were published in psychiatry and psychology journals between 2012 and 2017 [246]. Of 116 RCTs meeting the criteria, spin was identified in 56% of abstracts. Spin was found in 2 titles, 24 results sections, and conclusion sections. Industry funding was not associated with increased odds of spin in the abstract. Spin has similarly been reported in cardiovascular RCTs with statistically nonsignificant primary outcomes [247]. This systematic review of 93 RCTs from 6 high-impact journals found positive spin of statistically nonsignificant primary outcomes in 57% of abstracts and 67% of main text of the published articles. A related aspect of this problem is that articles involving a male first or last author were found to be more likely to present research findings positively in titles and abstracts compared with articles in which both the first and last authors were women, particularly in the highest-impact journals [248]. Positive presentation of research findings was associated with higher downstream citations.

Although scientific reporting of statistics has improved over the years, especially in top-tier journals, there is still a tendency to focus on p-values and not confidence intervals, Bayesian factors, or effect sizes that are also important for discerning the value of experimental outcomes [249]. Bayesian factors may be particularly important, as a study with a hypothesis that a priori is unlikely (or highly likely) will only have its probability of being correct increased a small (or large) amount when results from an experiment with a p-value indicating low likelihood of chance is obtained [250]. A related concern is the use of "*p*-hacking," where multiple variables are analyzed looking for results that achieve statistical significance [251]. These concerns have led for calls to reduce the threshold for statistical significance to $p < 0.005$, which would reduce the false-positive rate of rejecting the null hypothesis (i.e., study results being falsely accepted as true) [252, 253]. Some have argued for abandoning *p*-values entirely [254, 255].

It should be noted that even if statistical methods and results are reported correctly, readers will not necessarily understand them. A number of studies have found that professionals who read scientific journals tend to understand natural frequencies much better than probabilities [256]. Thus, these readers can calculate the risk of a disease better by using natural frequencies (e.g., 10 out of 100) than probabilities (e.g., 10%).

Even when studies result in statistically significant differences, there are still reporting problems that can overstate the value of the treatment being studied. Abola et al. reported on the frequency of "superlatives" in reporting cancer research in the media (e.g., "game changer" and "breakthrough") [257]. Krishnamurti et al. found that lay readers of medical studies were likely be influenced to view the results of a study positively by adding words such as "breakthrough" and "promising" as compared to not using them [258].

Also a problem in the literature is the manipulation of study design to achieve a beneficial outcome. Smith cataloged the ways that pharmaceutical companies and others have "gamed" studies to get good results [259]. He also provided "advice" on how to perform this process:

- Conduct a trial against a drug known to be inferior instead of the best current treatment.
- Conduct a trial against a competitor at too low (to get better result) or too high (to have less toxicity) of a dose.
- Conduct trials with samples too small to show a difference from competitor.
- Use multiple endpoints and select those that show best benefit.
- Do multicenter trials but only report results from centers that are favorable.
- Conduct subgroup analysis and only report those that are favorable.
- Report results most likely to impress, i.e., report relative rather than absolute risk reduction.

Smith also noted that the publication of a positive study can be lucrative, i.e., worth billions, for a drug that treats a common condition. Actual scientific papers look more "professional" than advertisements, and paper reprints of them passed out by sales representatives are a large source of revenue for journals, up to 70% profit margin. This has led Smith to call the medical journals and pharmaceutical companies "uneasy bedfellows" and advocate that medical journals not publish such studies but instead serve as a forum to review their findings and limitations [260].

One series of methodological manipulations gave critical mass to a major change by journals, namely, the requirement of clinical trial registration to prevent changes after the trial was started and insure complete reporting [261]. These manipulations were of studies of COX-2 inhibitors, touted as a "better" nonsteroidal anti-inflammatory drug (NSAID) for pain control that would reduce the known gastrointestinal complications of older drugs in this category (e.g., ibuprofen). In one study [262], researchers (from the manufacturer) omitted 6 months of data because they believed it was invalid [263]. This data was published on the Web site of the US Food and Drug Administration (FDA) and discovered by a number of researchers [264, 265], and when added to the data reported in the paper, the original conclusions of safety were no longer warranted [266]. The latter authors also noted that the paper had been cited by 169 other papers, and 30,000 reprints had been ordered before these problems came to light. In another study of a different COX-2 inhibitor [267], three patients suffering myocardial infarctions were excluded from the study despite the authors knowing about them, and their inclusion would have changed the conclusion of the paper to the agent being harmful [268].

The outrage over the changes in the NSAID trials being made after their inception increased previous long-standing calls for pre-trial registration. Long advocated by many EBM advocates to protect integrity of RCT conduct and reporting, registration requires those conducting RCTs to register them with details of hypotheses, methods, sample size calculations, and more [261]. Any changes to the original protocol must be documented and scrutinized. After the COX-2 and related (e.g., SSRI inhibitors and suicide, [269]) debacles, the ICMJE adopted a policy of requiring trial registration at inception of study [270]. Since then, RCTs have had to be registered in ClinicalTrials.gov [271] or other comparable databases [272] as a condition of publication in major journals.

All of these problems lead to what some call "waste" of research questions not being relevant to patients or physicians, design and methods not appropriate, reports never published, and some that are published being biased or not usable [273, 274]. A related concern is the "hypercompetitive" grant funding environment that has emerged in the United States, which results in younger scientists having difficulty establishing their careers, while older scientists may be less willing to pursue high-risk research that may be more difficult to get funded [275]. As such, the current environment of science favors scientists being conservative and incremental in areas they choose to perform research [276, 277].

There is also waste with regard to RCTs that are conducted poorly and/or never published. Discussing the former, Zarin et al. noted the existence of "uninformative" RCTs having small sample sizes, unimportant questions, or generally inapplicable results present a challenge to ethics, science, and medical practice [278]. They also note RCTs that never see publication, not only depriving society the results to potentially improve clinical care but also subjecting research subjects to experiments needlessly. There are other problems related to RCTs. One is that the success rate for researchers actually completing them is relatively low [279]. Another is that some types of studies have higher rates of protocol modification after inception of the study, which in one analysis was found to be higher for RCTs of dietary interventions than of drug studies [280].

Tatsioni et al. attempted to quantify the problem of unpublished studies [281]. They searched ClinicalTrials.gov for long unpublished, large RCTs that started after 2007 and were completed before 2012, focusing on the 500 trials with the largest number of participants. RCTs for which the investigators did not publish the study or report results at ClinicalTrials.gov were then further assessed. The authors identified 67 preregistered but unreported RCTs (13.4%), with a median enrollment of 765 (range, 511–11,000), which were unreported for a median of 9 years after completion. The total number of participants involved was 87,883.

Methodological concerns are not limited to clinical trials. With the growing success of machine learning, the incidence of errors in a sample of machine learning experiments in the domain of software defect prediction was 22 of 49 papers [282].

This has led to the description of methods to make machine learning models in healthcare more reproducible [283].

2.5.3.3 Reproducibility and Replicability

Another concern about science is the lack of reproducibility of research findings. This problem was brought to light by two pharmaceutical companies noting the declining success of phase II clinical trials for cancer chemotherapy [284]. Begley and Ellis found only 11–25% of published preclinical studies were reproducible [285], with similar results obtained by Prinz et al. [286]. The identification of these problems led to concerns in other fields, such as psychology [287]. A subsequent attempt to replicate 100 studies from psychology by the Open Science Collaboration found that only 36% achieved statistical significance, with the mean effect about one-half of the original studies [288]. One study has shown that just reproducing the data analysis overturned the results, making the case for more widespread availability of primary data from studies [289]. Ioannidis noted that the problem was more serious for preclinical than clinical research [290]. Coiera et al. pointed out that replication of studies can be challenging in biomedical and health informatics since many studies take place using systems and operational settings that themselves vary widely from study to study [291]. There have also been calls for reproducibility in the IR field, including advocacy for reproducible baselines upon which new experimentation can be based [292].

A survey of 1500 scientists in 2015 found that over half believed there was a "crisis" in reproducibility [293]. These results and concerns led to the reproducibility initiative, an effort to validate 50 landmark cancer biology studies[29] [294]. Early results have started to achieve publication [295, 296]. These problems also led the National Institutes of Health to require addressing of rigor and reproducibility in grant proposals.[30]

There are also informatics-related problems related to reproducibility of research. Many scientific researchers write code but are not always well-versed in best practices of testing and error detection [297]. Scientists have a history of relying on incorrect data or models [298]. In addition, they may also not be good about selection of best software packages for their work [299]. One example came from a widely used algorithm for interpreting functional magnetic resonance imaging (fMRI) whose errors led to questions about the validity of up to 40,000 studies that made use of fMRI [300]. Gene sequencing data, especially those which are older, may be inaccurate and undermine experiments [301].

Informatics can also play a role in helping to solve the reproducibility problem. For example, it may lead to approaches allowing the more precise identification of research resources (organisms, cell lines, genes, reagents, etc.) in the biomedical literature [302]. In the case of "omics" research, release of computer code can allow

[29] https://validation.scienceexchange.com/#/reproducibility-initiative

[30] https://www.nih.gov/research-training/rigor-reproducibility

inspection for validity [303]. Peng called for reproducible methods in all of the computational sciences [304]. Recent development of tools, such as Jupyter notebooks that allow runnable code and documentation around it [305] and the Reproducible Document Stack [306], could also serve as a new form of scientific publication, which would allow readers to see and understand computer code and its operation on underlying data [307].

Another approach is the development of a Rigor and Transparency Index, which is a metric of quality for assessing biological and medical science methods [308]. Papers are given a score based on the presence, when appropriate, of some or all of the following entities:

- Institutional Review Board Statement
- Consent statement
- Institutional animal care and use committee statement
- Randomization of subjects into groups
- Blinding of investigator or analysis
- Power analysis for group size
- Sex as a biological variable
- Cell line authentication
- Cell line contamination check

The Rigor and Transparency Index also includes a score for appropriate biological or computational entities:

- Antibody
- Organism
- Cell line
- Plasmid
- Oligonucleotide
- Software project/tool

The National Academy of Sciences (NAS) published a report in 2019 that reviewed the problem and made recommendations [309]. A first step was to distinguish between the reproducibility (computational reproducibility—obtaining consistent computational results using the same input data, computational steps, methods, code, and conditions of analysis) and replicability (obtaining consistent results across studies aimed at answering the same scientific question, each of which has obtained its own data). These differences are contextualized in Table 2.4, which

Table 2.4 Context of reproducibility and replicability based on whether the analysis or the data are different, adapted from The Turing Way[a]

	Data		
Analysis		Same	Different
	Same	Reproducible	Replicable
	Different	Robust	Generalizable

[a]https://the-turing-way.netlify.com/reproducibility/03/definitions.html

is adapted from a Web site devoted to reproducible data science called the Turing Way.[31]

Recommendations from the NAS report included:

- All researchers should include a clear, specific, and complete description of how the reported results were reached. Reports should include details appropriate for the type of research, including:
  - A clear description of all methods, instruments, materials, procedures, measurements, and other variables involved in the study
  - A clear description of the analysis of data and decisions for exclusion of some data or inclusion of other
  - For results that depend on statistical inference, a description of the analytic decisions and when these decisions were made and whether the study is exploratory or confirmatory
  - A discussion of the expected constraints on generality, such as which methodological features the authors think could be varied without affecting the result and which must remain constant
  - Reporting of precision or statistical power
  - Discussion of the uncertainty of the measurements, results, and inferences.
- Funding agencies and organizations should consider investing in research and development of open-source, usable tools and infrastructure that support reproducibility for a broad range of studies across different domains in a seamless fashion. Concurrently, investments would be helpful in outreach to inform and train researchers on best practices and how to use these tools.
- Journals should consider ways to ensure computational reproducibility for publications that make claims based on computations, to the extent ethically and legally possible.
- The National Science Foundation should take steps to facilitate the transparent sharing and availability of digital artifacts, such as data and code, for NSF-funded studies—including developing a set of criteria for trusted open repositories to be used by the scientific community for objects of the scholarly record and endorsing or considering the creation of code and data repositories for long-term archiving and preservation of digital artifacts that support claims made in the scholarly record based on NSF-funded research, among other actions.

Another challenge to replicable research is how to handle research with confidential data. This includes not only patient data but also email, search logs, and other data individuals want to keep private. One possible solution is to certify the research with a trusted third party [310]. Another approach that has been used is so-called Evaluation as a Service (EaaS), where researchers do not see the sensitive data but instead send their computer programs to the data and just receive aggregate results back [311, 312].

[31] https://the-turing-way.netlify.com/reproducibility/03/definitions.html

2.5.3.4 Reporting Issues in Primary Literature

Even if the methods of research are appropriate, another challenge to the primary literature is the reporting of methods. Most scientific papers follow the template of Introduction, Materials and Methods, Results, and Discussion and/or Conclusions. Some fields use alternatives to this format, but most experimental studies generally follow the pattern of pairing methods with results. In this writer's view, a good scientific study tells a story of why the research was important, what was done, what it showed, how it fits in the larger picture of what is known on the subject, and what should be done next.

Reporting methods and results, however, has been known to be incomplete and inconsistent. An early assessment identified 11 factors deemed important in the design and analysis of RCTs, such as eligibility criteria for admission to the trial, method of randomization used, and blinding, and found that only slightly over half of all studies in 4 major medical journals reported them adequately [313]. The problems in the reporting of methods and results in RCTs led to the formation of the Consolidated Standards of Reporting Trials (CONSORT) statement, which provided a checklist of 22 items to include when reporting an RCT [314]. Most of these elements were included because it has been known that their omission was associated with biased evidence favoring the treatment being studied. For example, studies not using masked assessments of the outcome (i.e., the person judging whether a patient got better did not know whether the patient had received the experimental or control intervention), studies rated as low quality, and studies not concealing the allocation of the patients to the experimental or control intervention, all had been found to have a higher average treatment effect than studies of better quality [315]. The use of the CONSORT statement was shown to result in improvements in the quality of reports of RCTs [316], although others noted that good reporting was not strictly correlated with good quality of the study itself [317]. The success of the CONSORT statement led to the development of a similar approaches for other types of studies, such as the Strengthening the Reporting of Observational Studies in Epidemiology (STROBE) statement [318]. The Enhancing the QUAlity and Transparency Of health Research (EQUATOR) Network[32] provides a clearinghouse for over 400 types of clinical studies.

Another limitation of articles about RCTs is inadequate reporting of adverse events. Chan et al. assessed 102 clinical trials and their clinical outcome measures that were approved by ethics committees in Denmark [319]. They found that 50% of the efficacy outcomes and 65% of the harm outcomes were incompletely reported. More recently, de Vries et al. found that journal publications of clinical trials were much less complete than in reporting adverse effects, especially serious ones, than FDA reviews of drugs [320]. Related to this problem is that RCTs in general tend to underreport adverse effects or not have text words or indexing terms that enable

[32] https://www.equator-network.org/

their retrieval [321–323]. This makes it vitally important that post-marketing surveillance of approved drugs occurs [324].

An additional limitation of RCTs is that some clinical interventions require training or skill that is not always taken into account. One way to address this has been proposed in "expertise"-based trials, where only those with enough training and skill to carry out the intervention do so [325]. Related to this is a problem for rapidly changing technologies, which includes informatics applications, such that the intervention becomes different due to improvements or other changes in the technology. For this reason, "tracker trials" that maintain the intervention but track its change have been advocated [326].

Another reporting-related issue is the understandability of benefits and risks of medical interventions by clinicians, other professionals such as policy-makers, and patients. In an overview of what is known, Politi et al. have noted that our understanding is incomplete, not only with regard to the meaning of various adjectives that are commonly used to quantify the level of risk (e.g., severe, minimal, etc.) but also concerning the uncertainty of our knowledge [327]. One challenge is a tendency for authors to report relative over absolute risks, which may make an intervention seem more effective than is warranted, especially when a condition is uncommon. For example, the relative risk reduction of a treatment that lowers mortality from 2/100 patients to 1/100 patients is 50%, although even the less effective treatment has a mortality of only 2%. This has led to calls for more standardized reporting of benefits and harms in the literature and communication of both relative risk and frequencies [328, 329].

With the growing access to medical information by patients, some have assessed the best ways to report scientific literature to nonprofessionals. One study compared various methods for presenting results to patients and found that relative and absolute risk reduction was more readily understood than number needed to treat (NNT), a common approach used to convey the magnitude of treatment benefit to clinicians [330]. However, in another study NNT was found to yield a higher consent rate for a treatment of known benefit than presenting the benefit as how long the treatment would postpone an adverse outcome [331].

Also found to be a problem in journal articles is incomplete reporting of past studies. Gotzsche and Olsen [332] found that subsequent references to seven RCTs of mammography screening tended to omit important limitations of the trials. They advocated that study protocols remain available on the Web after the results have been published. Clarke et al. [333] noted that only 2 of 25 RCTs where prior trials existed described the new results in the proper context of prior trials. Similarly, Tatsioni et al. documented the persistence of citing observational studies in the literature where results of large-scale clinical trials have superseded their conclusions [334].

A related concern to authorship is conflict of interest (COI). ICMJE guidelines do not prevent authors with a financial interest from publishing, requiring only that they disclose such interests. The ICMJE has developed a uniform format for disclosure of so-called competing interests [335]. The rationale is based on research showing that industry-sponsored drug trials are more likely to have positive outcomes in the face of no differences in study methods, leading to concern about selective methods, analysis, or reporting [336]. Dunn et al. found that for 22 systematic reviews of neuraminidase inhibitors, those with financial conflicts of interest were more likely to present evidence about neuraminidase inhibitors in a positive manner and recommend their use than reviewers without financial conflicts of interest [337].

In oncology, financial relationships between authors and the pharmaceutical industry have been purported to be common, expensive, and frequently undisclosed. In one study, while one-third of oncologist authors failed to completely disclose payments from the sponsor of the published clinical trial, one-quarter of authors did not receive any payments, which indicated that abstaining from industry payments during a clinical trial was possible [338]. Ornstein and Thomas documented a case of undisclosed payments of speaking fees and research support to José Baselga, Chief Medical Officer, Memorial Sloan Kettering Cancer Center, who had published in a number of prestigious medical journals [339].

This has led to views pro and con that medical journals stop publishing research funded by the pharmaceutical industry [340]. One group of contrarians, however, noted that there is no evidence that conflict of interest rules has prevented biased research from being published and that the effort around it is a waste of time and resources [341]. The International Society for Medical Publication Professionals has published a statement on Good Publication Practice for Communicating Company-Sponsored Medical Research [342]. Tierney et al. also note instances when interests of commercial sponsors of research and academic scientists could be aligned in areas such as medication adherence and post-marketing surveillance [343].

Of course, reporting COI for individual studies may not be enough. Although most high-impact medical journals require disclosure of authors' individual COI, few disclose those of their editorial teams [344]. Another more recent manifestation of the problem extends to social media. One study found that a majority of hematology-oncology physicians on Twitter with >$1000 financial COI were more likely to post frequent tweets mentioning specific drugs for which they had a conflict and almost none disclosed those financial ties [345].

Even when methods and results are adequately described, the writing may be problematic. One of the most critical areas for high-quality writing is the abstract, which may be the only part of the paper read and may be the only part seen if a user is searching a bibliographic database such as PubMed. One early innovation was the *structured abstract*, which requires information about the objective, design, setting, participants, intervention, main outcome, results, and conclusions from a study [346].

Journal articles may also have inaccuracies in citations and quotations. Unless noted by peer reviewers, these errors usually pass through the editorial process. One analysis found that citation errors occurred in 7 to 60% of journal articles, with 1 to 24% being so significant that the articles cannot be located based on the information given [347, 348]. This problem has also been found in the biomedical informatics literature [349]. Assessing the 5 biomedical informatics journals with the highest IFs for each journal's first issue of 2004, they found 311 errors in 225 of the 656 references (34.3%) in 37 articles. The percentage of articles with errors varied by journal, from 22.1% for *Journal of the American Medical Informatics Association* to 40.7% for *International Journal of Medical Informatics*. The most common element with an error was the author name (31%), followed by the title (17%), page (7.4%), and year (3.5%).

A new wrinkle to the problem of inadequate citations is Web references provided in scientific papers that are inaccessible or incorrect. This was first noted by Crichlow et al., who assessed URLs in the references of all original research papers in five major medical journals [350]. In 91 articles analyzed, there were 68 URLs in the references, 8.6% of which were inaccessible. These authors noted that de Lacey et al. had found a similar 8% overall rate of errors in citations in the paper-based journal literature in 1985 [351]. Another analysis found "reference rot," where URLs had become invalid and/or the content on the cited pages changed for about one-fifth of citations to URLs in scientific literature [352]. This led to the development of a now-defunct Web site Hiberlink, which aimed to preserve the content of Web pages cited in the scientific literature [353]. It is possible that efforts described in Chap. 6, such as the use of the Digital Object Identifier (DOI), will ameliorate this problem.

Another reporting-related problem in the biomedical literature is gene names. Some of these problems emanate from the use of the Microsoft Excel spreadsheet program, which may automatically convert gene names that appear to Excel to be dates (e.g., Apr-1), floating-point numbers (e.g., 2310009E13), and other types of data [354]. Byrne and Labbé developed a tool, Seek & Blastn, which discovers errors in gene identifiers and nucleotide sequences in scientific papers [355]. One application of the tool uncovered errors and probably fraud related to the human cancer cell line gene TPD52L2 [356, 357]. Another problem related to genes is that those that have been more highly annotated are more likely to be further studied in research than those with the strong supporting molecular data, leading to biases in research [358].

2.5.3.5 Publication Bias

An additional problem with the primary literature that has been known for decades [359] and still persists [360] is *publication bias*. Given studies of equal methodological rigor, those with "positive" results are more likely to be published. Publication bias tends to result because scientists want to report positive results and journal editors (and presumably their readers) want to read them. As will be seen in the next section, publication bias is also problematic for the conduct of meta-analysis, where the aggregation of studies presumes that individual studies represent the full spectrum of results.

The problem of publication bias was first noted by Sterling, who found that studies yielding statistically significant results were more likely to be published than those that did not, raising the possibility that studies with significant results may never be further verified [361]. Rosenthal labeled this the "file drawer" problem, in that researchers would let languish negative results from their research in their file drawers [362]. Analyses in other fields beyond biomedicine have also found evidence of publication bias [363, 364].

Dickersin was the first to note this problem with clinical trials, observing that studies approved by various institutional review boards and/or NIH funding agencies were more likely to be published if statistically significant results were achieved [365]. Another analysis found that studies with positive results were 2.3 times more likely to be published than those with negative results [366]. The likelihood of publication for clinical trials was even higher (3.1 times more likely). Studies with indeterminate results were even less likely to be published, while those measuring qualitative outcomes did not seem to reflect the influence of publication bias. Similar publication bias was also found to occur with studies submitted for presentation at scientific meetings [367]. Systematic reviews of studies assessing subsequent publication of abstracts presented at scientific meetings, with an average of only 44–46% ultimately achieving publication as a full paper [368, 369]. Studies in basic science and those having a positive outcome were more likely to eventually be published as papers. Abstracts were more likely to be published as papers if they were presented orally, at a small meeting, or at a US meeting. More recently, a study of 129 phase 3 RCT abstracts accepted to the Pediatric Academic Societies conference, 27.9% were not subsequently published, and 39.5% were never registered in ClinicalTrials.gov [370]. Previous trial registration and sample size were associated with greater likelihood of publication, with mean time to publication from study presentation of 26.5 months. There was also evidence of publication bias.

There are other manifestations of publication bias. An additional finding from Stern and Simes was that the median time to publication for studies with positive results was significantly shorter (4.7–4.8 vs. 8.0 years) [366]. Likewise, Ioannidis found that clinical trials not achieving statistical significance of the results in the treatment of human immunodeficiency virus (HIV) were likely to be published later than those that did [371]. Another aspect of publication bias is that researchers from non-English-speaking countries were more likely to publish their positive results more in English-language journals [372].

One highly investigated area of publication bias has come from psychiatry. Turner et al. identified 74 RCTs performed on 12 antidepressant drugs that were registered by the US Food and Drug Administration (FDA) to obtain approval to market the drug [373]. While nearly all of the studies with positive results were published (37 of 38), a majority of the negative were either not published (22 of 36) or published in a way that the authors believed conveyed a positive outcome (11 of 36). As a result, although 94% of trials appeared to be positive, only 51% were actually so. A meta-analysis done on patient-level data from these trials showed that the non-publication created an apparent 32% better (11–69% for individual drugs) effect size for the drugs than was warranted by all the data. These authors also assessed antipsychotic drugs and found a similar (though lower in magnitude) bias in positive clinical trial results being more likely to be published in medical journals [374]. There are still hurdles faced by negative trials after publication bias for trials of treatment for depression, including outcome reporting bias, spin, and citation bias [375]. These problems have led one major funder, Wellcome Trust in the United Kingdom, to self-publish all of its funded research [376].

Other research has shown that data from FDA reports does not always make it to appearing in drug label information for clinicians, such as information on harms, limited efficacy, and uncertainty [377]. In general, there are important data from study reports, and registries do not make it into journal publication [378]. All of these findings have led to improvement in how the FDA reports data submitted by drug manufacturers to obtain approval [379].

Another well-known instance that led to policy changes came from clinical trials of the drug oseltamivir (Tamiflu), which is used early in the course of influenza to reduce the severity and duration of symptoms. In performing a systematic review on the efficacy of this drug [380], authors found that 60% of data from clinical trials performed by the manufacturer (Roche) had never been released [381]. This led to calls by the BMJ to make all clinical trials data available (anonymized) in addition to publishing papers [382], building on previous efforts calling for such data to be available to peer reviewers [383]. The BMJ also developed a Web site that ultimately led Roche to release all the data on oseltamivir. A subsequent meta-analysis found that oseltamivir did hasten time to clinical symptom alleviation, lowered risk of lower respiratory tract complications and admittance to hospital, but also led to increased nausea and vomiting [384]. This led to the conclusion that the drug's harms did not outweigh its benefits and that probably a total of $20 billion was wasted by various countries in stockpiling the medication. This episode did lead drug companies to release data on other drugs from other clinical trials [385].

One method for overcoming publication bias has been the requirements for registration and timely publication of RCTs. One requirement of ClinicalTrials.gov, stipulated in the Food and Drug Administration Amendments Act (FDAAA) of 2007 and finalized in 2016, was that RCTs be published within 12 months of completion and provide summary results [386]. Unfortunately, the problem of unreported and unpublished RCTs has persisted despite the new law [387]. One analysis found that only 15 of 40 US academic medical centers were fully in compliance for all of the RCTs they performed [388]. Another analysis of studies completed in 2018–2019 found that only 40.9% of RCTs reported results within 1 year after completion as required and 63.8% never reported results [389]. An additional investigation not only replicated these findings but also determined that various details, such as all-cause mortality, were not reported in consistent manners [390].

Industry RCTs were more likely to be compliant than non-industry, non-US government sponsors. In addition, sponsors conducting large numbers of RCTs were more likely to be compliant than those carrying smaller numbers of trials. The FDAAA Trials Tracker site[33] tracks compliance in real time, allowing the data to be queried by organization, study sponsor, and other attributes.

Negative results or the inability to obtain statistical significance are not reasons not to publish, since in the case of clinical trials, for example, it is just as important

[33] http://fdaaa.trialstracker.net/

to know when a therapy is not more effective than the current standard or none at all. This is even more crucial with the current widespread use of meta-analysis, since data that should be part of a meta-analysis might not be used because it had never been published. Indeed, Chalmers has called failure to publish a clinical trial a form of "scientific misconduct" [391]. This view was recently reiterated [392].

In biomedical and health informatics, Friedman and Wyatt have also raised concern about publication bias, where system developers often perform evaluations and are less likely to publish unfavorable results about their systems, especially when such data may detract from future grant funding [393]. There has been shown to be publication bias in clinical trials of EHRs [394].

2.5.3.6 Fraud in Primary Literature

A final issue to discuss concerning primary literature is invalid or fraudulent science. This is one area where technology has probably played a helpful role, both in its detection as well as removal. As noted earlier, science is mostly based on honesty and trust, which makes fraud by nefarious characters relatively easy. Fraud was much harder to detect when data and its analysis were less digitally connected and was much more difficult to root out of the literature when most access was via many paper copies of articles. Having fewer "copies" of articles, accessed from central servers, makes the designation of retracted articles much easier in modern times.

The advent of MEDLINE launched the ability to indicate the retraction of incorrect or fraudulent literature [395]. But removing it from library shelves was considerably more difficult. A survey of 129 academic medical libraries in North America in the 1990s found that 59% had no policy or practices for calling retracted publications to the attention of their patrons [396]. Another study found that journals are inconsistent in how they identify retracted publications [397].

Although it was harder to detect in the past, there have been well-publicized instances of identified research fraud, with a conundrum on how to remove it from the literature. In an analysis of the work of John Darsee, a Harvard researcher who was later found to have fabricated experimental results, two researchers found that the other publications of Darsee, whose validity may never be known, were still cited by other researchers in a positive light [398]. A similar analysis of the publications of Robert Slutsky, another scientist guilty of fraud, found a similar phenomenon, though the rate of citation diminished as the case was publicized in the press [399]. Likewise, another scientist known to publish fraudulent work, Stephen Breuning, was also found to have positive citations of his work long after he had pleaded guilty to deception [400].

The continued problem of fraud has led to development of a Web site and blog, Retraction Watch, which tracks retractions and other instances of fraud in the scientific literature.[34] The site has a "Leaderboard" of scientists with the most retractions, with the

[34] https://retractionwatch.com/

top person having 183 papers retracted. The site also has a top-ten list of most highly cited retracted papers of all-time, with several having over 1000 citations after the retraction. It also publishes an annual list of the top retractions for a given year, providing insight into most egregious causes for retraction of scientific papers, e.g. [401]. Some of the sleuths who have contributed to rooting out incorrect or fraudulent science [402] and their methods [403] have been described. Grey et al. recently published a checklist to help readers of scientific papers identify possible scientific misconduct[35] [404].

Analysis of the Retraction Watch database has yielded a number of observations [405]. Although the absolute number of annual retractions has grown, the rate of increase has slowed. Much of the rise appears to reflect improved oversight at a growing number of journals, although the authors suggest that more editors should step up. Relatively few authors are responsible for a disproportionate number of retractions, as just 500 of more than 30,000 authors named in the retraction database (which includes co-authors) account for about one-quarter of the 10,500 retractions. Nations with smaller scientific communities have a bigger problem with retractions. A retraction does not always signal scientific misbehavior. About half of all retractions do appear to have involved fabrication, falsification, or plagiarism.

Some of the more current episodes of fraud, however, dwarf older ones described in earlier editions of this book. For example, an instance of massive "peer review and citation ring" was led by a Taiwanese scientist in the *Journal of Vibration and Control*, leading to retraction of 60 articles [406]. Another high-profile event leading to article retractions centered around a cancer researcher from Duke University, Anil Potti, whose work in using gene-expression arrays to predict drug response was found to be fraudulent [407]. An investigation by the Chinese government raised concerns that as many as 80% of all clinical drug trials performed in China had fraudulent results [408]. Carlisle documented data fabrication and other reasons for nonrandom sampling in 5087 RCTs in anesthesia and general medical journals [409]. More recently, a similar large-scale problem has been identified in Russia, where over 600 papers were retracted by academic journals, mainly due to plagiarism, self-plagiarism, and academics being designated as co-authors without having contributed work to the research [410].

Fraud has also been found to occur as a result of manipulation of the peer review process, where paper authors suggest peer reviewers who carried out bogus positive reviews [183]. This led the publishers Springer and BMC to retract dozens of papers. A similar exposure of peer review fraud came from the journal *Tumor Biology*, which ultimately retracted 107 papers [411]. Further problems were found with scientists being listed on the journal's editorial board without their consent or knowledge [412]. Dansinger reported the story of a paper of his that was republished (with title and author names changed but otherwise unchanged) by another scientist to whom the paper was sent for peer review [413]. The co-authors of the published paper retracted it [414]. Another reported instance of fraud in the peer review process was identified by the *Journal of Theoretical Biology*, where an editorial board member managing a peer review process was a colleague of an author and inappropriately

[35] http://resource-cms.springernature.com/springer-cms/rest/v1/content/17547550/data/v1

handled a number of reviews, including asking authors of submitted manuscripts to cite the work of himself and his colleagues [415]. The journal itself published an editorial describing its "editorial malpractice" in allowing the process to occur.

Analyses of some of the most highly retracted and otherwise problematic scientists have been explored. It is important to remember that these are the most extreme examples and not forget that the mostly honor-based scientific process allows them to occur. McHugh and Yentis analyzed 313 fraudulent papers by 3 scientists with very high levels of retraction: Scott Reuben, Joachim Boldt, and Yoshitaka Fujii [416]. They found that not all of their work had been retracted, and some of those that had did not adhere to Council on Publication Ethics (COPE) guidelines for retraction.[36] Additional work by Marcus and Oransky described how Fujii was discovered and caught [417]. Fujii has the highest number of retractions in the Retraction Watch database, with 183 retracted papers. Another scientist, Joachim Boldt, recently reached the 100 mark [418].

Another area of fraud has been image manipulation [419]. One analysis focused on 40 journals over 20 years, finding about 3.8% of images were problematic, about half of which appeared to be due to deliberate manipulation [420]. Another analysis of 960 papers published in *Molecular and Cellular Biology* from 2009 to 2016 found 59 (6.1%) to contain inappropriately duplicated images, leading to 41 corrections, 5 retractions, and 13 instances in which no action was taken [421]. While the majority of inappropriate image duplication resulted from errors during figure preparation that could be remedied by correction, about 10% of papers with inappropriate image duplication were retracted. If that proportion of retractions was representative of all scientific papers with images, it could mean that as many as 35,000 papers in the biomedical literature might be candidates for retraction due to inappropriate image duplication.

Additional examples of highly retracted scientists abound. One researcher whose work had received high visibility in the news media but turned out to be fraudulent was Brian Wansink. His work was found to be error-ridden [422] and employed data dredging and p-hacking [423]. Six of his papers were retracted from *JAMA* journals [424]. Another problematic scientist has been Piero Anversa, whose fraudulent work on cardiac stem cells led to clinical trials being launched to evaluate their efficacy [425]. Once discovered, this led NIH to discontinue trials based on them [426] and calls by his institution to retract all studies based on them [427]. Leaders in the field of cardiac stem cell therapeutic research published a perspective on ways for the field to learn from and move forward from this episode [428].

Even though journal sites have been good at indicating retraction of fraudulent articles, they continue to receive citations by other papers. One analysis found that the work of Scott Reuben, noted above, continued to be cited after exposure of his discredited research, with not all citations mentioning the fraud of his work [429]. In 1 analysis of 47 retracted radiation oncology articles, 92% of citations continued to reference the retracted article as legitimate work [430]. In addition, 3 practice guidelines and 15 systematic reviews and meta-analyses were also identified that cited

[36] https://publicationethics.org/retraction-guidelines

retracted articles as valid work. An analysis of the highly cited but retracted paper of Wakefield et al. [431] on a (discredited) link between vaccines and autism had several hundred citations after the retraction but only 72% mentioning the retraction [432]. Only about 38% of citing articles before the retraction were subsequently updated to mention the retraction. In a massive cause of fraud in psychology literature, with 56 retracted papers of Diederik Stapel, many papers in the literature prior to start of retractions, and some afterward, still cite his work positively [433]. Bakker and Riegelman assessed retracted publications in mental health literature across bibliographic platforms [434]. They found that for 812 retracted publications, about 40% did not indicate that the paper had been retracted on their site. They also looked at articles PDFs, finding that 26% did not indicate that the paper had been retracted.

Fraud in science has a number of other ramifications. Among scientists with multiple retractions due to fraud, publications have been found to decline rapidly after the first retraction, but a small minority continued to publish regularly [435]. Retractions impact meta-analyses, with articles retracted due to fraud rarely impacting results but due to data being removed causing reduce effect sizes [436].

Various other schemes are facilitated by the wide reach of the Internet. For example, Retraction Watch also uncovered a Russian site that sells production of first-author scholarly papers published in a reputable journal for a fee of $500 [437]. Byrne and Christopher described how journals and peer reviewers can identify submissions from so-called paper mills by requesting raw data, especially for images and figures, and checking for verifiable reagents and their identifiers [438]. A somewhat related form of fraud was noted in a study that found 56% of academic CVs with at least one publication listed at least one that was unverifiable or inaccurate in a self-promoting way [439].

Wang et al. reported on a survey of inappropriate requests to biostatisticians for manipulation of statistics [440]. At least 20% of the respondents reported requests such as removing or altering data records to better support the research hypothesis; interpreting the statistical findings on the basis of expectation, not actual results; not reporting key missing data that might bias the results; and ignoring violations of assumptions that would change results from positive to negative.

2.5.4 Systematic Reviews and Meta-Analysis

As noted earlier in the chapter, the scientific literature is fragmented, perhaps purposefully [30]. As will be seen in subsequent chapters, even experienced searchers have difficulty identifying all the relevant articles on a given topic. The proliferation of RCTs, particularly when they assess the same diseases and treatments, gave rise to the impetus for systematic reviews, which were introduced in Sect. 2.4. Systematic reviews are distinguished from traditional review articles, described in the next section, by their focused questions, exhaustive review of the literature, and use of evidence-based techniques [441]. When appropriate, systematic reviews involve the use of *meta-analysis*, where the results of appropriately similar trials are pooled to obtain a more comprehensive picture with greater statistical power. The term meta-analysis was coined by Glass [442], and the technique is used increasingly in assessing the results of clinical trials. Meta-analyses are not limited to RCTs and have been used with diagnostic test studies [443] and observational studies [444]. Per the Haynes 4S model, systematic reviews are "syntheses" that bring together all of the studies for a given scientific question [113].

There are some variations to systematic reviews. Recent years have seen the growth of *scoping reviews*, which aim to scope and map the evidence for a given question but not necessarily perform a comprehensive review [445, 446]. Another variation is the network meta-analysis, where three or more treatments are compared across multiple different studies [447].

Two of the largest producers of systematic reviews worldwide are the Cochrane Collaboration[37] [448] and the US Agency for Healthcare Research and Quality (AHRQ). The latter calls its systematic reviews "evidence reports"[38] [449]. There are also many systematic reviews scattered throughout the biomedical and health literature. The US Institute of Medicine published a guide of standards for the production of systematic reviews [450]:

- Standards for initiating reviews:
  - Establish team with sufficient expertise and experience
  - Ensure user and stakeholder input
  - Formulating topic and protocol
- Finding and assessing individual studies:
  - Documenting search
  - Managing data
- Synthesizing body of evidence:
  - Using prespecified methods
  - Qualitative and, where feasible, quantitative analysis
- Reporting:
  - Appropriate sections
  - Peer review
- (Managing bias and conflict of interest throughout)

A minimum set of items for reporting in systematic reviews and meta-analyses that is widely required by journals is the Preferred Reporting Items for Systematic Reviews and Meta-Analyses (PRISMA) statement[39] [451]. The standard for grading the quality of individual studies included in systematic reviews is the Grading of Recommendations Assessment, Development and Evaluation (GRADE) [452].

Systematic reviews have other benefits to science. They can also provide an inventory of the state of the science. They may also prevent unnecessary research. For example, 1 analysis found that the harm from the drug aprotinin was present after 12 RCTs, but a subsequent 52 RCTs just served to verify the finding [453].

[37] https://www.cochranelibrary.com/

[38] https://www.ahrq.gov/research/findings/evidence-based-reports/search.html

[39] http://www.prisma-statement.org/

This led the journal *Lancet* to require all reports of RCTs to include a clear summary of previous findings.

Meta-analysis makes use of summary measures to report its results. For dichotomous variables (i.e., events), the *odds ratio* (OR) or *relative risk/risk ratio* (RR) is typically used, while for continuous variables, the *mean difference* (MD) or *standardized mean difference* (SMD) is usually employed. In addition to knowing the point estimate of the treatment effect, one must know the precision of the value. That is, how likely is it that the point estimate from the patient sample represents the true value for the entire population? To determine the precision, the *confidence interval* (CI) is calculated, with the 95% CI representing the range of values in which the true value of the population has a 95% likelihood of falling.

The summary measures are commonly displayed graphically. For continuous variables, the OR or RR is typically configured so that an OR or RR < 1 (falling to the left of the OR or RR = 1 vertical line) indicates the intervention is beneficial (i.e., fewer events), whereas when the R or RR > 1 (falling to the right of the OR or RR = 1 vertical line) indicates it is detrimental. If the 95% CI does not touch the OR or RR = 1 line, the difference is statistically significant. The results of meta-analysis are typically displayed in a *forest plot*, with one row for the outcome of each study and the summary statistic at the bottom.

These concepts and the value of the meta-analysis are best demonstrated in the logo of the Cochrane Collaboration (see Fig. 2.5). The logo demonstrates an early meta-analysis that was done to assess whether steroids are beneficial to the fetus in premature labor. Of the seven trials identified at the time the logo was created, five showed statistically insignificant benefit (i.e., their CI crossed the OR = 1 line).

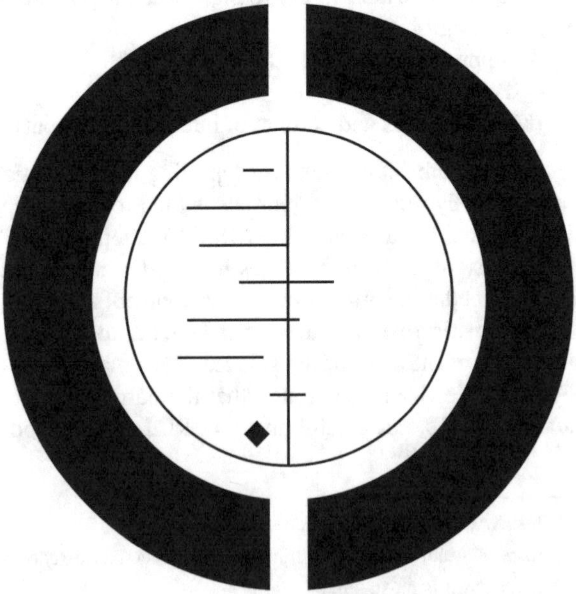

Fig. 2.5 Logo of the Cochrane Collaboration showing result of meta-analysis demonstrating benefit for use of corticosteroids in preterm labor. (Courtesy of the Cochrane Collaboration)

However, when all seven trials were included in a meta-analysis, the results unequivocally demonstrated benefit, with the CI well to the left of the OR = 1 line.

One of the challenges of meta-analysis is the variability of the studies that are used in the analysis. The problem of publication bias described above is likely to be amplified in meta-analysis, since the analysis relies on the full spectrum of results for a given research question to be published. But there may also be variation due to heterogeneity of the studies. There are several ways to assess heterogeneity. One involves the use of *funnel plots*, which are scatter plots of the treatment effect on the horizontal axis against a measure of the sample size on the vertical axis [454]. In general, an unbiased meta-analysis should show studies with small sample sizes having more scattered effect sizes than those with larger samples, that is, a funnel plot would appear as a symmetrical inverted funnel. Biased meta-analyses, however, are more likely to show asymmetrical funnel plots. This approach has been shown to explain why subsequent large RCTs contradict meta-analyses (i.e., the new large study added to the meta-analysis shows an asymmetrical funnel plot) and to demonstrate publication bias in meta-analyses [455]. Two hypothetical funnel plots are shown in Fig. 2.6.

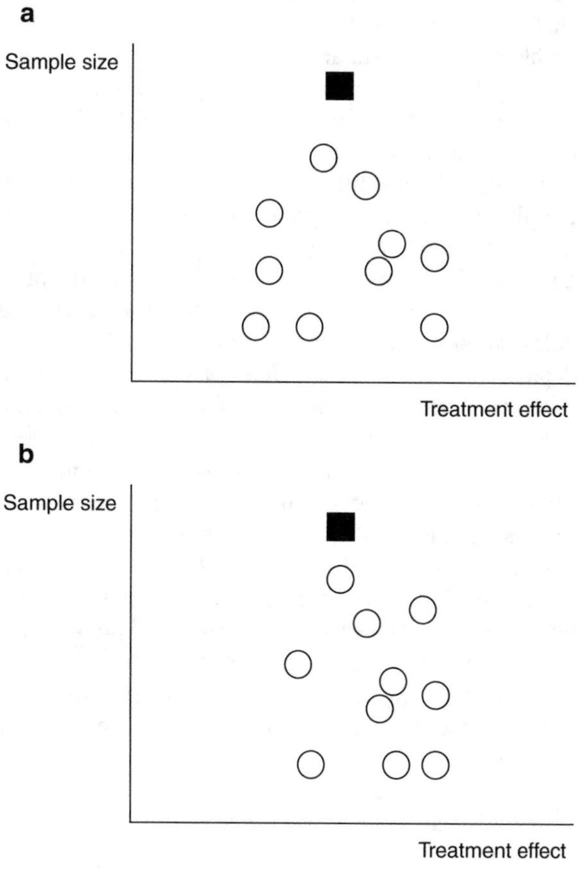

Fig. 2.6 Hypothetical funnel plots showing potentially (**a**) unbiased and (**b**) biased meta-analyses. (Courtesy of the Cochrane Collaboration)

A more quantitative approach is the I^2 statistic, which estimates the proportion of the variance in study estimates that is due to heterogeneity [456]. There are different interpretations of its meaning, but one approach is to consider values of 50% "concerning" [115].

Another challenge for systematic reviews has been developing methods for determining when they should be updated. Garner et al. developed a checklist, noting that the decision should consider whether the review has addressed a current question, employed valid methods, and was well conducted and whether there are new relevant methods, studies, or other information on existing included studies [457]. One possibility is the use of informatics methods, in particular machine learning methods to filter the literature [458], possibly augmented with a "crowdsourcing" approach [459].

Another limitation of systematic reviews is that some studies may not be published in the journal literature. One analysis found that the exclusion of so-called *grey literature* from meta-analyses was likely to exaggerate the benefit of interventions [125], although another found that published trials demonstrated an overall larger treatment effect [460]. The latter analysis also found that published trials were likely to be larger and of higher methodological quality. Grey literature most commonly consisted of either abstracts (49%) or unpublished data (33%). A related challenge, especially for meta-analysis, is duplicate publication (which is actually a problem beyond meta-analysis), since it results in single individuals being counted more than once, potentially effecting the results of the analysis [461].

Another problem with systematic reviews is their (probably excessive) proliferation. An analysis by Ioannidis found substantial numbers of systematic reviews and meta-analyses on similar topics that yielded disparate results [462]. He also found that the growth of systematic reviews and meta-analyses published was growing much larger than other types of papers. His analysis concluded that most topics addressed by meta-analyses of RCTs had overlapping, redundant meta-analyses, with same-topic meta-analyses sometimes exceeding 20. He also noted that some fields produce massive numbers of meta-analyses; e.g., 185 meta-analyses of antidepressants for depression were published between 2007 and 2014. These meta-analyses were often produced either by industry employees or by authors with industry ties, with results aligned with sponsor interests. In assessing Ioannidis' results, Page and Moher called for online systematic reviews, updated in real time [463]. To reduce the number of duplicate systematic reviews, the PROSPERO International Prospective Register of Systematic Reviews[40] has been established so potential authors can see if a systematic review is already being done on a given topic.

Page et al. analyzed the epidemiology and reporting characteristics of 300 systematic reviews published in February 2014 [464]. They found that their quality was highly variable. At least a third of the systematic reviews did not report use of a protocol, eligibility criteria relating to publication status, years of coverage of the search, a full Boolean search logic for at least one database, methods for data

[40] https://www.crd.york.ac.uk/PROSPERO/

extraction, methods for study risk of bias assessment, a primary outcome, an abstract conclusion that incorporated study limitations, or the funding source. Cochrane systematic reviews, which accounted for 15% of the sample, had more complete reporting than all other types of systematic reviews.

Other research has looked at other aspects of systematic reviews. One study found there continue to be differences between studies that are commonly included vs. excluded in systematic reviews. In one analysis of Cochrane meta-analyses, treatment effects were found to be larger in published than in unpublished trials [465]. In addition, for published trials, those in a language other than English were found to have larger treatment effects than those published in English. Some systematic reviews have been found to have a considerable delay between search and publication, but only 47% of systematic review abstracts stated the last search date and 60% stated the databases that had been searched [26].

2.5.5 *Secondary Literature*

The main purpose of the scientific literature is for researchers to communicate with other researchers. Most others who use the information and especially the knowledge in the primary literature, such as clinicians and consumers, need it in a more summarized form. In most professional fields, healthcare included, practitioners apply scientific information but do not necessarily generate it and are therefore less likely to understand the scientific esoterica described by researchers. This is especially so for nonexpert professionals, such as clinicians, who must make decisions that are, however, based on specialized scientific information.

Secondary literature historically consisted of review articles (which are often published in the same journals that contain primary literature), books, editorials, clinical practice guidelines, and other forms of publication in which original research information is reviewed. Some of the review articles occur in the voluminous number of the "throw-away" journals. These journals often serve as vehicles for pharmaceutical or other advertising but nonetheless often feature well-written and concise articles on clinically pertinent topics. In fact, one study found that although such publications are of lower methodological quality from a research perspective, they communicate their message better via use of tables, pictures, larger fonts, and easier readability [466]. Of course, these publications are often justly criticized because it is unknown how the vested interests of the advertisers influence the editorial content.

New technology has changed secondary literature similar to how it has impacted primary literature. Many secondary literature journals and other sources are now electronic. As we will discuss in Chap. 3, there are numerous biomedical and health Web sites, some of which cater to clinicians and others to patients. But this literature still has limitations that existed when it was predominantly paper-based.

One continued problem with secondary publication sources is their ability to keep up with the advance of primary literature. Banzi et al. assessed various online point-of-care summary sources for their speed of updating their evidence, finding that some were better than others in the speed of incorporating new evidence [467]. Ketchum et al. found similar variation in the amount and currency of evidence for four common clinical problems, with very little overlap in citations provided [468].

Another problem with secondary information sources is error. Two recent studies have found numerous errors in drug compendia, which physicians and other healthcare professionals use constantly for information on the drugs they prescribe and administer. One study found that across 270 drug summaries reviewed within 5 well-known drug compendia, the median total number of errors identified per source was 782, with the greatest number of errors occurring in the categories of dosage and administration, patient education, and warnings and precautions [469]. A majority of errors were classified as incomplete, with the remainder inaccurate and omitted. Another study assessed one company's prescription opioid products across 7 different compendia and discovered 859 errors, with the greatest percentage in safety and patient education categories. The authors reported errors to publishers of the compendia, but the complete or partial resolution of errors was only 34%, leaving about two-thirds of the identified errors remaining [470].

Conflict of interest is also a problem in secondary literature. One study of authors of six well-known medical textbooks found a large subset of authors had patents and received remuneration from medical product companies that was not disclosed to readers [471].

One specific type of secondary literature that grew in stature as efforts to standardize healthcare evolved is the clinical practice guidelines (CPG). These are, "systematically developed statements to assist practitioners and patient decisions about appropriate health care for specific clinical circumstances" [472]. CPGs are used as more than just documents for reading, for they also serve to guide documentation and provide decision logic for the provision of medical care [473].

One concern with CPGs is their sheer number. A study of British general medical practices found 855 difference CPGs had been sent to physicians in 65 different practices, which could be stacked nearly 70 cm tall [474]. Another concern with CPGs is that clinicians do not use them. Cabana et al. performed a systematic review assessing the reasons for lack of adherence to CPGs, finding a variety of factors often dependent on the unique characteristics of the locations where they were studied [475]. The major categories of barriers include awareness of CPGs, agreement with them, altered expectations of patient outcomes, inability to overcome the inertia of previous practice, and barriers to carry them out.

Another problem related with CPGs is that while the evidence in the underlying RCTs may be valid, the guideline may not be applicable to populations, interventions, or outcomes that are stated in the guideline recommendation [476]. One well-documented example is the exclusion of elderly patients from RCTs of heart failure management [477]. Bennett et al. assessed 11 practice guidelines on oral medication treatment for type 2 diabetes mellitus and found not only was there substantial variation in the consistency with known best evidence but that about a third rated low in editorial independence, which consisted either of a lack of independence from funding bodies or the presence of a conflict of interest [478]. Similar to other statements for standard and complete reporting, the Reporting Items for practice Guidelines in HealThcare (RIGHT) Statement has been developed for reporting on CPGs [479]. The quality of studies used in CPGs is typically assessed using the GRADE framework [452].

An additional problem with CPGs is that while they consist of logic for use in clinical care, they are typically published as textual documents. Even further, they may have ambiguities that prevent their being translated into logic for clinical decision support [480]. This has spawned efforts to develop standards for "computable knowledge" that maintains knowledge in logical forms that can be used by computer systems [481].

Another concern with guidelines is the conflict of interest between those who perform studies for the industry as well and also develop clinical practice guidelines. Neuman et al. identified 14 guidelines on screening and/or treatment for hypertension and/or diabetes mellitus [482]. Of 288 panel members on these guidelines, 138 (48%) were found to have declared a conflict of interest, while 8 (11%) more declared no conflicts but actually had them. Likewise, Mendelson et al. looked at 17 guidelines on cardiovascular conditions and identified 279 of 498 (56%) panelists having a research grant, being on a speaker's bureau, and/or receiving honoraria, varying from 13 to 87% per guideline [483]. A systematic analysis of guidelines in interventional medicine subspecialties also found that most failed to grade evidence, made use of lower-quality evidence when present, and failed to adequately disclose conflicts of interest [484]. Khan et al. found that for 18 practice guidelines making recommendations for 10 high-revenue medications, nearly 50% of authors had payments, with a substantial minority not disclosing them [485].

Ioannidis has advocated that professional societies should abstain from authorship of guidelines and disease definition statements [486]. The American College of Physicians, one producer of guidelines, requires those involved in their product to disclose all healthcare-related interests and manage conflicts in a manner that is transparent, proportional, and consistent. Any person involved in the development of an ACP clinical guideline or guidance statement must disclose all financial and intellectual interests related to healthcare from the previous 3 years [487].

These problems with guidelines led the Institute of Medicine (IOM) to publish a report calling for "trustworthy" clinical guidelines [488, 489]. AHRQ developed an instrument to discern the extend of adherence to these standards, the National Guideline Clearinghouse Extent of Adherence to Trustworthy Standards (NEATS) instrument [490].

2.6 Electronic Publishing

In the first edition of this book, IR systems were still viewed as a means to get to paper-based scientific journals. While it was noted that online full-text journals had been in existence since the 1980s, high cost, low-resolution displays, and bandwidth-limited networks precluded their routine access. In the second edition, we noted that many journals and other resources were increasingly available electronically. In the third edition, we saw that electronic publishing, at least for journals, was nearly ubiquitous. In this fourth edition, we note that while some journals are still produced on paper, the primary vehicle for biomedical and health publishing is electronic. In this section, we will raise the major issues for electronic publishing that sets the context for the state-of-the-art of IR systems that follow in the ensuing chapters, which then leads into their coverage more deeply when discussing digital libraries.

In the early days of electronic publishing, the ease of replicating, deleting, and altering information on the Web led the American Association for the Advancement of Science (AAAS) to define a "definitive publication" in science, especially in the context of the electronic environment [491]. Such a publication should be peer-reviewed; the following statements apply as well:

- The publication must be publicly available.
- The relevant community must be made aware of its existence.
- A system for long-term access and retrieval must be in place.
- The publication must not be changed (technical protection and/or certification are desirable).
- It must not be removed (unless legally unavoidable).
- It must be unambiguously identified (e.g., by some sort of identifier).
- It must have a bibliographic record (metadata) containing certain minimal information.
- There must be a plan for archiving and long-term preservation.

2.6.1 Electronic Scholarly Publication

As noted above, electronic publishing of scientific journals and other publications is nearly ubiquitous. In addition to available content, the Internet and Web environment makes possible all kinds of new capabilities, such as the ability to link directly to the full text of an article from its bibliographic record, and the linkage of sources that cite or make use of content in the resource. Another change is that journals can alter the form and quantity of what they publish, since editorial space, always at a premium in paper journals, is less constrained in electronic environments.

This new electronic environment may offer advantages to users, but it is not without new issues and challenges. In particular, the technical challenges to electronic scholarly publication have been replaced by economic and political ones [492, 493]. Printing and mailing, tasks no longer needed in electronic publishing, comprised a significant part of the "added value" from publishers of journals. Since the intellectual portion of the peer review process is carried out by scientists, the role of the publisher can be reduced or perhaps eliminated with electronic submission of manuscripts and their electronic distribution to peer reviewers. There is, however, still some value added by publishers, such as copyediting and production.

Even if publishing companies as they are known were to vanish, there would still be some cost to the production of journals. Thus, while the cost of producing journals electronically is likely to be less, it is not zero, and even if journal content is distributed "free," someone has to pay the production costs.

The ease of distribution on the Web has given rise to a new publishing model called *Open Access* [57]. This model is sometimes called "author pays" based on the notion that publishing should be a cost incurred in research, which is usually funded by grants or contracts. In open access publishing, after the article is accepted and the publishing cost paid, the article is then made freely available on the Web. We will describe the economics and related issues of publishing, including open access, in more detail in Chap. 6.

2.6.2 Consumer Health Information

Another phenomenon of the Internet and Web is the ability of nonprofessionals to seek and access information written not only for professionals but also for "lay" audiences. Indeed, as was noted in the last chapter, over 80% of Web users regularly search for personal health information [494]. As with electronic scholarly publication, this has led to new opportunities as well as challenges, the most serious of the latter being concern about the quality of information, i.e., whether it is correct or may mislead people, not only imperiling their health but also costing them money.

The Web is inherently democratic, allowing virtually anyone to post information. This is no doubt an asset in modern democratic societies. However, it is potentially at odds with the operation of a professional field, particularly one like healthcare, where practitioners are ethically bound and legally required to adhere to the highest standard of care. To the extent that misleading or incorrect information is posted on the Web, this standard is challenged.

Concern about the quality of health information on the Web has been present since its early days [495]. One early systematic review of studies assessing the quality of health information found that 55 of 79 studies concluded that quality of information was a problem [496]. In many of these studies, the sites evaluated were from academic medical centers or other prestigious medical institutions. Since academic sites are usually managed in a decentralized manner (i.e., individual departments and often individual faculty maintain their own pages), one cannot assume that quality checking persists down to each department and faculty member with a Web page like it does on highly controlled corporate Web sites. Subsequent research has shown this continues to be a problem and is somewhat exacerbated by new developments, such as social media. Some more recent studies identifying problematic information quality include:

- A study assessing the ability of Google to answer five common pediatric questions found that when the answer was available, 78% of sites gave correct advice, with government sites giving correct information 100% of the time, news sites

giving correct information 55% of the time, and sponsored sites never giving correct advice [497].
- Web sites promoting use of robotic surgery tended to overstate the evidence for the value of this type of surgery and downplay its risks [498].
- Quality varies by topic but continues to be a problem for Web information [499].
- US hospital Web sites that offer the procedure always tout the benefits of transcatheter aortic valve replacement but only about a quarter reported any of the known risks [500].
- Most Web sites devoted to breast cancer are insufficient in helping women actively participate in decision-making for breast cancer surgery [501].
- Twitter bots and Russian trolls have been found to spread misinformation about vaccination [502].
- Incorrect news can spread rapidly with today's Internet, as exemplified by the incorrect reporting that 7% of the DNA of US astronaut Scott Kelly and its subsequent amplification. In reality, it was gene expression that was altered, something that could (and did) likely occur in the space environment [503].
- An analysis of 115 highly viewed YouTube videos on prostate cancer, with a collective reach of over 6 million viewers, found that 77% contained potential misinformation or biased content within the video or in the comments section [504].
- Only 60% of Web sites regarding common acute pediatric complaints were accurate [505].

Another concern about health information Web sites is readability. Most patients [506–508] and parents of child patients [509] read at an average of a fifth- to sixth-grade level. Reading ability also declines with age [510]. Those who deliver consumer health information must therefore take readability into account. The standard measure of assessing readability is the Flesch-Kincaid score [511]. This measure calculates reading grade level (RGL) based on average sentence length (ASL, the number of words divided by the number of sentences) and average number of syllables per word (ASW, the number of syllables divided by the number of words):

$$RGL = (.39 * ASL) + (11.8 * ASW) - 15.59 \tag{2.6}$$

Early studies of readability of health information on the Web found that most of it was written well above the reading level of average citizens. Graber et al. found that a sample of patient education material from the Web was written at a tenth-grade level [512]. Berland et al. determined that no English-language site they evaluated had readability below the tenth-grade level, while over half were written at a college level and 11% at a graduate school level [513]. Over 86% of Spanish sites were also written at the high school level or above. Cheng and Dunn found that readability of Australian health Web sites was above the average Australian levels of reading [514]. Another study compared readability for sites on osteoarthritis compared with 15 years earlier and found slight increases in readability difficulty over time [515]. Over half of Web sites regarding common acute pediatric complaints were readable at or below an eighth-grade level [505].

An additional challenge is numeracy, not only for consumers but even clinicians. A study of adults in the United States and Germany found numeracy skills varied widely among adults, with a gap between those with high and low levels of education, especially in the United States [516]. Another study of young and elderly adults in Germany found that frequencies instead of single-event probabilities are much more consistently understood [517]. Even physicians have problems with understanding a number of statistical concepts, as shown in a survey where they tended to overstate benefits and understate harms of a number of common treatments [518]. One recent analysis explored the reasons why physicians tend to be drawn to treatments not supported by evidence [519].

Eysenbach and Diepgen identified that problems of poor-quality and hard-to-read information on the Web were exacerbated by a "context deficit" that makes poor-quality information more difficult to distinguish [520]. They noted there are fewer less clear "markers" of the type of document (e.g., professional textbook vs. patient handout) and that the reader of a specific page may not be aware of the "context" of a Web site that includes disclaimers, warnings, and so forth. Furthermore, information may be correct in one context but incorrect in another, and this difference may not be detectable on a random page within a Web site (e.g., the differences in treatment in children vs. adults or across different ethnic groups).

One important site for health information has been Wikipedia,[41] a mass collaborative attempt to build a distributed online encyclopedia. Although the authoring and monitoring process has become more rigorous over the years, some used to quip about Wikipedia, "If you don't like the facts in Wikipedia, you can change them" (source unknown), while another lamented it as a "faith-based encyclopedia" [521]. Although content can be edited by anyone, medical articles are primarily written by a core group of medical professionals, and processes have been proposed to improve its clinical content [522]. One solution has been to embed its editing in medical [523] and pharmacy [524] education.

More recent studies have assessed the content of Wikipedia. One study assessed drug information, finding that a traditionally edited database (in this case, Medscape Drug Reference) was more complete, broader in scope, and had fewer errors of omission [525]. Another analysis found that the accuracy and depth of Wikipedia was comparable to information in the Physician Data Query (PDQ) of the National Cancer Institute but that Wikipedia was less readable [526]. An additional study noted that Wikipedia articles covering the ten most costly medical conditions in the United States contained many errors when assessed against standard peer-reviewed sources [527]. Another analysis found that update of Wikipedia after new FDA drug warnings were issued occurred within 2 weeks for 41% of drugs (58% for those used in high-prevalence diseases) but the remainder remained un-updated for much longer [528].

The impact of poor-quality information is unclear. An early systematic review of whether harm resulted from information obtained on the Internet found 15 case

[41] https://www.wikipedia.org/

reports [529]. But many self-help advocates, led by the late by Tom Ferguson [530], argued that patients and consumers are savvy enough to understand the limits of quality of information on the Web and should be trusted to discern quality using their own abilities to consult different sources of information and communicate with healthcare practitioners and others who share their condition(s). Indeed, the ideal situation may be a partnership among patients and their healthcare practitioners, as it has been shown that patients desire that their practitioners be the primary source of recommendations for online information [531].

This concern over quality of information led a number of individuals and organizations to develop guidelines for assessing the quality of health information. These guidelines usually defined explicit criteria for a Web page that a reader could apply to determine whether a potential source of information has attributes consistent with high quality. One of the earliest and most widely quoted set of criteria was published in *JAMA* [495]. These criteria stated that Web pages should contain the following:

- The name, affiliation, and credentials of the author—readers may differ on the value of an individual's credentials, but the information should be listed to be assessed by all.
- References to the claims made—if health claims are made, they should contain references to legitimate scientific research documenting the claim.
- Explicit listing of any perceived or real conflict of interest—a conflict of interest does not disqualify someone from posting information, but all perceived or real conflict of interests must be disclosed, as is required of those who teach continuing education courses.
- Date of most recent update—health information becomes outdated quickly, and the date that a page was most recently updated should be listed.

Another early set of criteria was the Health on the Net (HON) codes,[42] a set of voluntary codes of conduct for health-related Web sites. Sites that adhere to the HON codes can display the HONcode logo. These principles to which sites must adhere (details on the HON Web site) include:

- Authoritative
- Complementarity
- Privacy
- Attribution
- Justifiability
- Transparency
- Financial disclosure
- Advertising policy

The HONcode continues to be used in a voluntary fashion to indicate adherence to quality principles but is limited to Web sites and not newer more dynamic

[42] https://www.hon.ch/

information sources, such as social media [532]. One analysis of Web sites for ten common orthopedic sports medicine diagnoses found that sites displaying the HONcode were more likely to have higher-quality information [533].

An additional effort for self-policing the Web comes from the Contract for the Web,[43] which outlines a set of principles for governments, companies, and citizens to "safeguard" the free and open Web. Governments should ensure everyone can connect, access it at all times, and respect fundamental privacy and data rights. Companies should make the Internet affordable and accessible, respect privacy and data rights, and develop technologies that "support the best in humanity and challenge the worst." Citizens should be creators and collaborators, build communities that "respect civil discourse and human dignity," and fight for the Web.

Some early research assessed whether Web "robots" might be able to automatically detect these criteria? Price and Hersh found that some quality criteria could be detected and the output from a search can be reordered to give more prominent ranking of higher-quality pages [534]. One observation from their small dataset used to evaluate the system was that the quality criteria listed earlier may not truly be associated with the actual quality of pages. They noted, for example, the low-quality pages were more easily identifiable from their exclamation points and "1–800" telephone prefixes to call to order products. A larger application of this approach found that a number of quality indicators could be detected with high accuracy [535].

Of course, misleading and inaccurate health information is not limited to consumer Web sites. Another source of sometimes inaccurate information is the news media, whose objective can often be to create sensational news stories and/or maintain the attention of their audience rather than go into the nuances of complex health-related information. Shuchman and Wilkes assessed the problems of health news reporting in the general press, noting four problem areas [536]:

1. Sensationalism—there are a variety of reasons for sensationalism, from the desire of media executives to sell newspapers or increase television viewing to the efforts of scientists or their institutions to garner publicity for prestige and/or funding.
2. Biases and conflicts of interest—reporters may be misled by incomplete presentation of information or undisclosed conflict of interest by scientists, institutions, or the pharmaceutical industry.
3. Lack of follow-up—the press often has a short attention span and does not continue its coverage on stories that are initially sensationalized.
4. Stories that are not covered—health-related stories compete with other stories for coverage in the press. There are also instances of scientists who have, sometimes unwittingly, signed agreements forbidding publication of research not approved by the sponsor. One well-known case involved a study showing that generic versions of a thyroid medication were comparable to a brand-name drug [537].

[43] https://contractfortheweb.org/

Other data supports these observations. One particular problem is news media reporting of findings, usually preliminary, presented at scientific research meetings. Schwartz et al. found that of 149 such presentations receiving substantial attention in the news media, 76% were nonrandomized, 25% had fewer than 30 subjects, and 15% were nonhuman studies [538]. Furthermore, half were not subsequently published in MEDLINE-indexed journals. A related concern is lack of news media coverage of retraction of studies, with 1 analysis of 50 retractions identified in the MEDLINE database finding that only 3 were reported in newspaper articles [539]. Another study analyzed 436 news reports of cancer from the United States and found that aggressive treatment and survival were frequently discussed but that treatment failure, adverse events, and end-of-life care were rarely discussed [540].

More recent studies show new dimensions of this problem. Yavchitz et al. noted about half of press releases and news reports of RCTs contained similar kinds of spin described above [541]. Downing et al. found that half of media reports of the ACCORD-Lipid trial did not correctly report the lack of value for adding the drug fenofibrate to statin therapy in hyperlipidemia [542]. Schwitzer analyzed 1889 news stories on various medical topics and found that drugs, medical devices, and other interventions were usually portrayed positively, with potential harms often minimized and costs ignored [543]. Also a source of problematic information is exaggeration in academic press releases, which lead to exaggerations in the news [544].

2.7 Use of Knowledge-Based Health Information

Information sources, print or computer, are approached for two reasons: the need to locate a particular item of information, such as a document, report, or book, or the need to obtain information on a particular subject. Lancaster and Warner defined *subject needs* [545], which may in modern parlance be called *use cases* [546] and fall into three categories:

- The need for help in solving a certain problem or making a decision
- The need for background information on a topic
- The need to keep up with information in a given subject area

The first two subject needs are called retrospective information needs, in that documents already published are sought, while the latter need is called a current awareness need, which is met by filtering new documents to identify those on a certain topic. Retrospective needs may also be classified by the amount of information needed [545]:

- A single fact.
- One or more documents but less than the entire literature on the topic.
- A comprehensive search of the literature.
- It will be seen later that the interaction with an information system varies based on these different needs.

Wilkinson and Fuller described four types of information needs for document collections [547]:

- Fact-finding—locating a specific item of information
- Learning—developing an understanding of a topic
- Gathering—finding material relevant to a new problem not explicitly stated
- Exploring—browsing material with a partially specified information need that can be modified as the content is viewed

Another perspective on the use of information classified the kinds of information needs characteristic of users of health information have. Gorman defined four states of information need [548]:

- Unrecognized need—clinician not aware of information need or knowledge deficit.
- Recognized need—clinician aware of need but may or may not pursue it.
- Pursued need—information seeking occurs but may or may not be successful.
- Satisfied need—information seeking successful.

Perhaps ironically, the volume of research assessing information needs has declined in recent years with the growth and ubiquity of the Internet. A great deal of research in this area was done in the 1990s and 2000s, and we may question its applicability to modern times. We know, for example, that physicians use computers much more than the occasional amounts they did during those earlier times [549].

2.7.1 Models of Physician Thinking

There was substantial research in the twentieth century focused on models of physician thinking. The traditional view was based upon the *hypothetico-deductive model* [550]. In this model, the physician begins forming hypotheses based upon the initial information obtained, usually the patient's chief complaint. The skilled physician already begins to focus on data-driven hypotheses, which subsequently lead to hypothesis-driven selection of the next data to be collected. The process is iterated until one or more diagnoses can account for all the observations (or at least the observations deemed necessary to explain).

An alternative model, not necessarily at odds with the hypothetico-deductive view, was proposed by Schmidt et al., who noted that one implication of the hypothetico-deductive model was that diagnostic failures arise from taking shortcuts or giving insufficient attention to details [551]. However, they observed that experienced clinicians actually gathered smaller amounts of data and were able to arrive at correct diagnoses with fewer hypotheses. This led them to theorize that medical knowledge was contained in "illness scripts," which were based not only on learned medical knowledge but also past (and especially recent) experience. These scripts were based on causal networks that represented objects and their relationships in the world. They noted that medical education consisted of building these causal networks in the mind. As the student progressed through medical education and attained clinical experience, the networks become compiled into higher level, simplified models that explain patient signs and symptoms under diagnostic labels.

There was considerable evidence for this model. First, the hypothetico-deductive model implied that those with the best problem-solving skills should consistently be the best diagnosticians. Yet studies in which physicians and medical students were given patient management problems (PMPs), which simulate the clinical setting, found that there was wide variation in performance on different problems by the same practitioners [550]. Additional supporting evidence was that experienced physicians were much better able than students to recall details of patient encounters when the findings are randomly reordered [551]. This is because more experienced practitioners attached specific patients to instances of the scripts. Another finding in support of this model came from Patel et al., who noted that experienced physicians tended to make minimal use of basic science in their diagnostic efforts; rather, they match patients to patterns of clinical presentations for various diseases [552]. This was consistent with advanced training leading to building high-level scripts based on clinical findings.

Some researchers expressed concern that clinicians relied too much on personal knowledge and experience and not enough on aggregated experience and/or published literature. Sox et al. noted an *availability heuristic*, where clinicians inflate the diagnostic probability of a disease based on recent or otherwise well-remembered cases [553]. Tanenbaum carried out an ethnographic study of physicians being exposed to outcomes and research data, finding that they often continued to rely on personal experience despite contrary data from outcomes research or the medical literature [554]. Some medical editors lamented that the journal literature was underused [555, 556], yet others pointed out that this resource was too fragmented and time-consuming to use [120, 557]. McDonald noted that there is often not enough evidence to inform clinical decisions and that clinicians rely on heuristics to guide their decision-making, advocating that such heuristics be improved when the robustness of evidence is sparse [558].

2.7.2 Physician Information Needs

A great deal of work was carried out assessing physician informatics in the 1980s and 1990s, yet as noted above, this work was done at a time when computers and the Internet were not as ubiquitous as they are now, not to mention smartphones not having been invented. Nonetheless, we can learn from the conceptual framework developed to assess these needs. As noted by Gorman, physicians may have information needs that they do not immediately recognize [548]. Some of these needs may become recognized, pursued, or satisfied. Understanding these needs is important to building healthcare IR systems.

2.7.2.1 Unrecognized Needs

One of the difficulties in characterizing unrecognized information needs derives from the physicians' lack of direct awareness of their existence. As such, these needs can be identified only indirectly through the measurement of knowledge dissemination, knowledge stores, and outcomes of clinical practice that reflect application of knowledge. A number of early studies documented the slow dissemination of new (at the time) technologies, such as photocoagulation in diabetic retinopathy [559] and benefits of treating hypertension [560]. Another study looked at six important then-recent medical advances and finding that anywhere from 20 to 50% of physicians were unaware of them [561]. Another line of evidence demonstrating lack of information came from physicians who take recertification examinations. The scores of family practitioners, who are required to recertify every 6 years, tend to decline with each recertification examination [562]. Likewise, when internists with various levels of experience were given an 81-question subset of the American Board of Internal Medicine examination, a direct correlation was found between score and years out of residency training [563].

2.7.2.2 Recognized Needs

Physicians and other healthcare practitioners do recognize they have unmet information needs. A number of studies have attempted to gain insight into the quantity and nature of questions asked in clinical practice. Many investigators have attempted to measure such needs, although their results differ as a result of variations in practice settings, types of physician studied, and how information need itself was defined [548]. Even though the results are not entirely consistent, they do reveal that physicians have significant unmet information needs.

The first study of this type, performed by Covell et al., found that while physicians thought they had an unmet information need for about 1 out of every 77 patients, they actually had an average of 2 unmet needs for every 3 patients (0.62 unanswered questions per patient) [564]. Using a similar methodology with different physicians, Gorman and Helfand found a nearly identical frequency (0.60 per patient) of unmet information needs [565]. The former study assessed urban internists and specialists in Los Angeles, while the latter focused on urban and rural primary care physicians in Oregon. Ely et al. observed family physicians in Iowa who were observed to have 0.32 questions per patient [566].

All of these studies found that information needs were highly specific to patient problems. Ely et al. developed a taxonomy of generic questions, finding 69 different types, the top 10 of which are listed in Table 2.5 [566]. This table also gives the percentage of asked questions that were pursued as well as pursued questions that were answered, showing in general that treatment questions were more likely to be pursued and answered than diagnostic ones. This taxonomy was refined and validated with questions from Oregon primary care practitioners, and question types were found to be assignable with moderate reliability (kappa = 0.53) [567].

Table 2.5 Questions most commonly asked, pursued, and answered by physicians, adapted from [566]

Generic question	How many asked? (%)	How many asked were pursued? (%)	How many pursued were answered? (%)
What is the cause of symptom X?	9	9	50
What is the dose of drug X?	8	85	97
How should I manage disease or finding X?	7	29	83
How should I treat finding or disease X?	7	33	72
What is the cause of physical finding X?	7	18	46
What is the cause of text finding X?	4	40	72
Could this patient have disease or condition X?	4	14	67
Is test X indicated in situation Y?	4	29	83
What is the drug of choice for condition X?	3	47	76
Is drug X indicated in situation Y?	3	25	78

2.7.2.3 Pursued Needs

One consistent finding in the studies of unmet information needs was that physicians decided against pursuing answers for a majority of the questions. Covell et al. [564], Gorman and Helfand [565], and Ely et al. [566] found that answers were pursued only 30 to 36% of the time, indicating that 64 to 70% of information needs remained unmet. These studies also consistently found that when information was pursued, the most common sources were other humans, followed closely by textbooks and drug compendia. The use of journal articles as well as computer sources was low.

Gorman and Helfand [565] attempted to define that factors that were most likely to be associated with the decision to pursue an answer to a question. They defined 11 attributes of clinical questions and used multiple logistic regression in an attempt to identify those most likely to correlate with an answer being sought, as shown in Table 2.6. The most likely factors to cause answer seeking were as follows: the question required an urgent answer, it was likely to be answerable, and it would help manage other patients besides the one who had generated the question. The potential for a question to benefit a physician's general knowledge or to reduce his or her liability risk was not associated with pursuit of an answer.

Covell et al. also attempted to identify the impediments to answer seeking found that physicians either were too busy or did not have immediate access to an answer [564]. Another significant impediment to information seeking was the disarray of

Table 2.6 Factors influencing a physician's decision to seek an answer to a question, adapted from [565]

Factors most associated with pursuit of an answer:
Urgency—the question had to be answered soon.
Answerability—the physician felt an answer was likely to exist.
Generalizability—n answer would help manage other patients.
Factors not associated with answer seeking:
Knowledge—how much was previously known about the problem?
Uneasiness—how uneasy did the physician feel about the problem?
Potential help—an answer could help the patient.
Potential harm—not having an answer could hurt the patient.
Edification—an answer would benefit the practitioner's general knowledge.
Liability—the problem involved liability risk.
Knowledge of peers—peers of the practitioner know the answer.
Difficulty—how difficult would it be to find the answer?

the typical practitioner's library, consisting of out-of-date textbooks and inadequately indexed journal collections.

Ely and colleagues also assessed obstacles to obtaining answers to clinical questions [568]. They identified a total of 59 obstacles to accessing information. These were organized into five steps in asking and answering questions: recognizing a gap in knowledge, formulating a question, searching for relevant information, formulating an answer, and using the answer to direct patient care. They noted six obstacles that were particularly prominent to themselves and the clinicians they observed, quoted as follows:

- The excessive time required to find information
- Difficulty modifying the original question, which could be vague and open to interpretation
- Difficulty selecting an optimal strategy to search for information
- Failure of a seemingly appropriate resource to cover the topic
- Uncertainty about how to know when all the relevant evidence has been found so that the search can stop
- Inadequate synthesis of multiple bits of evidence into a clinically useful statement

Ely et al. also looked at reasons for not pursuing answers to questions [569]:

- Doubted existence of relevant information—25%
- Readily available consultation leading to referral rather than pursuit—22%
- Lack of time to pursue—19%
- Not important enough to pursue answer—15%
- Uncertain where to look for answer—8%

They then followed up on the 237 questions from the 585 that these physicians pursued but were unable to answer [570]. They grouped the questions into 19 generic types but found that 3 of the types accounted for slightly more than half of the questions:

1. Questions about undiagnosed abnormal clinical findings
2. Questions containing subquestions qualifying otherwise simple questions, such as how to manage one disease given the presence of another
3. Questions about the association between two highly specific findings or diseases

A survey of clinicians at Mayo Clinic found that 48% of respondents performed online searches for more than half of their patient interactions, with 91% occurring either before or within three hours of the patient interaction [571]. About 57% of respondents preferred synthesized information sources as compared to 13% who preferred primary literature. About 82% of knowledge searches took place on a workstation or office computer, while just 10% were done from a mobile device or at home.

Del Fiol et al. published a systematic review of three decades of work of clinician questions posed at the point of care [572]. Reiterating individual study findings, they found that the mean frequency of questions raised was 0.57 per patient seen, with clinicians pursuing 51% of questions and findings answers to 78% of those pursued. The most common types of questions were of drug treatment (34%) and potential causes of a symptom, physical finding, or diagnostic test finding (24%). The main barriers to information seeking were lack of time and doubt that an answer existed.

2.7.2.4 Satisfied Needs

What information resources are most likely to satisfy an information need? In a study of knowledge resource preferences of family physicians, Curley et al. [573] found that "cost" variables (e.g., availability, searchability, understandability, clinical applicability) were more closely associated with the decision to use a resource than "benefit" variables, such as its extensiveness and credibility. As with the studies described earlier, the family physicians in this study were more likely to use textbooks, compendia, and colleagues for information seeking over journal literature and bibliographic resources [574].

These observations led Shaughnessy et al. [557] to propose a formula for the usefulness of information:

$$\text{Usefullness} = \frac{\text{Relevance} * \text{Validity}}{\text{Work}} \qquad (2.7)$$

That is, the value of information is proportional to its relevance and validity to the clinical situation and inversely proportional to how difficult it is to find and apply.

Aakre et al. performed a systematic review of the barriers and facilitators to information seeking and identified five key determinants of information-seeking behaviors [575]:

- Time—including subthemes of time availability, efficiency of information seeking, and urgency of information need

- Accessibility—including subthemes of hardware access, hardware speed, hardware portability, information restriction, and cost of resources
- Personal skills and attitudes—including subthemes of computer literacy, information-seeking skills, and contextual attitudes about information seeking
- Institutional attitudes, cultures, and policies—including subthemes describing external individual and institutional information-seeking influences
- Knowledge resource features—including subthemes describing information-seeking efficiency, information content, information organization, resource familiarity, information credibility, information currency, workflow integration, compatibility of recommendations with local processes, and patient educational support

2.7.3 *Information Needs of Other Healthcare Professionals*

The information needs and usage of nonphysician healthcare providers have been much less studied, and there are few studies from the modern era of ubiquitous information. One study looked at information needs and seeking of nurse practitioners (NPs) [576]. The findings were not much different than those noted for physicians. The most frequent information needs reported were somewhat more focused than physicians and on two specific areas: drug therapy (43%) and diagnosis (41%). Most commonly used information sources were supervising physicians, drug reference manuals, textbooks, journal articles, and other NPs. The generalness of a need was found to be a negative predictor of information seeking.

2.7.4 *Information Needs of Biomedical and Health Researchers*

Another group in the healthcare field whose information needs have been minimally assessed is researchers. Roberts and Hayes collected and classified information requests to a library of a large pharmaceutical company [577]. A total of 1131 search requests were classified by the biological entity being searched (e.g., drug, disease, gene, etc.) and, when specified, type of document sought (e.g., scientific literature, business intelligence, patent record). The most common entities for which information was sought were drugs (31.3%), diseases (27.4%), genes (26.3%), companies (17.0%), methods (10.6%), authors (7.9%), geographic regions (5.7%), and drug sales (5.0%). About 36% of queries sought information on more than one of these entities, with the most common pair-wise combinations being drug-disease, drug-company, and drug-sales. The type of document sought varied by search entity, with queries on genes most commonly seeking patent information, queries on diseases seeking journal articles, and queries on drugs seeking business intelligence. Of course, the searching in a pharmaceutical company is likely to have different characteristics than other sites for biomedical research. Hemminger et al. studied academic scientists and found that they made substantial use of electronic resources, from accessing journal articles on the Web to communicating mostly electronically and making few visits to the physical library [578].

2.7.5 Information Needs of Consumers

Roberts and Demner-Fushman analyzed large corpora of online questions from clinicians and consumers and found that the form of consumer questions was highly dependent upon the individual online resource, especially in the amount of background information provided [579]. In contrast, they found that clinicians provided very little background information and often asked much shorter questions. The content of consumer questions was also highly dependent upon the resource. They also noted that while clinician questions commonly were about treatments and tests, consumer questions focused more on symptoms and diseases. In addition, consumers placed far more emphasis on certain types of health problems, such as sexual health. A survey of 13–18-year-olds in the United States found that 86% searched for health information online, with 25% searching for such information (in their language) "a lot" [580]. However, more common sources of information were parents, school health classes, and health professionals.

2.8 Summary

Clearly there are many issues in biomedical and health information that go beyond IR systems. Ioannidis et al. describe the "Medical Misinformation Mess," which consists of the following problems [581]:

- A good deal of published medical research is not reliable or is of uncertain reliability, offering no benefit to patients and not being useful to decision-makers.
- Most healthcare professionals lack awareness of this problem.
- Healthcare professionals also lack the skills to evaluate the reliability and usefulness of medical evidence.
- Patients and consumers also often lack relevant, accurate medical evidence and skilled guidance at the time they need to make medical decisions.

References

1. Blum B. Information systems for patient care. New York: Springer; 1984.
2. Rowley J. The wisdom hierarchy: representations of the DIKW hierarchy. J Inf Sci. 2007;33:163–80.

3. Losee R. The science of information. San Diego, CA: Academic Press; 1990.
4. Stone J. Information theory – a tutorial introduction. Sebtel Press; 2015.
5. Shannon C, Weaver W. The mathematical theory of communication. Urbana, IL: University of Illinois Press; 1949.
6. Robison R. How big is the human genome? Medium. 2014 January 5, 2014.
7. Bar-Hillel Y, Carnap R. Semantic information. Br J Philos Sci. 1953;4:147–57.
8. Belis M, Guiasu S. A quantitative-qualitative measure of information in cybernetic systems. IEEE Trans Inf Theory. 1968;14:593–4.
9. Price D. Little science, big science. New York: Columbia University Press; 1963.
10. Pao M. Concepts of information retrieval. Englewood, CO: Libraries Unlimited; 1989.
11. Molyneux R. ACRL University Library Statistics. Chicago: Association of Research Libraries; 1989.
12. Jinha A. Article 50 million: an estimate of the number of scholarly articles in existence. Learned Publishing. 2010;23:258–63.
13. Ware M, Mabe M. The STM report. An overview of scientific and scholarly journal publishing. Oxford: International Association of Scientific, Technical and Medical Publishers2009 September, 2009.
14. Bastian H, Glasziou P, Chalmers I. Seventy-five trials and eleven systematic reviews a day: how will we ever keep up? PLoS Med. 2010;7(9):e1000326.
15. Durack D. The weight of medical knowledge. N Engl J Med. 1978;298:773–5.
16. Madlon-Kay D. The weight of medical knowledge: still gaining. N Engl J Med. 1989;321:908.
17. Larsen P, von Ins M. The rate of growth in scientific publication and the decline in coverage provided by Science Citation Index. Scientometrics. 2010;84:575–603.
18. Bornmann L, Mutz R. Growth rates of modern science: a bibliometric analysis based on the number of publications and cited references. J Am Soc Inf Sci Technol. 2015;66:2215–22.
19. King C. Multiauthor papers: onward and upward. Science Watch 2012 July, 2012.
20. Weber M. The effects of listing authors in alphabetical order: a review of the empirical evidence. Research Evaluation. 2018;27:238–45.
21. Ioannidis J, Klavans R, Boyack K. The scientists who publish a paper every five days. Nature. 2018;561:167–9.
22. Littenberg B. Technology assessment in medicine. Acad Med. 1992;67:424–8.
23. Arnett D, Blumenthal R, Albert M, Michos E, Buroker A, Williams K, et al. 2019 ACC/AHA guideline on the primary prevention of cardiovascular disease. J Am Coll Cardiol. 2019;140:e596–646.
24. Poynard T, Munteanu M, Ratziu V, Benhamou Y, Martino VD, Taieb J, et al. Truth survival in clinical research: an evidence-based requiem? Ann Intern Med. 2002;136:888–95.
25. Shojania K, Sampson M, Ansari M, Ji J, Doucette S, Moher D. How quickly do systematic reviews go out of date? A survival analysis. Ann Intern Med. 2007;147:224–33.
26. Beller E, Chen J, Wang U, Glasziou P. Are systematic reviews up-to-date at the time of publication? Syst Rev. 2013;2:36.
27. McLellan F. 1966 and all that – when is a literature search done? Lancet. 2001;358:646.
28. Antman E, Lau J, Kupelnick B, Mosteller F, Chalmers T. A comparison of results of meta-analyses of randomized controlled trials and recommendations of clinical experts: treatments for myocardial infarction. J Am Med Assoc. 1992;268:240–8.
29. Balas E, Boren S. Managing clinical knowledge for health care improvement. In: van Bemmel J, McCray A, editors. Yearbook of medical informatics. Stuttgart: Schattauer; 2000. p. 65–70.
30. Ziman J. Information, communication, knowledge. Nature. 1969;224:318–24.
31. Refinetti R. In defense of the least publishable unit. FASEB J. 1991;4:128–9.
32. Bornmann L, Daniel H. Multiple publication on a single research study: does it pay? The influence of number of research articles on total citation counts in biomedicine. J Am Soc Inf Sci Technol. 2007;58:1100–7.
33. Casadevall A, Fang F. Field science—the nature and utility of scientific fields. mBio. 2015;6(5):e01259–15.

34. Varga A. Shorter distances between papers over time are due to more cross-field references and increased citation rate to higher-impact papers. Proc Natl Acad Sci. 2019;116:22094–9.
35. Anonymous. Bibliometrics: an overview. Leeds, England: University of Leeds 2014 July, 2014.
36. Berger J, Baker C. Bibliometrics: an overview. RGUHS J Pharmaceut Sci. 2014;4(3):81–92.
37. Garfield E. "Science Citation Index" – a new dimension in indexing. Science. 1964;144:649–54.
38. Price D. Networks of scientific papers. Science. 1965;149:510–5.
39. Adam D. The counting house. Nature. 2002;415:726–8.
40. Ioannidis J, Boyack K, Small H, Sorensen A, Klavans R. Bibliometrics: is your most cited work your best? Nature. 2014;514:561–2.
41. Teplitskiy M, Duede E, Menietti M, Lakhani K. Citations systematically misrepresent the quality and impact of research articles: survey and experimental evidence from thousands of citers. arXivorg. 2020:arXiv:2002.10033.
42. Lawrence S. Free online availability substantially increases a paper's impact. Nature. 2001;411:521.
43. Antelman K. Do open-access articles have a greater research impact? Coll Res Libr. 2004;65:372–82.
44. Eysenbach G. Citation advantage of open access articles. PLoS Biol. 2006;4(5):e157.
45. Piwowar H, Day R, Fridsma D. Sharing detailed research data is associated with increased citation rate. PLoS One. 2007;2(3).
46. Craig I, Plume A, McVeigh M, Pringle J, Amin M. Do open access articles have greater citation impact? A critical review of the literature. J Informet. 2007;1:239–48.
47. Aksnes D. Characteristics of highly cited papers. Res Eval. 2003;12:159–70.
48. Aksnes D. Citation rates and perceptions of scientific contribution. J Am Soc Inf Sci Technol. 2006;57:169–87.
49. Lozano G, Larivière V, Gingras Y. The weakening relationship between the impact factor and papers' citations in the digital age. J Am Soc Inf Sci Technol. 2011;63:2140–5.
50. Acharya A, Verstak A, Suzuki H, S Henderson, Iakhiaev M, Chiung YuLin C et al. Rise of the rest: the growing impact of non-elite journals. arXivorg. 2014:arXiv:1410.2217.
51. Bornmann L, Ye A, Ye F. Identifying landmark publications in the long run using field-normalized citation data. J Doc. 2018;74:278–88.
52. Letchford A, Moat H, Preis T. The advantage of short paper titles. R Soc Open Sci. 2015;2(8):150266.
53. Letchford A, Preis T, Moat H. The advantage of simple paper abstracts. J Inform. 2016;10:1–8.
54. Greenberg S. How citation distortions create unfounded authority: analysis of a citation network. Br Med J. 2009;339:b2680.
55. Trinquart L, Johns D, Galea S. Why do we think we know what we know? A metaknowledge analysis of the salt controversy. Int J Epidemiol. 2016;45:251–60.
56. Vucetic S, Chanda A, Zhang S, Bai T, Maiti A. Peer assessment of CS doctoral programs shows strong correlation with faculty citations. Commun ACM. 2018;61(9):70–6.
57. Piwowar H, Priem J, Larivière V, Alperin J, Matthias L, Norlander B, et al. The state of OA: a large-scale analysis of the prevalence and impact of open access articles. PeerJ. 2018; 6:e4375.
58. Larivière V, Gong K, Sugimoto C. Citations strength begins at home. Nature Index2018.
59. Leung P, Macdonald E, Stanbrook M, Dhalla IA, Juurlink D. A 1980 letter on the risk of opioid addiction. N Engl J Med. 2017;376:2194–5.
60. Porter J, Jick H. Addiction rare in patients treated with narcotics. N Engl J Med. 1980;302:123.
61. Koberlein B. The tale of a 1986 experiment that proved Einstein wrong. Forbes 2018 April 6, 2018.
62. Silvertooth E. Special relativity. Nature. 1986;322:590.
63. Silvertooth E. Experimental detection of the ether. Specul Sci Technol. 1986;10(1):3–7.
64. Dubin D. The most influential paper Gerard Salton never wrote. Libr Trends. 2004;52:748–64.
65. Pao M. An empirical examination of Lotka's law. J Am Soc Inf Sci. 1986;37:26–33.

66. Bradford S. Documentation. Crosby Lockwood: London; 1948.
67. Urquhart J, Bunn R. A national loan policy for science serials. J Doc. 1959;15:21–5.
68. Trueswell R. Some behavioral patterns of library users: the 80/20 rule. Wilson Libr Bull. 1969;43:458–61.
69. Bates M. After the dot-bomb: getting Web information right this time. First Monday. 2002;7:7.
70. Self P, Filardo T, Lancaster F. Acquired immunodeficiency syndrome (AIDS) and the epidemic growth of its literature. Scientometrics. 1989;17:49–60.
71. Wilczynski N, Garg A, Haynes B, editors. A method for defining a journal subset for a clinical discipline using the bibliographies of systematic reviews. MEDINFO 2007 – Proceedings of the Twelfth World Congress on Health (Medical) Informatics; 2007; Brisbane: IOS Press.
72. Nash-Stewart C, Kruesi L, DelMar C. Does Bradford's Law of Scattering predict the size of the literature in Cochrane Reviews? J Med Libr Assoc. 2012;100:135–8.
73. Venable G, Shepherd B, Loftis C, McClatchy S, Roberts M, Fillinger M, et al. Bradford's law: identification of the core journals for neurosurgery and its subspecialties. J Neurosurg. 2016;124:569–79.
74. Garfield E. The impact factor. Current Contents. 1994;25:3–7.
75. West R. Impact factors need to be improved. Br Med J. 1996;313:1400.
76. Smith R. Commentary: the power of the unrelenting impact factor – is it a force for good or harm? Int J Epidemiol. 2006;35:1129–30.
77. Warraich H. Impact factor and the future of medical journals. Atlantica 2014 January 10, 2014.
78. Lee K, Schotland M, Bacchetti P, Bero L. Association of journal quality indicators with methodological quality of clinical research articles. J Am Med Assoc. 2002;287:2805–8.
79. Saha S, Saint S, Christakis D. Impact factor: a valid measure of journal quality? J Med Libr Assoc. 2003;91:42–6.
80. McKibbon K, Wilczynski N, Haynes R. What do evidence-based secondary journals tell us about the publication of clinically important articles in primary healthcare journals. BMC Med. 2004;2:33.
81. Garfield E. The history and meaning of the journal impact factor. J Am Med Assoc. 2006;295:90–3.
82. Dong P, Loh M, Mondry A. The "impact factor" revisited. Biomed Digi Libraries. 2005;2:7.
83. Browman H, Stergiou K. Factors and indices are one thing, deciding who is scholarly, why they are scholarly, and the relative value of their scholarship is something else entirely. Ethics Sci Environ Politics. 2008;8:1–3.
84. Simons K. The misused impact factor. Science. 2008;322:165.
85. Lawrence P. Lost in publication: how measurement harms science. Ethics Sci Environ Politics. 2008;8:9–11.
86. Radicchi F. In Science "there is no bad publicity": Papers criticized in comments have high scientific impact. Scientific Reports. 2012;2:815.
87. Eyre-Walker A, Stoletzki N. The assessment of science: the relative merits of post-publication review, the impact factor, and the number of citations. PLoS Biol. 2013;11:e1001675.
88. Ingwersen P. The calculation of web impact factors. J Doc. 1998;54:236–43.
89. Noruzi A. The Web Impact Factor: a critical review. Electron Libr. 2006;24:490–500.
90. Thelwall M. What is this link doing here? Beginning a fine-grained process of identifying reasons for academic hyperlink creation. Inf Res. 2003;8:3.
91. Hirsch J. An index to quantify an individual's scientific research output. Proc Natl Acad Sci. 2005;102:16569–72.
92. Hersh W, Buckley C, Leone T, Hickam D, editors. OHSUMED: an interactive retrieval evaluation and new large test collection for research. Proceedings of the 17th Annual International ACM SIGIR Conference on Research and Development in Information Retrieval; 1994; Dublin: Springer.

93. Kulkarni A, Aziz B, Shams I, Busse J. Comparisons of citations in Web of Science, Scopus, and Google Scholar for articles published in general medical journals. J Am Med Assoc. 2009;302:1092–6.
94. Delgado-López-Cózar E, Robinson-García N, Torres-Salinas D. The Google Scholar experiment: how to index false papers and manipulate bibliometric indicators. J Am Soc Inf Sci Technol. 2014;65:446–54.
95. Egghe L. Theory and practise of the g-index. Scientometrics. 2006;69:131–52.
96. Callahan A, Winnenburg R, Shah N. U-Index, a dataset and an impact metric for informatics tools and databases. Scientific Data. 2018;5:180043.
97. Ioannidis J, Baas J, Klavans R, Boyack K. A standardized citation metrics author database annotated for scientific field. PLoS Biol. 2019;17(8):e3000384.
98. Hutchins B, Yuan X, Anderson J, Santangelo G. Relative citation ratio (RCR): a new metric that uses citation rates to measure influence at the article level. PLoS Biol. 2016;14(9):e1002541.
99. Hutchins B, Baker K, Davis M, Diwersy M, Haque E, Harriman R, et al. The NIH Open Citation Collection: a public access, broad coverage resource. PLoS Biol. 2019;70(10):e3000385.
100. Lauer M, Roychowdhury D, Patel K, Walsh R, Pearson K. Marginal returns and levels of research grant support among scientists supported by the National Institutes of Health. bioRxiv. 2017.
101. Hall N. The Kardashian index: a measure of discrepant social media profile for scientists. Genome Biol. 2014;15:424.
102. Andrews J. An author co-citation analysis of medical informatics. J Med Libr Assoc. 2003;91:47–56.
103. Eggers S, Huang Z, Chen H, Yan L, Larson C, Rashid A, et al. Mapping medical informatics research. In: Chen H, Fuller S, Friedman C, Hersh W, editors. Medical informatics: knowledge management and data mining in biomedicine. New York, NY: Springer; 2005. p. 36–62.
104. Zerhouni E. The NIH Roadmap Science 2003;302:63–4, 72.
105. Trujillo C, Long T. Document co-citation analysis to enhance transdisciplinary research. Sci Adv. 2018;4(1):e1701130.
106. Chamberlain S. Consuming article-level metrics: observations and lessons. Inf Stand Quart. 2013;25(2):4–13.
107. Lin J, Fenner M. Altmetrics in evolution: defining & redefining the ontology of article-level metrics. Inf Stand Quart. 2013;25(2):20–6.
108. Yan K, Gerstein M. The spread of scientific information: insights from the web usage statistics in PLoS article-level metrics. PLoS One. 2011;6(5):e19917.
109. Warren H, Raison N, Dasgupta P. The rise of altmetrics. J Am Med Assoc. 2017;317:131–2.
110. Ioannidis J. Neglecting major health problems and broadcasting minor, uncertain issues in lifestyle science. J Am Med Assoc. 2019;322:2069–70.
111. Dawkins R. The selfish gene. New York: Oxford University Press; 1976.
112. Scheufele D, Krause N. Science audiences, misinformation, and fake news. Proc Natl Acad Sci. 2019;116:7662–9.
113. Haynes R. Of studies, syntheses, synopses, and systems: the "4S" evolution of services for finding current best evidence. ACP J Club. 2001;134:A11–A3.
114. Guyatt G, Rennie D, Meade M, Cook D, editors. Users' guides to the medical literature: a manual for evidence-based clinical practice. 3rd ed. New York, NY: McGraw-Hill; 2014.
115. Guyatt G, Rennie D, Meade M, Cook D, editors. Users' guides to the medical literature: essentials of evidence-based clinical practice. 3rd ed. New York, NY: McGraw-Hill; 2015.
116. Haynes R. Of studies, syntheses, synopses, summaries, and systems: the "5S" evolution of information services for evidence-based healthcare decisions. Evid Based Med. 2006;11:162–4.
117. DiCenso A, Bayley L, Haynes R. ACP Journal Club. Editorial: Accessing preappraised evidence: fine-tuning the 5S model into a 6S model. Annals of Internal Medicine. 2009;151(6):JC3–2, JC3.

118. Sackett D, Richardson W, Rosenberg W, Haynes R. Evidence-based medicine: how to practice and teach EBM. New York, NY: Churchill Livingstone; 2000.
119. Buckley D, Ansari M, Butler M, Soh C, Chang C. The refinement of topics for systematic reviews: lessons and recommendations from the Effective Health Care Program. J Clin Epidemiol. 2014;67:425–32.
120. Hersh W. "A world of knowledge at your fingertips": the promise, reality, and future directions of on-line information retrieval. Acad Med. 1999;74:240–3.
121. Slawson D, Shaughnessy A. Teaching evidence-based medicine: should we be teaching information management instead? Acad Med. 2005;80:685–9.
122. Kuhn T. The structure of scientific revolutions. Chicago: University of Chicago Press; 1962.
123. Fouad Y, Aanei C. Revisiting the hallmarks of cancer. Am J Cancer Res. 2017;7:1016–36.
124. Bourne P. Ten simple rules for getting published. PLoS Comput Biol. 2005;1(5):e57.
125. McAuley L, Pham B, Tugwell P, Moher D. Does the inclusion of grey literature influence estimates of intervention effectiveness reported in meta-analyses? Lancet. 2000;356:1228–31.
126. Yarborough M, Nadon R, Karlin D. Point of View: four erroneous beliefs thwarting more trustworthy research. elife. 2019;8:e45261.
127. Anonymous. Uniform Requirements for Manuscripts Submitted to Biomedical Journals: Writing and Editing for Biomedical Publication: International Committee of Medical Journal Editors 2006.
128. Davidoff F, DeAngelis C, Drazen J, Hoey J, Hojgaard L, Hortin R, et al. Sponsorship, authorship, and accountability. Ann Intern Med. 2001;135:463–6.
129. Taichman D, Backus J, Baethge C, Bauchner H, Flanagin A, Florenzano F, et al. A disclosure form for work submitted to medical journals – a proposal from the International Committee of Medical Journal Editors. J Am Med Assoc. 2020;323:1050–1.
130. Taichman D, Sahni P, Pinborg A, Peiperl L, Laine C, James A, et al. Data sharing statements for clinical trials: a requirement of the International Committee of Medical Journal Editors. Ann Intern Med. 2017;167:63–5.
131. Kempner J, Perlis C, Merz J. Forbidden knowledge. Science. 2005;307:854.
132. Dzau V, Leshner A. Public health research on gun violence: long overdue. Ann Intern Med. 2018;168:876–7.
133. Fischetti M. Government attempts to silence science are revealed in detail – a tracker reveals more than 300 government attempts to suppress knowledge. Sci Am 2019 May, 2019.
134. Nost E. EPA Discontinues Updates to Climate Change Websites: Environmental Data & Governance Initiative Website Monitoring Report2018 October 31, 2018.
135. Salas R, Laden F, Jacobs W, Jha A. The U.S. Environmental Protection Agency's proposed transparency rule threatens health. Ann Intern Med. 2019;170:197–8.
136. Anonymous. APLU, Other Higher Ed & Research Groups Send EPA Letter Expressing Concerns with Proposed Rule on Research-based Rulemaking. Association of Public and Land-grant Universities; 2019.
137. Dal-Ré R, Janiaud P, Ioannidis J. Real-world evidence: How pragmatic are randomized controlled trials labeled as pragmatic? BMC Med. 2018;16(1):49.
138. Sox H, Lewis R. Pragmatic trials – practical answers to "real world" questions. J Am Med Assoc. 2016;316:1205–6.
139. Smith R. Why scientists should be held to a higher standard of honesty than the average person. Thebmjopinion 2014.
140. Moynihan R, Bero L, Hill S, Johansson M, Lexchin J, Macdonald H, et al. Pathways to independence: towards producing and using trustworthy evidence. Br Med J. 2019;367:l6576.
141. Jamieson K, McNutt M, Kiermer V, Sever R. Signaling the trustworthiness of science. Proc Natl Acad Sci. 2019;116:19231–6.
142. Prasad V, Vandross A, Toomey C, Cheung M, Rho J, Quinn S, et al. A decade of reversal: an analysis of 146 contradicted medical practices. Mayo Clin Proc. 2013;88:790–8.

143. Djulbegovic B, Kumar A, Glasziou P, Perera R, Reljic T, Dent L, et al. New treatments compared to established treatments in randomized trials. Cochrane Database Syst Rev. 2012;10:MR000024.
144. Prasad V, Cifu A. Ending medical reversal: improving outcomes, saving lives. Baltimore, MD: Johns Hopkins University Press; 2015.
145. Herrera-Perez D, Haslam A, Crain T, Gill J, Livingston C, Kaestner V, et al. A comprehensive review of randomized clinical trials in three medical journals reveals 396 medical reversals. elife. 2019;8:e45183.
146. Hooper M. Scholarly review, old and new. J Sch Publ. 2019;1:53–75.
147. Hargens L. Variation in journal peer review systems: possible causes and consequences. J Am Med Assoc. 1990;263:1348–52.
148. Purcell G, Donovan S, Davidoff F. Changes to manuscripts during the editorial process: characterizing the evolution of a clinical paper. J Am Med Assoc. 1998;280:227–8.
149. Garfunkel J, Lawson E, Hamrick H, Ulshen M. Effect of acceptance or rejection on the author's evaluation of peer review of medical manuscripts. J Am Med Assoc. 1990;263:1376–8.
150. Jefferson T, Wager E, Davidoff F. Measuring the quality of editorial peer review. J Am Med Assoc. 2002;287:2786–90.
151. Peters D, Ceci S. Peer-review practices of psychological journals: the fate of published articles, submitted again. Behav Brain Sci. 1982;5:187–255.
152. Ingelfinger F. Peer review in biomedical publication. Am J Med. 1974;56:686–92.
153. Garfunkel J, Ulshen M, Hamrick H, Lawson E. Problems identified by secondary review of accepted manuscripts. J Am Med Assoc. 1990;263:1369–71.
154. Emerson G, Warme W, Wolf F, Heckman J, Brand R, Leopold S. Testing for the presence of positive-outcome bias in peer review: a randomized controlled trial. Arch Intern Med. 2010;170:1934–9.
155. Siler K, Lee K, Bero L. Measuring the effectiveness of scientific gatekeeping. Proc Natl Acad Sci. 2015;112:360–5.
156. Tomkins A, Zhang M, Heavlina W. Reviewer bias in single- versus double-blind peer review. Proc Natl Acad Sci. 2017;114:12708–13.
157. Nicholson J. Nope! 8 Rejected Papers That Won the Nobel Prize. Authorea 2016.
158. Italie H. Not so fast: many Nobel winners endured initial rejections. AP News 2019 October 14, 2019.
159. Haug C. The downside of open-access publishing. N Engl J Med. 2013;368:791–3.
160. Beall J. Predatory journals exploit structural weaknesses in scholarly publishing. 4Open. 2018;1.
161. Grant A. The proliferation of questionable conferences. Phys Today. 2018;
162. Readings B. Caught in the net: notes from the electronic underground. Surfaces. 1994;4:9–10.
163. Young N, Ioannidis J, Al-Ubaydli O. Why current publication practices may distort science. PLoS Med. 2008;5(10):e201.
164. Schooler J. Unpublished results hide the decline effect. Nature. 2011;470:437.
165. Smith R. Classical peer review: an empty gun. Breast Cancer Res. 2010;12(Suppl 4):S13.
166. Smith R. A better way to publish science. BMJ Opinions 2015.
167. Stumpf W. "Peer" review. Science. 1980;207:822–3.
168. Li D, Agha L. Big names or big ideas: do peer-review panels select the best science proposals? Science. 2015;348:434–8.
169. Fang F, Bowen A, Casadevall A. NIH peer review percentile scores are poorly predictive of grant productivity. elife. 2016;2016(5):e13323.
170. Pier E, Brauer M, Filut A, Kaatz A, Raclaw J, Nathan M, et al. Low agreement among reviewers evaluating the same NIH grant applications. Proc Natl Acad Sci. 2018;115:2952–7.
171. Wang Y, Jones B, Wang D. Early-career setback and future career impact. Nat Commun. 2019;10:4331.
172. Smaldino P, Turner M, Andrés P, Kallens C. Open science and modified funding lotteries can impede the natural selection of bad science. OSF Preprints. 2019.

173. Smith S. The Jordan Rules. New York, NY: Pocket Books; 1994.
174. Kaplan D. How to fix peer review. The Scientist. 2005;19(11):10.
175. Bourne P, Korngreen A. Ten simple rules for reviewers. PLoS Comput Biol. 2006;2(9):e110.
176. Stossel T. Reviewer status and review quality: experience of the Journal of Clinical Investigation. N Engl J Med. 1985;312:658–9.
177. Evans A, McNutt R, Fletcher S, Fletcher R. The characteristics of peer reviewers who produce good quality reviews. J Gen Intern Med. 1993;8:422–8.
178. Nylenna M, Riis P, Karlsson Y. Multiple blinded reviews of the same two manuscripts: effect of referee characteristics and publication language. J Am Med Assoc. 1994;272:149–51.
179. Black N, van Rooyen S, Godlee F, Smith R, Evans S. What makes a good reviewer and a good review for a general medical journal? J Am Med Assoc. 1998;280:231–3.
180. Callaham M, Baxt W, Waeckerie J, Wears R. Reliability of editors' subjective quality ratings of peer reviews of manuscripts. J Am Med Assoc. 1998;280:229–31.
181. Schroter S, Tite L, Hutchings A, Black N. Differences in review quality and recommendations for publication between peer reviewers suggested by authors or by editors. J Am Med Assoc. 2006;295:314–7.
182. Wager E, Parkin E, Tamber P. Are reviewers suggested by authors as good as those chosen by editors? Results of a rater-blinded, retrospective study. BMC Med. 2006;4:13.
183. Haug C. Peer-review fraud—hacking the scientific publication process. N Engl J Med. 2015;373:2393–5.
184. Normile D. China cracks down after investigation finds massive peer-review fraud. Sci News. 2017.
185. Garrow J, Butterfield M, Marshall J, Williamson A. The reported training and experience of editors in chief of specialist clinical medical journals. J Am Med Assoc. 1998;280:286–7.
186. Moher D, Galipeau J, Alam S, Barbour V, Bartolomeos K, Baskin P, et al. Core competencies for scientific editors of biomedical journals: consensus statement. BMC Med. 2017;15:167.
187. Anonymous. Transparent peer review one year on. Nature Communications. 2016;7:13626.
188. Cosgrove A, Cheifet B. Transparent peer review trial: the results. Genome Biol. 2018;19:206.
189. Polka J, Kiley R, Konforti B, Stern B, Vale R. Publish peer reviews. Nature. 2018;560:545–7.
190. Ingelfinger F. Annual discourse: swinging copy and sober science. N Engl J Med. 1969;281:526–32.
191. Angell M, Kassirer J. The Ingelfinger rule revisited. N Engl J Med. 1991;325:1371–3.
192. Calcagno V, Demoinet E, Gollner K, Guidi L, Ruths D, de Mazancourt C. Flows of research manuscripts among scientific journals reveal hidden submission patterns. Science. 2012;338:1065–9.
193. Chen J, Konstan J. Conference paper selectivity and impact. Commun ACM. 2010;53(6):79–83.
194. Niles M, Schimanski L, McKiernan E, Alperin J. Why we publish where we do: faculty publishing values and their relationship to review, promotion and tenure expectations. bioRxiv. 2019.
195. Chiarelli A, Johnson R, Pinfield S, Richens E. Accelerating scholarly communication: The transformative role of preprints Zenodo2019 September 24, 2019.
196. Sever R, Eisen M, Inglis J. Plan U: universal access to scientific and medical research. PLoS Biol. 2019;17(6):e3000273.
197. Abdill R, Blekhman R. Tracking the popularity and outcomes of all bioRxiv preprints. bioRxiv. 2018.
198. Maslove D. Medical preprints—a debate worth having. J Am Med Assoc. 2018;391:443–4.
199. Sheldon T. Preprints could promote confusion and distortion. Nature. 2018;559:445.
200. Oakden-Rayner L, Beam A, Palmer L. Medical journals should embrace preprints to address the reproducibility crisis. Int J Epidemiol. 2018;47:1363–5.
201. Chambers C. The registered reports revolution - lessons in cultural reform. Significance. 2019;16(4):23–7.

202. Ebrahim S, Sohani Z, Montoya L, Agarwal A, Thorlund K, Mills E, et al. Reanalyses of randomized clinical trial data. J Am Med Assoc. 2014;312:1024–32.
203. Ross J, Krumholz H. Ushering in a new era of open science through data sharing: the wall must come down. J Am Med Assoc. 2013;309:1355–6.
204. Mazor K, Richards A, Gallagher M, Arterburn D, Raebel M, Nowell W, et al. Stakeholders' views on data sharing in multicenter studies. J Compar Effective Res. 2017;6:537–47.
205. Mello M, Lieou V, Goodman S. Clinical trial participants' views of the risks and benefits of data sharing. N Engl J Med. 2018;378:2202–11.
206. Mello M, Francer J, Wilenzick M, Teden P, Bierer B, Barnes M. Preparing for responsible sharing of clinical trial data. N Engl J Med. 2013;369:1651–8.
207. Alsheikh-Ali A, Qureshi W, Al-Mallah M, Ioannidis J. Public availability of published research data in high-impact journals. PLoS One. 2011;6(9):e24357.
208. Longo D, Drazen J. Data sharing. N Engl J Med. 2016;374:276–7.
209. Berger B, Gaasterland T, Lengauer T, Orengo C, Gaeta B, Markel S, et al. ISCB's initial reaction to The New England Journal of Medicine Editorial on data sharing. PLoS Comput Biol. 2016;12(3):e1004816.
210. Greene C, Garmire L, Gilbert J, Ritchie M, Hunter L. Celebrating parasites. Nat Genet. 2017;49:483–4.
211. Rosenbaum L. Bridging the data-sharing divide—seeing the devil in the details, not the other camp. N Engl J Med. 2017;376:2201–3.
212. Grossman R, Heath A, Ferretti V, Varmus H, Lowy D, Kibbe W, et al. Toward a shared vision for cancer genomic data. N Engl J Med. 2016;379:1109–12.
213. Collins F, Varmus H. A new initiative on precision medicine. N Engl J Med. 2015;372:793–5.
214. Kesselheim A, Avorn J. New "21st Century Cures" legislation: speed and ease vs science. J Am Med Assoc. 2017;317:581–2.
215. Fleurence R, Curtis L, Califf R, Platt R, Selby J, Brown J. Launching PCORnet, a national patient-centered clinical research network. J Am Med Inform Assoc. 2014;21:578–82.
216. Hripcsak G, Duke J, Shah N, Reich C, Huser V, Schuemie M, et al. Observational Health Data Sciences and Informatics (OHDSI): opportunities for observational researchers. Stud Health Technol Inform. 2015;216:574–8.
217. Dalerba P, Sahoo D, Paik S, Guo X, Yothers G, Song N, et al. CDX2 as a prognostic biomarker in stage II and stage III colon cancer. N Engl J Med. 2016;374:211–22.
218. Anonymous. Toward fairness in data sharing. N Engl J Med. 2016;375:405–7.
219. Merson L, Gaye O, Guerin P. Avoiding data dumpsters—toward equitable and useful data sharing. N Engl J Med. 2016;374:2414–5.
220. Rockhold F, Nisen P, Freeman A. Data sharing at a crossroads. N Engl J Med. 2016;375:1115–7.
221. Strom B, Buyse M, Hughes J, Knoppers B. Data sharing—is the juice worth the squeeze? N Engl J Med. 2016;375:1608–9.
222. Read K, Sheehan J, Huerta M, Knecht L, Mork J, Humphreys B. Sizing the problem of improving discovery and access to NIH-funded data: a preliminary study. PLoS One. 2015;10(7):e0132735.
223. Kush R, Goldman M. Fostering responsible data sharing through standards. N Engl J Med. 2014;370:2163–5.
224. Tenenbaum J, Avillach P, Benham-Hutchins M, Breitenstein M, Crowgey E, Hoffman M, et al. An informatics research agenda to support precision medicine: seven key areas. J Am Med Inform Assoc. 2016;23:791–5.
225. Khera R, Angraal S, Couch T, Welsh J, Nallamothu B, Girotra S, et al. Adherence to methodological standards in research using the National Inpatient Sample. J Am Med Assoc. 2017;318:2011–8.
226. Bierer B, Crosas M, Pierce H. Data authorship as an incentive to data sharing. N Engl J Med. 2017;376:1684–7.
227. Pierce H, Dev A, Statham E, Bierer B. Credit data generators for data reuse. Nature. 2019;570:30–2.

228. Lo B, DeMets D. Incentives for clinical trialists to share data. N Engl J Med. 2016;375:1112–5.
229. Shanahan D. Clinical trial data and articles linked for the first time. CrossRef Blog 2016.
230. Hersh W, Boone K, Totten A. Data from: Characteristics of the healthcare information technology workforce in the HITECH era: underestimated in size, still growing, and adapting to advanced uses. In: Repository DD, editor. 2018.
231. Federer L, Belter C, Joubert D, Livinski A, Lu Y, Snyders L, et al. Data sharing in PLOS ONE: an analysis of data availability statements. PLoS One. 2018;13(5):e0194768.
232. Naudet F, Sakarovitch C, Janiaud P, Cristea I, Fanelli D, Moher D, et al. Data sharing and reanalysis of randomized controlled trials in leading biomedical journals with a full data sharing policy: survey of studies published in The BMJ and PLOS Medicine. Br Med J. 2018;360:k400.
233. Tannenbaum S, Ross J, Krumholz H, Desai N, Ritchie J, Lehman R, et al. Early experiences with journal data sharing policies: a survey of published clinical trial investigators. Ann Intern Med. 2018;169:586–8.
234. Fletcher R, Fletcher S. Clinical research in general medical journals: a 30-year perspective. N Engl J Med. 1979;301:180–3.
235. Ioannidis J. Contradicted and initially stronger effects in highly cited clinical research. J Am Med Assoc. 2005;294:218–28.
236. Ioannidis J. Why most published research findings are false. PLoS Med. 2005;2(8):e124.
237. Montori V, Devereaux P, Adhikari N, Burns K, Eggert C, Briel M, et al. Randomized trials stopped early for benefit: a systematic review. J Am Med Assoc. 2005;294:2203–9.
238. Mueller P, Montori V, Bassler D, Koenig B, Guyatt G. Ethical issues in stopping randomized trials early because of apparent benefit. Ann Intern Med. 2007;146:878–81.
239. Allison D, Brown A, George B, Kaiser K. A tragedy of errors. Nature. 2016;530:27–9.
240. Glantz S. Biostatistics: how to detect, correct, and prevent errors in the medical literature. Circulation. 1980;61:1–7.
241. Moher D, Dulberg C, Wells G. Statistical power, sample size, and their reporting in randomized controlled trials. J Am Med Assoc. 1994;272:122–4.
242. Halpern S, Karlawish J, Berlin J. The continuing unethical conduct of underpowered clinical trials. J Am Med Assoc. 2002;288:358–62.
243. Georgescu C, Wren J. Algorithmic identification of discrepancies between published ratios and their reported confidence intervals and P-values. Bioinformatics. 2017;34:1758–66.
244. Boutron I, Dutton S, Ravaud P, Altman D. Reporting and interpretation of randomized controlled trials with statistically nonsignificant results for primary outcomes. J Am Med Assoc. 2010;303:2058–64.
245. Ochodo E, de Haan M, Reitsma J, Hooft L, Bossuyt P, Leeflang M. Overinterpretation and misreporting of diagnostic accuracy studies: evidence of "spin". Radiology. 2013;267:581–8.
246. Jellison S, Roberts W, Bowers A, Combs T, Beaman J, Wayant C, et al. Evaluation of spin in abstracts of papers in psychiatry and psychology journals. BMJ Evid Based Med. 2019:Epub ahead of print.
247. Khan M, Lateef N, Siddiqi T, Rehman K, Alnaimat S, Khan S, et al. Level and prevalence of spin in published cardiovascular randomized clinical trial reports with statistically nonsignificant primary outcomes – a systematic review. JAMA Netw Open. 2019;2(5):e192622.
248. Lerchenmueller M, Sorenson O, Jena A. Gender differences in how scientists present the importance of their research: observational study. Br Med J. 2019;367:l6573.
249. Chavalarias D, Wallach J, Li A, Ioannidis J. Evolution of reporting p values in the biomedical literature, 1990–2015. J Am Med Assoc. 2016;315:1141–8.
250. Nuzzo R. Scientific method: statistical errors. Nature. 2014;506:150–2.
251. Head M, Holman L, Lanfear R, Kahn A, Jennions M. The extent and consequences of p-hacking in science. PLoS Biol. 2015;13:e1002106.
252. Benjamin D, Berger J, Johannesson M, Nosek B, Wagenmakers E, Winship C, et al. Redefine statistical significance. Nat Hum Behav. 2018;2:6–10.

253. Ioannidis J. The proposal to lower p value thresholds to .005. J Am Med Assoc. 2018;319:1429–30.
254. Amrhein V, Greenland S, McShane B. Retire statistical significance. Nature. 2019;567:305–7.
255. Goodman S. Why is getting rid of p-values so hard? Musings on science and statistics. Am Stat. 2019;73:26–30.
256. Hoffrage U, Lindsey S, Hertwig R, Gigerenzer G. Communicating statistical information. Science. 2000;290:2261–2.
257. Abola M, Prasad V. The use of superlatives in cancer research. JAMA Oncol. 2016;2: 139–41.
258. Krishnamurti T, Woloshin S, Schwartz L, Fischhoff B. A randomized trial testing US Food and Drug Administration "breakthrough" language. JAMA Intern Med. 2015;175:1856–8.
259. Smith R. Medical journals are an extension of the marketing arm of pharmaceutical companies. PLoS Med. 2005;2(5):e138.
260. Smith R. Medical journals and pharmaceutical companies: uneasy bedfellows. Br Med J. 2003;326:1202–5.
261. Dickersin K, Rennie D. Registering clinical trials. J Am Med Assoc. 2003;290:516–23.
262. Silverstein F, Faich G, Goldstein J, Simon L, Pincus T, Whelton A, et al. Gastrointestinal toxicity with celecoxib vs nonsteroidal anti-inflammatory drugs for osteoarthritis and rheumatoid arthritis: the CLASS study: a randomized controlled trial. J Am Med Assoc. 2000;284:1247–55.
263. Silverstein F, Simon L, Faich G. Reporting of 6-month vs 12-month data in a clinical trial of celecoxib – in reply. J Am Med Assoc. 2001;286:2399–400.
264. Hrachovec J, Mora M. Reporting of 6-month vs 12-month data in a clinical trial of celecoxib. J Am Med Assoc. 2001;286:2398.
265. Wright J, Perry T, Bassett K, Chambers K. Reporting of 6-month vs 12-month data in a clinical trial of celecoxib. J Am Med Assoc. 2001;286:2398–9.
266. Jüni P, Rutjes A, Dieppe P. Are selective COX 2 inhibitors superior to traditional non steroidal anti-inflammatory drugs? Br Med J. 2002;324:1287–8.
267. Bombardier C, Laine L, Reicin A, Shapiro D, Burgos-Vargas R, Davis B, et al. Comparison of upper gastrointestinal toxicity of rofecoxib and naproxen in patients with rheumatoid arthritis. N Engl J Med. 2000;343:1520–8.
268. Curfman G, Morrissey S, Drazen J. Expression of concern: Bombardier et al., "Comparison of upper gastrointestinal toxicity of rofecoxib and naproxen in patients with rheumatoid arthritis". N Engl J Med. 2005;353:2318–9.
269. Anonymous. Is GSK guilty of fraud? Lancet. 2004;363:1919.
270. DeAngelis C, Drazen J, Frizelle F, Haug C, Hoey J, Horton R, et al. Clinical trial registration: a statement from the International Committee of Medical Journal Editors. J Am Med Assoc. 2004;292:1363–4.
271. Zarin D, Tse T, Ide N. Trial Registration at ClinicalTrials.gov between May and October 2005. N Engl J Med. 2005;353:2779–87.
272. Haug C, Gotzsche P, Schroeder T. Registries and registration of clinical trials. N Engl J Med. 2005;353:2811–2.
273. Chalmers I, Glasziou P. Avoidable waste in the production and reporting of research evidence. Lancet. 2009;374:86–9.
274. Macleod M, Michie S, Roberts I, Dirnagl U, Chalmers I, Ioannidis J, et al. Biomedical research: increasing value, reducing waste. Lancet. 2014;383:101–4.
275. Alberts B, Kirschner M, Tilghman S, Varmus H. Rescuing US biomedical research from its systemic flaws. Proc Natl Acad Sci. 2014;111:5773–7.
276. Rzhetsky A, Foster J, Foster I, Evans J. Choosing experiments to accelerate collective discovery. Proc Natl Acad Sci. 2015;112:14569–74.
277. Smaldino P, McElreath R. The natural selection of bad science. R Soc Open Sci. 2016;3(9):160384.

278. Zarin D, Goodman S, Kimmelman J. Harms from uninformative clinical trials. J Am Med Assoc. 2019;322:813–4.
279. Wong C, Siah K, Lo A. Estimation of clinical trial success rates and related parameters. Biostatistics. 2019;20:273–86.
280. Ludwig D, Ebbeling C, Heymsfield S. Discrepancies in the registries of diet vs drug trials. JAMA Netw Open. 2019;2(11):e1915360.
281. Tatsioni A, Karassa F, Goodman S, Zarin D, Fanelli D, Ioannidis J. Lost evidence from registered large long-unpublished randomized controlled trials: a survey. Ann Intern Med. 2019;171:300–1.
282. Shepperd M, Guo Y, Li N, Arzoky M, Capiluppi A, Counsell S et al. The prevalence of errors in machine learning experiments. arXivorg. 2019:1909.04436.
283. Beam A, Manrai A, Ghassemi M. Challenges to the reproducibility of machine learning models in health care. J Am Med Assoc. 2020;323:305–6.
284. Arrowsmith J. Trial watch: Phase II failures: 2008–2010. Nat Rev Drug Discov. 2011;10:328–9.
285. Begley C, Ellis L. Raise standards for preclinical cancer research. Nature. 2012;483:531–3.
286. Prinz F, Schlange T, Asadullah K. Believe it or not: how much can we rely on published data on potential drug targets? Nat Rev Drug Discov. 2011;10:712.
287. Yong E. Replication studies: bad copy. Nature. 2012;485:298–300.
288. Anonymous. Estimating the reproducibility of psychological science. Science. 2015;349:aac4716.
289. LeNoury J, Nardo J, Healy D, Jureidini J, Raven M, Tufanaru C, et al. Restoring Study 329: efficacy and harms of paroxetine and imipramine in treatment of major depression in adolescence. Br Med J. 2015;351:h4320.
290. Ioannidis J. Acknowledging and overcoming nonreproducibility in basic and preclinical research. J Am Med Assoc. 2017;317:1019–20.
291. Coiera E, Ammenwerth E, Georgiou A, Magrabi F. Does health informatics have a replication crisis? J Am Med Inform Assoc. 2018;25:963–8.
292. Lin J, Crane M, Trotman A, Callan J, Chattopadhyaya I, Foley J, et al., editors. Toward reproducible baselines: the open-source IR reproducibility challenge. European Conference on Information Retrieval; 2016.
293. Baker M. Is there a reproducibility crisis? Nature. 2016;533:452–4.
294. Errington T, Iorns E, Gunn W, Tan F, Lomax J, Nosek B. Science forum: an open investigation of the reproducibility of cancer biology research. elife. 2014;3:e04333.
295. Nosek B, Errington T. Reproducibility in cancer biology: making sense of replications. elife. 2017;2017(6):e23383.
296. Anonymous. Reproducibility in cancer biology: the challenges of replication. eLife. 2017;2017(6):e23693.
297. Merali Z. Computational science: …Error. Nature. 2010;467:775–7.
298. Sainani K. Error! – What biomedical computing can learn from its mistakes. Biomed Comput Rev 2011 September 1, 2011.
299. Joppa L, McInerny G, Harper R, Salido L, Takeda K, O'Hara K, et al. Troubling trends in scientific software use. Science. 2013;340:814–5.
300. Eklund A, Nichols T, Knutsson H. Cluster failure: why fMRI inferences for spatial extent have inflated false-positive rates. Proc Natl Acad Sci. 2016;113:7900–5.
301. Baptista R, Kissinger J. Is reliance on an inaccurate genome sequence sabotaging your experiments? PLoS Pathog. 2019;15(9):e1007901.
302. Vasilevsky N, Brush M, Paddock H, Ponting L, Tripathy S, Larocca G, et al. On the reproducibility of science: unique identification of research resources in the biomedical literature. PeerJ. 2013;5(1):e148.
303. Baggerly K, Coombes K. What information should be required to support clinical "omics" publications? Clin Chem. 2011;57:688–90.
304. Peng R. Reproducible research in computational science. Science. 2011;334:1226–7.

305. Perkel J. By Jupyter, It all makes sense. Nature. 2018;563:145–6.
306. Maciocci G, Tsang E, Bentley N, Aufreiter M. Reproducible Document Stack: towards a scalable solution for reproducible articles. elife. 2019;
307. Somers J. The scientific paper is obsolete. The Atlantic. 2018 April 5, 2018.
308. Menke J, Roelandse M, B Ozyurt, Martone M, Bandrowski A. Rigor and Transparency Index, a new metric of quality for assessing biological and medical science methods. Biorxiv. 2020.
309. Anonymous. Reproducibility and Replicability in Science. Washington, DC: National Academies Press; 2019.
310. Pérignon C, Gadouche K, Hurlin C, Silberman R, Debonnel E. Certify reproducibility with confidential data. Science. 2019;6449:127–8.
311. Hanbury A, Müller H, Balog K, Brodt T, Cormack G, Eggel I, et al. Evaluation-as-a-service: overview and outlook. arXivorg. 2015:arXiv:1512.07454.
312. Roegiest A, Cormack G, editors. An architecture for privacy-preserving and replicable high-recall retrieval experiments. Proceedings of the 39th International ACM SIGIR conference on Research and Development in Information Retrieval; 2016; Pisa, Italy.
313. DerSimonian R, Charette L, McPeek B, Mosteller F. Reporting on methods in clinical trials. N Engl J Med. 1982;306:1332–7.
314. Moher D, Schulz K, Altman D. The CONSORT statement: revised recommendations for improving the quality of reports of parallel-group randomized trials. Ann Intern Med. 2001;134:657–62.
315. Moher D, Pham B, Jones A, Cook D, Jadad A, Moher M, et al. Does quality of reports of randomised trials affect estimates of intervention efficacy reported in meta-analyses? Lancet. 1998;352:609–13.
316. Moher D, Jones A, Lepage L. Use of the CONSORT statement and quality of reports of randomized trials: a comparative before-and-after evaluation. J Am Med Assoc. 2001;285:2006–7.
317. Huwiler-Müntener K, Juni P, Junker C, Egger M. Quality of reporting of randomized trials as a measure of methodologic quality. J Am Med Assoc. 2002;287:2801–4.
318. von Elm E, Altman D, Egger M, Pocock S, Gøtzsche P, Vandenbroucke J. The Strengthening the Reporting of Observational Studies in Epidemiology (STROBE) statement: guidelines for reporting observational studies. Ann Intern Med. 2007;147:573–7.
319. Chan A, Hrobjartsson A, Haahr M, Gotzsche P, Altman D. Empirical evidence for selective reporting of outcomes in randomized trials: comparison of protocols to published articles. J Am Med Assoc. 2004;291:2457–65.
320. de Vries Y, Roest A, Beijers L, Turner E, de Jonge P. Bias in the reporting of harms in clinical trials of second-generation antidepressants for depression and anxiety: a meta-analysis. Eur Neuropsychopharmacol. 2016;26:1752–9.
321. Derry S, Loke Y, Aronson J. Incomplete evidence: the inadequacy of databases in tracing published adverse drug reactions in clinical trials. BMC Med Res Methodol. 2001;1:7.
322. Fromme E, Eilers K, Mori M, Hsieh Y, Beer T. How accurate is clinician reporting of chemotherapy adverse effects? A comparison with patient-reported symptoms from the Quality-of-Life Questionnaire C30. J Clin Oncol. 2004;22:3485–90.
323. Golder S, McIntosh H, Duffy S, Glanville J. Developing efficient search strategies to identify reports of adverse effects in MEDLINE and EMBASE. Health Inf Libr J. 2006;23:3–12.
324. Fontanarosa P, Rennie D, DeAngelis C. Postmarketing surveillance – lack of vigilance, lack of trust. J Am Med Assoc. 2004;292:2647–50.
325. Devereaux P, Bhandari M, Clarke M, Montori V, Cook D, Yusuf S, et al. Need for expertise based randomised controlled trials. Br Med J. 2005;330:88.
326. Lilford R, Braunholtz D, Greenhalgh R, Edwards S. Trials and fast changing technologies: the case for tracker studies. Br Med J. 2000;320:43–6.
327. Politi M, Han P, Col N. Communicating the uncertainty of harms and benefits of medical interventions. Med Decis Mak. 2007;27:681–95.
328. Sedrakyan A, Shih C. Improving depiction of benefits and harms: analyses of studies of well-known therapeutics and review of high-impact medical journals. Med Care. 2007;45:S23–S8.

329. Sawaya G, Guirguis-Blake J, LeFevre M, Harris R, Petitti D. Update on the methods of the U.S. Preventive Services Task Force: estimating certainty and magnitude of net benefit. Ann Intern Med. 2007;147:871–5.
330. Sheridan S, Pignone M, Lewis C. A randomized comparison of patients' understanding of number needed to treat and other common risk reduction formats. J Gen Intern Med. 2003;18:884–92.
331. Berry D, Knapp P, Raynor T. Expressing medicine side effects: assessing the effectiveness of absolute risk, relative risk, and number needed to harm, and the provision of baseline risk information. Patient Educ Couns. 2006;63:89–96.
332. Gotzsche P, Olson O, editors. Misleading publications of major mammography screening trials in major medical journals. Fourth International Congress on Peer Review in Biomedical Publication; 2001; Barcelona: American Medical Association.
333. Clarke M, Alderson P, Chalmers I. Discussion sections in reports of controlled trials published in general medical journals. J Am Med Assoc. 2002;287:2799–801.
334. Tatsioni A, Bonitsis N, Ioannidis I. Persistence of contradicted claims in the literature. J Am Med Assoc. 2007;298:2517–26.
335. Drazen J, VanDerWeyden M, Rosenberg S, Marusic A, Laine C, Kotzin S, et al. Uniform format for disclosure of competing interests in ICMJE journals. N Engl J Med. 2009;361:1896–7.
336. Lundh A, Sismondo S, Lexchin J, Busuioc O, Bero L. Industry sponsorship and research outcome. Cochrane Database Syst Rev. 2012;12:MR000033.
337. Dunn A, Arachi D, Hudgins J, Tsafnat G, Coiera E, Bourgeois F. Financial conflicts of interest and conclusions about neuraminidase inhibitors for influenza – an analysis of systematic reviews. Ann Intern Med. 2014;161:513–8.
338. Wayant C, Turner E, Meyer C, Sinnett P, Vassar M. Financial conflicts of interest among oncologist authors of reports of clinical drug trials. JAMA Oncol. 2018;4:1426–8.
339. Ornstein C, Thomas K. Top cancer researcher fails to disclose corporate financial ties in major research journals. New York, NY: ProPublica2018 September 8, 2018.
340. Smith R, Gøtzsche P, Groves T. Should journals stop publishing research funded by the drug industry? Br Med J. 2014;348:g171.
341. Barton D, Stossel T, Stell L. After 20 years, industry critics bury skeptics, despite empirical vacuum. Int J Clin Pract. 2014;68:666–73.
342. Battisti W, Wager E, Baltzer L, Bridges D, Cairns A, Carswell C, et al. Good publication practice for communicating company-sponsored medical research: GPP3. Ann Intern Med. 2015;163:461–4.
343. Tierney W, Meslin E, Kroenke K. Industry support of medical research: important opportunity or treacherous pitfall? J Gen Intern Med. 2016;23:544–52.
344. Dal-Ré R, Caplan A, Marusic A. Editors' and authors' individual conflicts of interest disclosure and journal transparency – a cross-sectional study of high-impact medical specialty journals. BMJ Open. 2019;9:e029796.
345. Kaestner V, Brown A, Tao D, Prasad V. Conflicts of interest in Twitter. Lancet Hematol. 2017;4:e408–e9.
346. Haynes R, Mulrow C, Huth E, Altman D, Gardner M. More informative abstracts revisited. Ann Intern Med. 1990;113:69–76.
347. Riesenberg L, Dontineni S, editors. Review of reference inaccuracies. Fourth International Congress on Peer Review in Biomedical Publication; 2001; Barcelona: American Medical Association.
348. Wager E, Middleton P, editors. Reference accuracy in peer-reviewed journals: a systematic review. Fourth International Congress on Peer Review in Biomedical Publication; 2001; Barcelona: American Medical Association.
349. Aronsky D, Ransom J, Robinson K. Accuracy of reference in five biomedical informatics journals. J Am Med Inform Assoc. 2005;12:225–8.
350. Crichlow R, Winbush N, Davies S. The accessibility and accuracy of Web references in five major medical journals. J Am Med Assoc. 2004;292:2723–4.

351. de Lacey G, Record C, Wade J. How accurate are quotations and references in medical journals? Br Med J. 1985;291:884–6.
352. Klein M, VandeSompel H, Sanderson R, Shankar H, Balakireva L, Zhou K, et al. Scholarly context not found: one in five articles suffers from reference rot. PLoS One. 2014;9(12):e115253.
353. Perkel J. The trouble with reference rot. Nature. 2015;521:111–2.
354. Ziemann M, Eren Y, El-Osta A. Gene name errors are widespread in the scientific literature. Genome Biol. 2016;17:177.
355. Byrne J, Labbé C, editors. Fact checking nucleotide sequences in life science publications: the Seek & Blastn Tool. Eighth International Congress on Peer Review and Scientific Publication; 2017; Chicago, IL.
356. Byrne J, Labbé C. Striking similarities between publications from China describing single gene knockdown experiments in human cancer cell lines. Scientometrics. 2017;110:1471–93.
357. Phillips N. Tool spots DNA errors in papers. Nature. 2017;551:422–3.
358. Haynes W, Tomczak A, Khatri P. Gene annotation bias impedes biomedical research. Sci Rep. 2018;8:1362.
359. Dickersin K. The existence of publication bias and risk factors for its occurrence. J Am Med Assoc. 1990;263:1385–9.
360. Dwan K, Gamble C, Williamson P, Kirkham J. Systematic review of the empirical evidence of study publication bias and outcome reporting bias – an updated review. PLoS One. 2013;8(7):e66844.
361. Sterling T. Publication decisions and their possible effects on inferences drawn from tests of significance - or vice versa. J Am Stat Assoc. 1959;54:30–4.
362. Rosenthal R. The "file drawer problem" and tolerance for null results. Psychol Bull. 1979;86:638–41.
363. Fanelli D. Negative results are disappearing from most disciplines and countries. Scientometrics. 2012;90:891–904.
364. Franco A, Malhotra N, Simonovits G. Publication bias in the social sciences: unlocking the file drawer. Science. 2014;345:1502–5.
365. Dickersin K, Min Y. Publication bias: a problem that won't go away. Ann N Y Acad Sci. 1993;703:135–48.
366. Stern J, Simes R. Publication bias: evidence of delayed publication in a cohort study of clinical research projects. Br Med J. 1997;315:640–5.
367. Callaham M, Wears R, Weber E, Barton C, Young G. Positive-outcome bias and other limitations in the outcome of research abstracts submitted to a scientific meeting. J Am Med Assoc. 1998;280:254–7.
368. Scherer R, Langenberg P, editors. Full publication of results initially presented in abstracts: revisited. Fourth International Congress on Peer Review in Biomedical Publication; 2001; Barcelona: American Medical Association.
369. von Elm E, Costanza M, Walder B, Tramer M. More insight into the fate of biomedical meeting abstracts: a systematic review. BMC Med Res Methodol. 2003;3:12.
370. Crockett L, Okoli G, Neilson C, Rabbani R, Abou-Setta A, Klassen T. Publication of randomized clinical trials in pediatric research – a follow-up study. JAMA Netw Open. 2018;1(1):e180156.
371. Ioannidis J. Effect of statistical significance of results on the time to completion and publication of randomized efficacy trials. J Am Med Assoc. 1998;279:281–6.
372. Egger M, Zellweger-Zahner T, Schneider M, Junker C, Lengeler C, Antes G. Language bias in randomised controlled trials published in English and German. Lancet. 1997;350:326–9.
373. Turner E, Matthews A, Linardatos E, Tell R, Rosenthal R. Selective publication of antidepressant trials and its influence on apparent efficacy. N Engl J Med. 2008;358:252–60.
374. Turner E, Knoepflmacher D, Shapley L. Publication bias in antipsychotic trials: an analysis of efficacy comparing the published literature to the US Food and Drug Administration Database. PLoS Med. 2012;9:3.

375. de Vries Y, Roest A, de Jonge P, Cuijpers P, Munafò M, Bastiaansen J. The cumulative effect of reporting and citation biases on the apparent efficacy of treatments: the case of depression. Psychol Med. 2018;48:2453–5.
376. Bohannon J. U.K. research charity will self-publish results from its grantees. Science Insider 2016.
377. Schwartz L, Woloshin S. Lost in transmission – FDA drug information that never reaches clinicians. N Engl J Med. 2009;361:1717–20.
378. Wieseler B, Kerekes M, Vervoelgyi V, McGauran N, Kaiser T. Impact of document type on reporting quality of clinical drug trials: a comparison of registry reports, clinical study reports, and journal publications. Br Med J. 2012;344:d8141.
379. Turner E. How to access and process FDA drug approval packages for use in research. Br Med J. 2013;347:f5992.
380. Jefferson T, Jones M, Doshi P, DelMar C. Neuraminidase inhibitors for preventing and treating influenza in healthy adults: systematic review and meta-analysis. Br Med J. 2009;339:b5106.
381. Doshi P, Jefferson T, DelMar C. The imperative to share clinical study reports: recommendations from the Tamiflu experience. PLoS Med. 2012;9(4):e1001201.
382. Godlee F. Clinical trial data for all drugs in current use. Br Med J. 2012;345:e7304.
383. Godlee F. Goodbye PubMed, hello raw data. Br Med J. 2011;342:d212.
384. Abbasi K. The missing data that cost $20bn. Br Med J. 2014;348:g2695.
385. Strom B, Buyse M, Hughes J, Knoppers B. Data sharing, year 1 – access to data from industry-sponsored clinical trials. N Engl J Med. 2014;371:2052–4.
386. Zarin D, Tse T, Williams R, Carr S. Trial reporting in ClinicalTrials.gov – the final rule. N Engl J Med. 2016;375:1998–2004.
387. Piller C. FDA and NIH let clinical trial sponsors keep results secret and break the law. Sci News. 2020;
388. Bruckner T. Clinical trial transparency at US universities – Compliance with U.S. law and global best practices. Washington, DC: Transpari MED2019 March 25, 2019.
389. DeVito N, Bacon S, Goldacre B. Compliance with legal requirement to report clinical trial results on ClinicalTrials.gov: a cohort study. Lancet. 2020;395:361–9.
390. Zarin D, Fain K, Dobbins H, Tse T, Williams R. 10-year update on study results submitted to ClinicalTrials.gov. N Engl J Med. 2019;381:1966–74.
391. Chalmers I. Under-reporting scientific research is scientific misconduct. J Am Med Assoc. 1990;263:1405–8.
392. Wallach J, Krumholz H. Not reporting results of a clinical trial is academic misconduct. Ann Intern Med. 2019;171:293–4.
393. Friedman C, Wyatt J. Publication bias in medical informatics. J Am Med Inform Assoc. 2001;8:189–91.
394. Vawdrey D, Hripcsak G. Publication bias in clinical trials of electronic health records. J Biomed Inform. 2013;46:139–41.
395. Colaianni L. Retraction, comment, and errata policies of the U.S. National Library of Medicine. Lancet. 1992;340:536–7.
396. Hughes C. Academic medical libraries' policies and procedures for notifying library users of retracted scientific publications. Med Ref Serv Q. 1998;17(2):37–40.
397. Friedman P. Correcting the literature following fraudulent publication. J Am Med Assoc. 1990;263:1416–9.
398. Kochen C, Budd J. The persistence of fraud in the literature: The Darsee case. J Am Soc Inf Sci. 1992;43:488–93.
399. Whitely W, Rennie D, Hafner A. The scientific community's response to evidence of fraudulent publication: the Robert Slutsky case. J Am Med Assoc. 1994;272:170–3.
400. Garfield E, Welljams-Dorof A. The impact of fraudulent research on the scientific literature: the Stephen Breuning case. J Am Med Assoc. 1990;1990:1424–6.
401. Anonymous. The Top Retractions of 2019 The Scientist. 2019 December 16, 2019.

402. Anonymous. Meet the scientific sleuths: More than a dozen who've had an impact on the scientific literature. Retraction Watch 2018.
403. Marcus A, Oransky I. Meet the 'data thugs' out to expose shoddy and questionable research. Retraction Watch 2018.
404. Grey A, Avenell A, Klein A, Gunsalus C. Check for publication integrity before misconduct. Nature. 2020;577:167–9.
405. Brainard J, You J. Rethinking retractions. Science. 2018;362:390–3.
406. Anonymous. Retraction Notice. J Vibrat Control. 2014;20:1601–4.
407. Reich E. Cancer trial errors revealed. Nature. 2011;469:139–40.
408. Woodhead M. 80% of China's clinical trial data are fraudulent, investigation finds. Br Med J. 2016;355:i5396.
409. Carlisle J. Data fabrication and other reasons for non-random sampling in 5087 randomised, controlled trials in anaesthetic and general medical journals. Anaesthesia. 2017;72: 944–52.
410. Chawla D. Russian journals retract more than 800 papers after 'bombshell' investigation. Science. 2020;
411. Stigbrand T. Retraction note to multiple articles in Tumor Biology. Tumor Biol 2017.
412. Feldwisch-Drentrup H. Journal that holds record for retracted papers also has a problem with editorial board members Science News 2017.
413. Dansinger M. Dear plagiarist: a letter to a peer reviewer who stole and published our manuscript as his own. Ann Intern Med. 2017;166:143.
414. Finelli C, Crispino P, Gioia S, LaSala N, D'amico L, LaGrotta M, et al. Retraction: The improvement of large High-Density Lipoprotein (HDL) particle levels, and presumably HDL metabolism, depend on effects of low-carbohydrate diet and weight loss. EXCLI J. 2016;15:570.
415. Chaplain M, Kirschner D, Iwasa Y. JTB editorial malpractice: a case report. J Theor Biol. 2020;488:110171.
416. McHugh U, Yentis S. An analysis of retractions of papers authored by Scott Reuben. Joachim Boldt and Yoshitaka Fujii Anaesthesia. 2018;74:17–21.
417. Marcus A, Oransky I. How the Biggest Fabricator in Science Got Caught. Nautilus 2015.
418. Marcus A. Anesthesiologist joins the 100-retraction club. Retraction Watch 2020.
419. Milne G. This science vigilante calls out bogus results in prestigious journals. Medium. 2019 November;5:2019.
420. Bik E, Casadevall A, Fang F. The prevalence of inappropriate image duplication in biomedical research publications. mBio. 2016;7(3):e00809–16.
421. Bik E, Fang F, Kullas A, Davis R, Casadevall A. Analysis and correction of inappropriate image duplication: the Molecular and Cellular Biology experience. Mol Cel Biol. 2018;38:e00309–18.
422. Bauchner H, Fontanarosa P, Flanagin A, Thornton J. Scientific misconduct and medical journals. J Am Med Assoc. 2018;320:1985–7.
423. O'Connor A. More evidence that nutrition studies don't always add up. New York Times 2018 September 29, 2018.
424. Bauchner H. Notice of retractions: "first foods most: after 18-hour fast, people drawn to starches first and vegetables last," "fattening fasting: hungry grocery shoppers buy more calories, not more food," and "watch what you eat: action-related television content increases food intake" by Brian Wansink. JAMA Intern Med. 2018;178:1450.
425. Drazen J. Expression of Concern: Beltrami AP et al. Evidence that human cardiac myocytes divide after myocardial infarction. N Engl J Med 2001;344:1750–7 and Quaini F et al. Chimerism of the transplanted heart. N Engl J Med 2002;346:5–15. N Engl J Med. 2018;379:1870.
426. Anonymous. Statement on NHLBI decision to pause the CONCERT-HF trial. Bethesda, MD: National Institutes of Health 2018 October 29, 2018.

427. Keown A. Harvard, Brigham and Women's Hospital Seek retraction of 31 articles with falsified data. BioSpace 2018.
428. Chien K, Frisén J, Fritsche-Danielson R, Melton D, Murry C, Weissman I. Regenerating the field of cardiovascular cell therapy. Nat Biotechnol. 2019;37:232–7.
429. Bornemann-Cimenti H, Szilagyi I, Sandner-Kiesling A. Perpetuation of retracted publications using the example of the Scott S. Reuben case: incidences, reasons and possible improvements. Sci Eng Ethics. 2015;22:1063–72.
430. Hamilton D. Continued citation of retracted radiation oncology literature – do we have a problem? Int J Radiat Oncol Biol Phys. 2018;103:1036–42.
431. Anonymous. Retraction—ileal-lymphoid-nodular hyperplasia, non-specific colitis, and pervasive developmental disorder in children. Lancet. 2010;375:445.
432. Suelzer E, Deal J, Hanus K, Ruggeri B, Sieracki R, Witkowski E. Assessment of citations of the retracted article by Wakefield et al with fraudulent claims of an association between vaccination and autism. JAMA Netw Open. 2019;2(11):e1915552.
433. Fernández L, Vadillo M. Retracted papers die hard: Diederik Stapel and the enduring influence of flawed science. PsyArVix 2019.
434. Bakker C, Riegelman A. Retracted publications in mental health literature: discovery across bibliographic platforms. J Librarianship Scholar Commun. 2018;6:eP2199.
435. Mistry V, Grey A, Bolland M. Publication rates after the first retraction for biomedical researchers with multiple retracted publications. Accountab Res – Policies Qual Assur. 2019;26:277–87.
436. Fanelli D, Moher D. What difference do retractions make? An estimate of the epistemic impact of retractions on recent meta-analyses. bioRxiv. 2019:https://doi.org/10.1101/734137.
437. Marcus A. Exclusive: Russian site says it has brokered authorships for more than 10,000 researchers. Retraction Watch 2019.
438. Byrne J, Christopher J. Digital magic, or the dark arts of the 21st century—how can journals and peer reviewers detect manuscripts and publications from paper mills? FEBS Lett. 2020;594:583–9.
439. Phillips T, Saunders R, Cossman J, Heitman E. Assessing trustworthiness in research: a pilot study on CV verification. J Empir Res Hum Res Ethics. 2019;14:353–64.
440. Wang M, Yan A, Katz R. Researcher requests for inappropriate analysis and reporting: a U.S. survey of consulting biostatisticians. Ann Intern Med. 2018;169:554–8.
441. Nelson H, editor. Systematic reviews to answer health care questions. Baltimore, MD: Lippincott Williams & Wilkins; 2014.
442. Glass G. Primary, secondary, and meta-analysis of research. Educ Res. 1976;10:3–8.
443. Glasziou P, Irwig L. Meta-analysis of diagnostic tests. In: Armitage P, Colton T, editors. Encyclopaedia of biostatistics, vol. 4. Chichester: Wiley; 1998. p. 2579–85.
444. Stroup D, Berlin J, Morton S, Olkin L, Williamson G, Rennie D, et al. Meta-analysis of observational studies in epidemiology: a proposal for reporting. J Am Med Assoc. 2000;283:2008–12.
445. Pham M, Rajić A, Greig J, Sargeant J, Papadopoulos A, McEwen S. A scoping review of scoping reviews: advancing the approach and enhancing the consistency. Res Synth Methods. 2014;5:371–85.
446. Munn Z, Peters M, Stern C, Tufanaru C, McArthur A, Aromataris E. Systematic review or scoping review? Guidance for authors when choosing between a systematic or scoping review approach. BMC Med Res Methodol. 2018;18:143.
447. Tonin F, Rotta I, Mendes A, Pontarolo R. Network meta-analysis: a technique to gather evidence from direct and indirect comparisons. Pharm Pract. 2017;15:943.
448. Friedrich M. The Cochrane Collaboration turns 20: assessing the evidence to inform clinical care. J Am Med Assoc. 2013;309:1881–2.
449. Clancy C, Slutsky J. Advancing excellence in health care: getting to effectiveness. J Investig Med. 2005;53:65–6.

450. Anonymous. Finding what works in health care: standards for systematic reviews. Washington, DC: Institute of Medicine 2011 March 23, 2011.
451. Moher D, Liberati A, Tetzlaff J, Altman D. Preferred reporting items for systematic reviews and meta-analyses: the PRISMA statement. Ann Intern Med. 2009;151:264–9.
452. Guyatt G, Oxman A, Akl E, Kunz R, Vist G, Brozek J, et al. GRADE guidelines: 1. Introduction-GRADE evidence profiles and summary of findings tables. J Clin Epidemiol. 2011;64:383–94.
453. Fergusson D, Glass K, Hutton B, Shapiro S. Randomized controlled trials of aprotinin in cardiac surgery: could clinical equipoise have stopped the bleeding? Clin Trials. 2005;2: 218–29.
454. Copas J, Shi J. Meta-analysis, funnel plots and sensitivity analysis. Biostatistics. 2000;1:247–62.
455. Egger M, Smith G, Schneider M, Minder C. Bias in meta-analysis detected by a simple, graphical test. Br Med J. 1997;315:629–34.
456. Higgins J, Thompson S. Quantifying heterogeneity in a meta-analysis. Stat Med. 2002;21:1539–58.
457. Garner P, Hopewell S, Chandler J, MacLehose H, Akl E, Trivella M, et al. When and how to update systematic reviews: consensus and checklist. Br Med J. 2016;354:i3507.
458. Shekelle P, Shetty K, Newberry S, Maglione M, Motala A. Machine learning versus standard techniques for updating searches for systematic reviews: a diagnostic accuracy study. Ann Intern Med. 2017;167:213–5.
459. Martin P, Surian D, Bashir R, Bourgeois F, Dunn A. Trial2rev: combining machine learning and crowd-sourcing to create a shared space for updating systematic reviews. JAMIA Open. 2019;1:15–22.
460. Hopewell S, McDonald S, Clarke M, Egger M. Grey literature in meta-analyses of randomized trials of health care interventions. In: Cochrane Library. Update Software. 2003. http://www.cochrane.org/cochrane/mrabstr/mr000010.htm.
461. von Elm E, Poglia G, Walder B, Tramer M. Different patterns of duplicate publication: an analysis of articles used in systematic reviews. J Am Med Assoc. 2004;291:974–80.
462. Ioannidis J. The mass production of redundant, misleading, and conflicted systematic reviews and meta-analyses. Milbank Q. 2016;94:485–514.
463. Page M, Moher D. Mass production of systematic reviews and meta-analyses: an exercise in mega-silliness? Milbank Q. 2016;94:515–9.
464. Page M, Shamseer L, Altman D, Tetzlaff J, Sampson M, Tricco A, et al. Epidemiology and reporting characteristics of systematic reviews of biomedical research: a cross-sectional study. PLoS Med. 2016;13(5):e1002028.
465. Dechartres A, Atal I, Riveros C, Meerpohl J, Ravaud P. Association between publication characteristics and treatment effect estimates – a meta-epidemiologic study. Ann Intern Med. 2018;169:385–93.
466. Rochon P, Bero L, Bay A, Gold J, Dergal J, Binns M, et al. Comparison of review articles published in peer-reviewed and throwaway journals. J Am Med Assoc. 2002;287: 2853–6.
467. Banzi R, Cinquini M, Liberati A, Moschetti I, Pecoraro V, Tagliabue L, et al. Speed of updating online evidence based point of care summaries: prospective cohort analysis. Br Med J. 2011;343:d5856.
468. Ketchum A, Saleh A, Jeong K. Type of evidence behind point-of-care clinical information products: a bibliometric analysis. J Med Internet Res. 2011;13(1):e21.
469. Randhawa A, Babalola O, Henney Z, Miller M, Nelson T, Oza M, et al. A collaborative assessment among 11 pharmaceutical companies of misinformation in commonly used online drug information compendia. Ann Pharmacother. 2016;50:352–9.
470. Talwar S, Randhawa A, Dankiewicz E, Crudele N, Haddox J. Caveat emptor: erroneous safety information about opioids in online drug-information compendia. J Opioid Manag. 2016;12:281–8.

471. Piper B, Lambert D, Keefe R, Smukler P, Selemon N, Duperry Z. Undisclosed conflicts of interest among biomedical textbook authors. AJOB Empirical Bioethics. 2018;9(2):59–68.
472. Field M, Lohr K, editors. Clinical practice guidelines: directions for a new program. Washington, DC: National Academies Press; 1990.
473. Shiffman R, Brandt C, Liaw Y, Corb G. A design model for computer-based guideline implementation based on information management services. J Am Med Inform Assoc. 1999;6:99–103.
474. Hibble A, Kanka D, Penchion D, Pooles F. Guidelines in general practice: the new Tower of Babel? Br Med J. 1998;317:862–3.
475. Cabana M, Rand C, Powe N, Wu A, Wilson M, Abboud P, et al. Why don't physicians follow clinical practice guidelines? A framework for improvement. J Am Med Assoc. 1999;282:1458–65.
476. McAlister F, van Diepen S, Padwal R, Johnson J, Majumdar S. How evidence-based are the recommendations in evidence-based guidelines? PLoS Med. 2007;4(8):e250.
477. Cherubini A, Oristrell J, Pla X, Ruggiero C, Ferretti R, Diestre G, et al. The persistent exclusion of older patients from ongoing clinical trials regarding heart failure. Arch Intern Med. 2011;171:550–6.
478. Bennett W, Odelola O, Wilson L, Bolen S, Selvaraj S, Robinson K, et al. Evaluation of guideline recommendations on oral medications for type 2 diabetes mellitus: a systematic review. Ann Intern Med. 2012;156:27–36.
479. Chen Y, Yang K, Marušić A, Qaseem A, Meerpohl J, Flottorp S, et al. A reporting tool for practice guidelines in health care: the RIGHT statement. Ann Intern Med. 2017;166:128–32.
480. Maviglia S, Zielstorff R, Paterno M, Teich J, Bates D, Kuperman G. Automating complex guidelines for chronic disease: lessons learned. J Am Med Inform Assoc. 2003;10:154–65.
481. Friedman C, Flynn A. Computable knowledge: an imperative for learning health systems. Learn Health Syst. 2019;3(4):e10203.
482. Neuman J, Korenstein D, Ross J, Keyhani S. Prevalence of financial conflicts of interest among panel members producing clinical practice guidelines in Canada and United States: cross sectional study. Br Med J. 2011;343:d5621.
483. Mendelson T, Meltzer M, Campbell E, Caplan A, Kirkpatrick J. Conflicts of interest in cardiovascular clinical practice guidelines. Arch Intern Med. 2011;171:577–84.
484. Feuerstein J, Akbari M, Gifford A, Hurley C, Leffler D, Sheth S, et al. Systematic analysis underlying the quality of the scientific evidence and conflicts of interest in interventional medicine subspecialty guidelines. Mayo Clin Proc. 2014;89:16–24.
485. Khan R, Scaffidi M, Rumman A, Grindal A, Plener I, Grover S. Prevalence of financial conflicts of interest among authors of clinical guidelines related to high-revenue medications. JAMA Intern Med. 2018;178:1712–5.
486. Ioannidis J. Professional societies should abstain from authorship of guidelines and disease definition statements. Circ Cardiovasc Qual Outcomes. 2018;11(10):e004889.
487. Qaseem A, Wilt T. Disclosure of interests and management of conflicts of interest in clinical guidelines and guidance statements: methods from the Clinical Guidelines Committee of the American College of Physicians. Ann Intern Med. 2019;171:354–61.
488. Laine C, Taichman D, Mulrow C. Trustworthy clinical guidelines. Ann Intern Med. 2011;154:774–5.
489. Graham R, Mancher M, Wolman D, Greenfield S, Steinberg E. Clinical practice guidelines we can trust. Washington, DC: National Academies Press 2011 March 23, 2011.
490. Jue J, Cunningham S, Lohr K, Shekelle P, Shiffman R, Robbins C, et al. Developing and testing the Agency for Healthcare Research and Quality's National Guideline Clearinghouse Extent of Adherence to Trustworthy Standards (NEATS) instrument. Ann Intern Med. 2019;170:480–7.
491. Frankel M, Elliot R, Blume M, Bourgois J, Hugenholtz B, Lundquist M, et al. Defining and certifying electronic publication in science. American Association for the Advancement

of Science 2000. http://www.aaas.org/spp/dspp/sfrl/projects/epub/define.htm. Accessed July 1, 2002.
492. Hersh W, Rindfleisch T. Electronic publishing of scholarly communication in the biomedical sciences. J Am Med Inform Assoc. 2000;7:324–5.
493. Anonymous. The future of the electronic scientific literature. Nature. 2001;413:1–3.
494. Fox S, Duggan M. Health Online 2013. Washington, DC: Pew Internet & American Life Project 2013 January 15, 2013.
495. Silberg W, Lundberg G, Musacchio R. Assessing, controlling, and assuring the quality of medical information on the Internet: caveat lector et viewor – let the reader and viewer beware. J Am Med Assoc. 1997;277:1244–5.
496. Eysenbach G, Powell J, Kuss O, Sa E-R. Empirical studies assessing the quality of health information for consumers on the world wide web: a systematic review. J Am Med Assoc. 2002;287:2691–700.
497. Scullard P, Peacock C, Davies P. Googling children's health: reliability of medical advice on the internet. Arch Dis Child. 2010;95:580–2.
498. Mirkin J, Lowrance W, Feifer A, Mulhall J, Eastham J, Elkin E. Direct-to-consumer Internet promotion of robotic prostatectomy exhibits varying quality of information. Health Aff. 2012;31:760–9.
499. Kitchens B, Harle C, Li S. Quality of health-related online search results. Decis Support Syst. 2014;57:454–62.
500. Kincaid M, Fleisher L, Neuman M. Presentation on US hospital websites of risks and benefits of transcatheter aortic valve replacement procedures. JAMA Intern Med. 2015;175:440–1.
501. Bruce J, Tucholka J, Steffens N, Neuman H. Quality of online information to support patient decision-making in breast cancer surgery. J Surg Oncol. 2015;112:575–80.
502. Broniatowski D, Jamison A, Qi S, AlKulaib L, Chen T, Benton A, et al. Weaponized health communication: Twitter bots and Russian trolls amplify the vaccine debate. Am J Public Health. 2018;108:1378–84.
503. Koren M. How Did Astronaut DNA become 'Fake News'? The Atlantic 2018 March 16, 2018.
504. Loeb S, Sengupta S, Butaney M, Macaluso J, Czarniecki S, Robbins R, et al. Dissemination of misinformative and biased information about prostate cancer on YouTube. Eur Urol. 2018;75:564–7.
505. Rothrock S, Rothrock A, Swetland S, Pagane M, Isaak S, Romney J, et al. Quality, trustworthiness, readability, and accuracy of medical information regarding common pediatric emergency medicine-related complaints on the Web. J Emerg Med. 2019;57:469–77.
506. Overland J, Hoskins P, McGill M. Low literacy: a problem in diabetes education. Diab Med. 1993;10:847–50.
507. Foltz A, Sullivan J. Reading level, learning presentation preference, and desire for information among cancer patients. J Cancer Educ. 1996;11:32–8.
508. Williams D, Counselman F, Caggiano C. Emergency department discharge instructions and patient literacy: a problem of disparity. Am J Emerg Med. 1996;14:19–22.
509. Murphy P. Reading ability of parents compared with reading level of pediatric patient education materials. Pediatrics. 1994;93:460–8.
510. Gazmararian J, Baker D, Williams M, Parker R, Scott T, Green D, et al. Health literacy among Medicare enrollees in a managed care organization. J Am Med Assoc. 1999;281:545–51.
511. Flesch R. A new readability yardstick. J Appl Psychol. 1948;32:221–33.
512. Graber M, Roller C, Kaeble B. Readability levels of patient education material on the World Wide Web. J Fam Pract. 1999;48:58–61.
513. Berland G, Elliott M, Morales L, Algazy J, Kravitz R, Broder M, et al. Health information on the Internet: accessibility, quality, and readability in English and Spanish. J Am Med Assoc. 2001;285:2612–21.
514. Cheng C, Dunn M. Health literacy and the Internet: a study on the readability of Australian online health information. Aust N Z J Public Health. 2015;39:309–14.

515. Murray K, Murray T, O'Rourke A, Low C, Veale D. Readability and quality of online information on osteoarthritis: an objective analysis with historic comparison. Internact J Med Res. 2019;8(3):e12855.
516. Galesic M, Garcia-Retamero R. Statistical numeracy for health: a cross-cultural comparison with probabilistic national samples. Arch Intern Med. 2010;170:462–8.
517. Gigerenzer G, Galesic M. Why do single event probabilities confuse patients? Br Med J. 2010;344:e245.
518. Krouss M, Croft L, Morgan D. Physician understanding and ability to communicate harms and benefits of common medical treatments. JAMA Intern Med. 2016;176:1565–7.
519. Epstein D. When evidence says no, but doctors say yes ProPublica 2017 February 22, 2017.
520. Eysenbach G, Diepgen T. Towards quality management of medical information on the internet: evaluation, labelling, and filtering of information. Br Med J. 1998;317:1496–502.
521. McHenry R. The faith-based encyclopedia tech central station 2004 November 15, 2004.
522. Shafee T, Masukume G, Kipersztok L, Das D, Häggström M, Heilman J. Evolution of Wikipedia's medical content: past, present and future. J Epidemiol Commun Health. 2017;71(11):1122.
523. Tackett S, Gaglani S, Heilman J, Azzam A. The reCAPTCHA of medical education. Med Teach. 2017;41:598–600.
524. Apollonio D, Broyde K, Azzam A, DeGuia M, Heilman J, Brock T. Pharmacy students can improve access to quality medicines information by editing Wikipedia articles. BMC Med Educ. 2018;18:265.
525. Clauson K, Polen H, Boulos M, Dzenowagis J. Scope, completeness, and accuracy of drug information in Wikipedia. Ann Pharmacother. 2008;42:1814–21.
526. Rajagopalan M, Khanna V, Leiter Y, Stott M, Showalter T, Dicker A, et al. Patient-oriented cancer information on the Internet: a comparison of Wikipedia and a professionally maintained database. J Oncol Pract. 2011;7:319–23.
527. Hasty R, Garbalosa R, Barbato V, Valdes P, Powers D, Hernandez E, et al. Wikipedia vs peer-reviewed medical literature for information about the 10 most costly medical conditions. J Am Osteopath Assoc. 2014;114:368–73.
528. Hwang T, Bourgeois F, Seeger J. Drug safety in the digital age. N Engl J Med. 2014;370:2460–2.
529. Crocco A, Villasis-Keever M, Jadad A. Analysis of cases of harm associated with use of health information on the internet. J Am Med Assoc. 2002;287:2869–71.
530. Ferguson T. From patients to end users: quality of online patient networks needs more attention than quality of online health information. Br Med J. 2002;324:555–6.
531. Tang P, Newcomb C, Gorden S, Kreider N, editors. Meeting the information needs of patients: results from a patient focus group. Proceedings of the 1997 AMIA Annual Fall Symposium; 1997; Nashville, TN: Hanley & Belfus.
532. Boyer C, Baujard V, Geissbuhler A. Evolution of health web certification through the HONcode experience. Stud Health Technol Inform. 2011;169:53–7.
533. Starman J, Gettys F, Capo J, Fleischli J, Norton H, Karunakar M. Quality and content of Internet-based information for ten common orthopaedic sports medicine diagnoses. J Bone Joint Surg. 2010;92:1612–8.
534. Price S, Hersh W, editors. Filtering Web pages for quality indicators: an empirical approach to finding high quality consumer health information on the World Wide Web. Proceedings of the AMIA 1999 Annual Symposium; 1999; Washington, DC: Hanley & Belfus.
535. Wang Y, Liu Z. Automatic detecting indicators for quality of health information on the Web. Int J Med Inform. 2007;76:575–82.
536. Shuchman M, Wilkes M. Medical scientists and health news reporting: a case of miscommunication. Ann Intern Med. 1997;126:976–82.
537. Rennie D. Thyroid storm. J Am Med Assoc. 1997;277:1238–43.
538. Schwartz L, Woloshin S, Baczek L. Media coverage of scientific meetings: too much, too soon? J Am Med Assoc. 2002;287:2859–63.

539. Rada R. Retractions, press releases and newspaper coverage. Health Inf Libr J. 2007;24:210–5.
540. Fishman J, Have T, Casarett D. Cancer and the media: how does the news report on treatment and outcomes? Arch Intern Med. 2010;170:515–8.
541. Yavchitz A, Boutron I, Bafeta A, Marroun I, Charles P, Mantz J, et al. Misrepresentation of randomized controlled trials in press releases and news coverage: a cohort study. PLoS Med. 2012;9(9):e1001308.
542. Downing N, Cheng T, Krumholz H, Shah N, Ross J. Descriptions and interpretations of the ACCORD-Lipid trial in the news and biomedical literature: a cross-sectional analysis. JAMA Intern Med. 2014;174:1176–82.
543. Schwitzer G. A guide to reading health care news stories. JAMA Intern Med. 2014;174:1183–6.
544. Sumner P, Vivian-Griffiths S, Boivin J, Williams A, Venetis C, Davies A, et al. The association between exaggeration in health related science news and academic press releases: retrospective observational study. Br Med J. 2014;349:g7015.
545. Lancaster F, Warner A. Information retrieval today. Arlington, VA: Information Resources Press; 1993.
546. Cockburn A. Writing effective use cases. Boston: Addison-Wesley; 2001.
547. Wilkinson R, Fuller M. Integration of information retrieval and hypertext via structure. In: Agosti M, Smeaton A, editors. Information retrieval and hypertext. Norwell, MA: Kluwer; 1996. p. 257–71.
548. Gorman P. Information needs of physicians. J Am Soc Inf Sci. 1995;46:729–36.
549. Anonymous. From Screen to Script: The Doctor's Digital Path to Treatment. New York, NY: Manhattan Research; Google 2012.
550. Elstein A, Shulman L, Sprafka S. Medical problem solving: an analysis of clinical reasoning. Cambridge, MA: Harvard University Press; 1978.
551. Schmidt H, Norman G, Boshuizen H. A cognitive perspective on medical expertise: theory and implications. Acad Med. 1990;65:611–21.
552. Patel V, Evans D, Groen G. Biomedical knowledge and clinical reasoning. In: Evans D, Patel V, editors. Cognitive science in medicine: biomedical modeling. Cambridge, MA: MIT Press; 1989. p. 53–112.
553. Sox H, Blatt M, Higgins M, Marton K. Medical decision making. Boston, MA: Butterworths; 1988.
554. Tanenbaum S. Knowing and acting in medical practice: the epistemological politics of outcomes research. J Health Polit Policy Law. 1994;19:27–44.
555. Huth E. The underused medical literature. Ann Intern Med. 1989;110:99–100.
556. Kassirer J. Too many books, too few journals. N Engl J Med. 1992;326:1427–8.
557. Shaughnessy A, Slawson D, Bennett J. Becoming an information master: a guidebook to the medical information jungle. J Fam Pract. 1994;39:489–99.
558. McDonald C. Medical heuristics: the silent adjudicators of clinical practice. Ann Intern Med. 1996;124:56–62.
559. Stross J, Harlan W. The dissemination of new medical information. J Am Med Assoc. 1979;241:2622–4.
560. Stross J, Harlan W. Dissemination of relevant information on hypertension. J Am Med Assoc. 1981;246:360–2.
561. Williamson J, German P, Weiss R, Skinner E, Bowes F. Health science information management and continuing education of physicians. Ann Intern Med. 1989;110:151–60.
562. Leigh T, Young P, Haley J. Performances of family practice diplomates on successive mandatory recertification examinations. Acad Med. 1993;68:912–21.
563. Ramsey P, Carline J, Inui T, Larson E, LoGerfo J, Norcini J, et al. Changes over time in the knowledge base of practicing internists. J Am Med Assoc. 1991;266:1103–8.
564. Covell D, Uman G, Manning P. Information needs in office practice: are they being met? Ann Intern Med. 1985;103:596–9.
565. Gorman P, Helfand M. Information seeking in primary care: how physicians choose which clinical questions to pursue and which to leave unanswered. Med Decis Mak. 1995;15:113–9.

566. Ely J, Osheroff J, Ebell M, Bergus G, Levy B, Chambliss M, et al. Analysis of questions asked by family doctors regarding patient care. Br Med J. 1999;319:358–61.
567. Ely J, Osheroff J, Gorman P, Ebell M, Chambliss M, Pifer E, et al. A taxonomy of generic clinical questions: classification study. Br Med J. 2000;321:429–32.
568. Ely J, Osheroff J, Ebell M, Chambliss M, Vinson D, Stevermer J, et al. Obstacles to answering doctors' questions about patient care with evidence: qualitative study. Br Med J. 2002;324:710–3.
569. Ely J, Osheroff J, Chambliss M, Ebell M, Rosenbaum M. Answering physicians' clinical questions: obstacles and potential solutions. J Am Med Inform Assoc. 2005;12:217–24.
570. Ely J, Osheroff J, Maviglia S, Rosenbaum M. Patient-care questions that physicians are unable to answer. J Am Med Inform Assoc. 2007;14:407–14.
571. Ellsworth M, Homan J, Cimino J, Peters S, Pickering B, Herasevich V. Point-of-care knowledge-based resource needs of clinicians: a survey from a large academic medical center. Appl Clin Inform. 2015;6:305–17.
572. DelFiol G, Workman T, Gorman P. Clinical questions raised by clinicians at the point of care: a systematic review. JAMA Intern Med. 2014;174:710–8.
573. Curley S, Connelly D, Rich E. Physicians use of medical knowledge resources: preliminary theoretical framework and findings. Med Decis Mak. 1990;10:231–41.
574. Connelly D, Rich E, Curley S, Kelly J. Knowledge resource preferences of family physicians. J Fam Pract. 1990;30:353–9.
575. Aakre C, Maggio L, DelFiol G, Cook D. Barriers and facilitators to clinical information seeking: a systematic review. J Am Med Inform Assoc. 2019;26:1129–40.
576. Cogdill K. Information needs and information seeking in primary care: a study of nurse practitioners. J Med Libr Assoc. 2003;91:203–14.
577. Roberts P, Hayes W, editors. Information needs and the role of text mining in drug development. Pacific Symposium on Biocomputing; 2008; Big Island, Hawaii: World Scientific Press.
578. Hemminger B, Lu D, Vaughan K, Adams S. Information seeking behavior of academic scientists. J Am Soc Inf Sci Technol. 2007;58:2205–25.
579. Roberts K, Demner-Fushman D. Interactive use of online health resources: a comparison of consumer and professional questions. J Am Med Inform Assoc. 2015;23:802–11.
580. Wartella E, Rideout V, Zupancic H, Beaudoin-Ryan L, Lauricella A. Teens, health, and technology – a national survey. Evanston, IL: Center on Media and Human Development, Northwestern University 2015 June, 2015.
581. Ioannidis J, Stuart M, Brownlee S, Strite S. How to survive the medical misinformation mess. Eur J Clin Investig. 2017;47:795–802.

Chapter 3
Content

In the first edition of this book in the mid-1990s, describing the content available in IR systems was relatively simple. Access to the Internet was mostly via telephone modem, and thus very slow, meaning that mostly only textual information could be transmitted. For the most part, IR systems were used to identify paper-based content (e.g., journals and textbooks) that could be retrieved from institutional or personal library shelves. Some computers had graphical display capabilities and could provide access to a wider range of content via CD-ROM disks, including images, though at resolutions much lower than today. By the second edition in the early 2000s, use of the Web was becoming widespread, although a substantial amount of material (i.e., journals and books) was still paper-based. By the third edition in the late 2000s, the knowledge world had become substantially electronic. At present, essentially all journal articles, textbooks, and other resources are available electronically, and an increasing amount of material is distributed only in electronic format.

This chapter is the first of several that explore the "state of the art" of information retrieval (IR) systems. This chapter focuses on content, i.e., what biomedical and health information resources are available. Our goal is not to be exhaustive, but rather representative, covering the diversity of content that is available. We will approach this via a classification scheme for content. This will be followed in subsequent chapters by coverage of indexing, retrieval, and digital libraries.

3.1 Classification of Health and Biomedical Information Content

The classification schema is shown in Table 3.1. It is not a pure schema, for some of the subcategories represent type of content (e.g., literature reference databases) while others describe its subject (e.g., the -omics databases). Nonetheless, the schema does cover the major types of health and biomedical information available

W. Hersh, *Information Retrieval: A Biomedical and Health Perspective*, Health Informatics, https://doi.org/10.1007/978-3-030-47686-1_3

Table 3.1 Classification of health and biomedical information content

1. Bibliographic
a. Literature reference databases
b. Web catalogs and feeds
c. Specialized registries
2. Full text
a. Periodicals
b. Books and reports
c. Web collections
3. Annotated
a. Images and videos
b. Citations
c. Evidence-based medicine resources
d. Molecular biology and -omics
e. Linked data
f. Other
4. Aggregations
a. Consumer health
b. Professional content
c Body of knowledge
d. Model organism databases

electronically, even if the boundaries between the categories have some areas of fuzziness. The classification will be revisited again in Chap. 5 when we cover approaches to searching various resources.

The first category consists of *bibliographic* content. It includes what was for decades the mainstay of IR systems, *literature reference databases*. Even with essentially the entire scientific publishing enterprising online, literature reference databases are still in widespread use as an entry point into the scientific literature (especially since many publishers want to direct people to their resources that require a fee to use). A second, more modern type of bibliographic content includes *Web catalogs and feeds*. There are fewer Web catalogs, which consist of Web pages that contain mainly links to other Web pages and sites, in modern times. Web feeds are bibliographic-like streams of information that inform users of new content on Web sites and in other databases. The final type of bibliographic content is the *specialized registry*. This resource is very close to a literature reference database except that it indexes more diverse content than journal and proceedings abstracts and articles.

The second category is *full-text* content. A large component of this content consists of the online versions of periodicals, books, and reports. As already noted, essentially all of this content, from journals to textbooks, is now available electronically. The electronic versions may be enhanced by measures ranging from the provision of supplemental data in a journal article to Web linkages or multimedia content in a textbook. Another type of content in this category is what we call the Web collection. Admittedly the diversity of information on Web collections is enormous, and they may include every other type of content described in this chapter. However, in the context of this category, "Web collection" refers to the vast number of static and dynamic Web pages that reside at a discrete Web location.

A third category consists of *annotated* content. We make the distinction between this content and bibliographic content by virtue of the annotation being tightly integrated with the content as opposed to being in a separate bibliographic database. Annotated content includes images and videos, citation databases, structured evidence-based medicine (EBM) resources, and biomedical research data. The latter are particularly prevalent in molecular biology and the -omics (e.g., genomics, proteomics, etc.), which consist of nucleotide or protein sequences, chromosome maps, and biological pathways. All these types of content are usually annotated with some amount of metadata, usually in textual form, and searched with IR-like systems, although the content itself may be predominantly nontextual or text that is nonnarrative.

The final category consists of *aggregations* of the first three categories. A number of Web sites consist of collections of different types of content, aggregated to form a coherent resource. We will look at examples in biomedical research, clinical content, and consumer content. In one sense, the entire Web can be viewed as one big aggregation, but as we will see, there are plenty of more confined aggregations that provide value within their (not always distinct) boundaries.

3.2 Bibliographic Content

Bibliographic content consists of references or citations to complete resources. It tends to be richer than other content in metadata, in this case data about the complete article, report, book, etc. [1]. This is not surprising, since bibliographic databases in essence consist of metadata. The original IR databases from the 1960s were bibliographic databases that typically contained references to literature on library shelves. Library card catalogs are also a type of bibliographic database, with the electronic version usually called an *online public access catalog* (OPAC). Bibliographic databases were designed to steer the searcher to printed resources, not to provide the information itself. Most have fields not only for the subject matter, such as the title, abstract, and indexing terms, but also other attributes, such as author name(s), publication date, publication type, and grant identification number.

In this section, we begin our discussion with literature reference databases, followed by descriptions of Web catalogs and feeds and then specialized registries. Although not typically thought of as bibliographic databases, many Web catalogs and feeds can be viewed as bibliographic in that they provide links to other information sources. Indeed, some modern bibliographic databases offer direct linkage to the literature they are referencing and hence are becoming similar to Web catalogs.

3.2.1 Literature Reference Databases

As already noted, the literature reference database MEDLINE may be the best-known IR application in all of health and biomedicine. Produced by the National Center for Biotechnology Information (NCBI)[1] within the National Library of Medicine (NLM),[2] MEDLINE was virtually synonymous with online searching for healthcare topics for many years. Some use the terms MEDLINE and PubMed synonymously, but as noted below, PubMed is a search system used to access MEDLINE on the NLM Web site, although its database includes more than just MEDLINE, as also noted below. There are also a substantial number of other bibliographic databases, some of which are produced by the NLM and others produced by additional information providers. A technical resource for all NLM resources is the *NLM Technical Bulletin*.[3] As noted later, NCBI produces a great deal of other information resources [2].

3.2.1.1 MEDLINE

MEDLINE contains bibliographic references to all the biomedical articles, editorials, letters to the editors, and other content in over 5200 scientific journals.[4] The journals are chosen for inclusion by the Literature Selection Technical Review Committee (LSTRC) of the National Institutes of Health[5] based on their meeting a critical number of standards for quality, peer review, and other standards. The number of records added to MEDLINE each year continues to grow, with over 900,000 added in 2019, bringing the total number to over 25 million.[6] The language of origin of over 95% of the citations is English, although journals representing 29 other languages are indexed.[7] About 88% of the records have abstracts, including some non-English articles, although an English translation is always provided. MEDLINE is updated daily.

The MEDLINE database is the electronic version of *Index Medicus*, the print publication that was the most common way to access medical literature for over a century. *Index Medicus* was founded in the nineteenth century by Dr. John Shaw Billings, who headed the forerunner of the NLM, the Library of the Surgeon General's Office from 1865 to 1895 [3]. Billings was the first to diligently catalog the literature of medicine, culminating in the first volume of *Index Medicus* published in 1879. In 2004, the NLM "retired" the print version of *Index Medicus* [4]. One enduring value

[1] https://www.ncbi.nlm.nih.gov/

[2] https://www.nlm.nih.gov/

[3] https://www.nlm.nih.gov/pubs/techbull/tb.html

[4] https://www.nlm.nih.gov/bsd/medline.html

[5] https://www.nlm.nih.gov/lstrc/jsel.html

[6] https://www.nlm.nih.gov/bsd/medline_pubmed_production_stats.html

[7] https://www.nlm.nih.gov/bsd/medline_lang_distr.html

of *Index Medicus* was that it allowed searching of pre-1966 literature, although NLM now maintains a database called OLDMEDLINE that contains citations from before the official 1966 "start date" of MEDLINE. OLDMEDLINE continues to grow and now has over two million references dating back to the 1940s.[8]

MEDLINE has evolved over the years. Beginning in 1975, the NLM began adding abstracts for all references that contained them. The Medical Subject Headings (MeSH) vocabulary, used to index MEDLINE and other NLM resources and covered in the next chapter, has expanded to over 23,000 terms. Additional attributes have been added to MEDLINE, such as the secondary source identifier (SI), which provides a link to records in other databases, such as the GenBank database of gene sequences and the ClinicalTrials.gov database of clinical trials. Other attributes have been enhanced, such as publication type (PT), which lists, for example, whether the article is a `meta-analysis`, `practice guideline`, `review article`, or `randomized controlled trial`. Another feature of MEDLINE that has been retired is the old MEDLINE UI (unique identifier), which has been replaced by the PMID as the unique identifier for MEDLINE and OLDMEDLINE citations [5].

The current MEDLINE record contains over 50 fields, the most important of which are listed in Table 3.2.[9] Table 3.3 contains the special tags that NLM uses for comments and corrections, such as when an article has an editorial or letter to the editor or has a correction or retraction.[10] A clinician may only be interested in just a handful of MEDLINE fields, such as the title, abstract, and indexing terms. But other fields contain specific information that may be of great importance to a more focused audience. For example, a genomics researcher might be highly interested in the SI field to link to genomic databases. Even the clinician may, however, derive benefit from some of the other fields. For example, the PT field can help in the application of EBM, such as when one is searching for a practice guideline or a randomized controlled trial. The PubMed status subset (SB) field allows searches to be limited to MEDLINE, in-process citations, publisher-supplied citations, and several subject subsets, all of which are listed in Table 3.4.[11] A sample MEDLINE record is shown in Fig. 3.1.

The major way that most users access MEDLINE is via the PubMed system[12] at the NLM, which provides access to other NLM databases as well and is free of charge. Although some people use the terms MEDLINE and PubMed synonymously, strictly speaking the former refers to the database and the latter to the search system. In addition, PubMed includes some additional material beyond just MEDLINE, including[13]:

---

[8] https://www.nlm.nih.gov/databases/databases_oldmedline.html

[9] https://www.nlm.nih.gov/bsd/mms/medlineelements.html

[10] https://www.nlm.nih.gov/bsd/policy/errata.html

[11] https://www.ncbi.nlm.nih.gov/books/NBK3827/table/pubmedhelp.T.journalcitation_subsets/

[12] http://pubmed.gov

[13] https://www.nlm.nih.gov/bsd/difference.html

Table 3.2 Fields in MEDLINE (Courtesy of NLM)

Field	Abbreviation
Abstract	AB
Copyright Information	CI
Affiliation	AD
Investigator Affiliation	IRAD
Article Identifier	AID
Author	AU
Author Identifier	AUID
Full Author	FAU
Book Title	BTI
Collection Title	CTI
Comments/Corrections	
Conflict of Interest Statement	COIS
Corporate Author	CN
Create Date	CRDT
Date Completed	DCOM
Date Created	DA
Date Last Revised	LR
Date of Electronic Publication	DEP
Date of Publication	DP
Edition	EN
Editor and Full Editor Name	ED FED
Entrez Date	EDAT
Gene Symbol	GS
General Note	GN
Grant Number	GR
Investigator Name and Full Investigator Name	IR FIR
ISBN	ISBN
ISSN	IS
Issue	IP
Journal Title Abbreviation	TA
Journal Title	JT
Language	LA
Location Identifier	LID
Manuscript Identifier	MID
MeSH Date	MHDA
MeSH Terms	MH
NLM Unique ID	JID
Number of References	RF
Other Abstract	OAB
Other Copyright Information	OCI
Other ID	OID
Other Term	OT
Other Term Owner	OTO

Table 3.2 (continued)

Field	Abbreviation
Owner	OWN
Pagination	PG
Personal Name as Subject	PS
Full Personal Name as Subject	FPS
Place of Publication	PL
Publication History Status	PHST
Publication Status	PST
Publication Type	PT
Publishing Model	PUBM
PubMed Central Identifier	PMC
PubMed Central Release	PMCR
PubMed Unique Identifier	PMID
Registry Number/EC Number	RN
Substance Name	NM
Secondary Source ID	SI
Source	SO
Space Flight Mission	SFM
Status	STAT
Subset	SB
Title	TI
Transliterated Title	TT
Volume	VI
Volume Title	VTI

Table 3.3 Comments and corrections in the MEDLINE Database (Courtesy of NLM)

Comment or correction type	MEDLINE display field tag	Description
Comment in	CIN	Cite reference containing a commentary about the article
Comment on	CON	Cites reference upon which the article comments
Erratum in	EIN	Cites published erratum to the article (appears on citation for original article)
Erratum for	EFR	Cites original article for which there is a published erratum
Corrected and Republished in	CRI	Cites final, correct version of a corrected and republished article (appears on citation for original article)
Corrected and Republished from	CRF	Cites original article subsequently corrected and republished
Dataset described in	DDIN	Cites description of a dataset

(continued)

Table 3.3 (continued)

Comment or correction type	MEDLINE display field tag	Description
Dataset use reported in	DRIN	Cites articles reporting results or use of a dataset
ExpressionOfConcernIn	ECI	Cites expression of concern (appears on citation for original article)
ExpressionOfConcernFor	ECF	Cites original article for which there is an expression of concern
Republished in	RPI	Cites subsequent (and possibly abridged) version of a republished article (appears on citation for original article)
Republished from	RPF	Cites first, originally published article
Retraction in	RIN	Cites retraction of the article (appears on citation for original article)
Retraction of	ROF	Cites article(s) being retracted
Update in	UIN	Cites updated version of the article (appears on citation for original article)
Update of	UOF	Cites article being updated; limited use
Summary for patients in	SPIN	Cites patient summary article
Original report in	ORI	Cites scientific article associated with a patient summary

Table 3.4 PubMed subsets (Courtesy of NLM)

Subset code	Journal/citation subset
AIM	Abridged Index Medicus is a list created in 1970 of approximately 120 core clinical English-language journals
D	Dentistry journals
E	Citations from bioethics journals or selected bioethics citations from other journals
H	Health administration journals, non-Index Medicus
IM	Index Medicus journals
K	Consumer health journals
N	Nursing journals
Q	History of medicine journals and selected citations from other journals
QIS	Citations from non-Index Medicus journals in the field of history of medicine
S	Citations from space life sciences journals and selected space life sciences citations from other journals
T	Health technology assessment journals, non-Index Medicus
X	AIDS/HIV journals (selected citations from other journals 1980–2000)

```
PMID  - 3675956
OWN   - NLM
STAT  - MEDLINE
DCOM  - 19871231
LR    - 20161021
IS    - 0889-7190 (Print)
IS    - 0889-7190 (Linking)
VI    -  33
IP    - 3
DP    - 1987 Jul-Sep
TI    - Effects of 25 (OH)-vitamin D3 in hypocalcemic patients on chronic hemodialysis.
PG    - 289-92
FAU   - Kronfol, N O
AU    - Kronfol NO
AD    - Department of Medicine, College of Medicine, University of Illinois, Chicago.
FAU   - Hersh, W R
AU    - Hersh WR
FAU   - Barakat, M M
AU    - Barakat MM
LA    - eng
PT    - Comparative Study
PT    - Journal Article
PL    - United States
TA    - ASAIO Trans
JT    - ASAIO transactions
JID   - 8611947
RN    - 0 (Parathyroid Hormone)
RN    - 27YLU75U4W (Phosphorus)
RN    - EC 3.1.3.1 (Alkaline Phosphatase)
RN    - FXC9231JVH (Calcitriol)
RN    - SY7Q814VUP (Calcium)
SB    - IM
MH    - Alkaline Phosphatase/blood
MH    - Calcitriol/*therapeutic use
MH    - Calcium/blood
MH    - Humans
MH    - Hypocalcemia/*drug therapy/etiology
MH    - Parathyroid Hormone/blood
MH    - Phosphorus/blood
MH    - Renal Dialysis/*adverse effects
EDAT  - 1987/07/01 00:00
MHDA  - 1987/07/01 00:01
CRDT  - 1987/07/01 00:00
PHST  - 1987/07/01 00:00 [pubmed]
PHST  - 1987/07/01 00:01 [medline]
PHST  - 1987/07/01 00:00 [entrez]
PST   - ppublish
SO    - ASAIO Trans. 1987 Jul-Sep;33(3):289-92.
```

Fig. 3.1 Sample MEDLINE record (Courtesy of NLM)

- In-process citations, which provide records for articles before they are indexed with MeSH or converted to out-of-scope status
- Citations to articles that are out-of-scope from certain MEDLINE journals, primarily general science and general chemistry journals, for which only the life sciences articles are indexed with MeSH
- *Ahead of print* citations that precede the article's final publication in a MEDLINE indexed journal
- Citations that precede the date that a journal was selected for MEDLINE indexing
- Pre-1966 citations that have not yet been updated with current MeSH and converted to MEDLINE status
- Citations to some additional life sciences journals that submit full text to PubMed Central (PMC) and receive a qualitative review by NLM
- Citations to author manuscripts of articles published by National Institutes of Health (NIH)-funded researchers
- Citations for books available on the NCBI Bookshelf

PubMed also defines various sets of journals as Journal/Citation subsets.[14] Some of these subsets replace former subject-specific databases that used to be maintained by NLM, such as AIDSLINE and CANCERLIT. An important subset remains *Abridged Index Medicus*, a list created in 1970 of approximately 120 core clinical English-language journals that represent "core clinical journals" for clinicians. There is overview page for all MEDLINE and PubMed documentation.[15]

There are other ways to access MEDLINE. Some information vendors, such as Ovid Technologies[16] and Aries Systems,[17] license the content for a free and provide value-added services that can be accessed for a fee by individuals and institutions.

3.2.1.2 Other NLM Bibliographic Resources

MEDLINE is only one of many databases produced by the NLM [2]. Not only are a number of more specialized databases also available, but they are also accessed from a variety of interfaces. While most of these databases are bibliographic, some provide full text (described in Sect. 3.3). Over the years, NLM has consolidated its bibliographic databases into MEDLINE and then provided "subsets" to narrow searching. The OPAC for NLM's books, serials, and AV materials is LocatorPlus,[18] which also contains some materials which do not reside at the NLM, such as those owned by the regional libraries of the National Network of Libraries of Medicine or other organizations that have agreements with NLM.

Historically, the NLM did not index scientific meeting abstracts except in a few specific subject areas and continues to not do so generally. This is because, in general,

---

[14] https://www.ncbi.nlm.nih.gov/books/NBK3827/table/pubmedhelp.T.journalcitation_subsets/

[15] https://www.nlm.nih.gov/bsd/pmresources.html

[16] https://www.ovid.com/product-details.901.html

[17] https://www.kfinder.com/kfinder/

[18] https://locatorplus.gov

conference proceedings publications are thought to be less critically peer-reviewed than journal publications as well as of less interest to searchers outside the specialty from which they were generated. However, some conference proceedings abstracts are in MEDLINE, including those from the field of biomedical and health informatics from conferences of the American Medical Informatics Association (AMIA).

3.2.1.3 Non-NLM Bibliographic Databases

The NLM is not the sole producer of bibliographic databases. A number of other entities, public and private, produce a wide variety of databases. Many of these databases used to be available from the two largest online information vendors, BRS (assets now owned by Ovid) and Dialog (Dialog Corp.).[19] Now, however, many information producers provide access to their bibliographic databases directly on their own Web sites. In the discussion that follows, we consider non-NLM bibliographic databases that we group into those of large general coverage, subject specific, and content-type specific.

Another long-standing biomedical and health bibliographic database is EMBASE,[20] which is complementary to MEDLINE [6]. EMBASE has a more international focus, including more non-English-language journals. These journals are often important for those carrying out systematic reviews and meta-analyses, who need access to all the studies done across the world [7].

The modern era of journals being published on the Web, even if their full-text content is behind a paywall, has led to a number of bibliographic databases discovered by Web crawling. The first of these was Google Scholar,[21] which indexes scientific publications discovered in the Google's larger Web-crawling effort. Other similar efforts include Microsoft Academic,[22] Semantic Scholar,[23] and Scopus.[24] All of these databases include links to the full text of articles as well as cited and citing documents. Their content goes beyond scientific articles to also include reports, presentations, patents, scientific Web pages, and more.

A variety of subject-specific bibliographic databases have existed for several decades although have evolved in the modern era. Some come from other US government agencies. For example, the Department of Education produces the ERIC (*Educational Resources Information Center*) database,[25] which has citations from education-related literature. Others come from private companies. For example, the major database for the nursing and allied health fields is CINAHL (*Cumulative Index to Nursing and Allied Health Literature*),[26] which covers nursing, physical

[19] https://dialog.com/

[20] https://www.elsevier.com/solutions/embase-biomedical-research

[21] https://scholar.google.com/

[22] https://academic.microsoft.com/home

[23] https://www.semanticscholar.org/

[24] https://www.elsevier.com/solutions/scopus

[25] https://eric.ed.gov/

[26] https://health.ebsco.com/products/the-cinahl-database

therapy, occupational therapy, laboratory technology, health education, physician assistants, and other allied health fields. Another prominent subject-specific database is PsycINFO,[27] which is produced by the American Psychological Association. A database of peer-reviewed journal literature for the complementary and alternative medicine field is the *Manual Alternative and Natural Therapy Index System* (MANTIS).[28]

A number of computer and information science bibliographic resources are valuable for the biomedical and health informatics field. These include:

- The Collection of Computer Science Bibliographies (CSB)[29]
- Digital Bibliography & Library Project (DBLP)[30]
- ACM Guide to Computing Literature[31]

Other bibliographic databases provide access to online resources. For medical educators, the Association of American Medical Colleges (AAMC) has developed MedEdPORTAL,[32] a database of peer-reviewed medical education resources. Each record in the database contains metadata about the resource, such as its educational objectives and document type. A more general database of learning objects is MERLOT (*Multimedia Educational Resource for Learning and Online Teaching*).[33] Likewise, for computer programmers, a bibliographic resource of computer code is Krugle.[34] Although a commercial product, a database of open-source computer code is available for free.

A database of all available books is *Books in Print*.[35] Of course, the major online booksellers such as Amazon.com[36] and Barnes & Noble[37] also can be considered to maintain bibliographic databases of books (that they sell). Another important database is ProQuest Dissertations & Theses Global (formerly *Dissertation Abstracts*),[38] which provides a curated collection of dissertations and theses from around the world dating back for North American universities to 1861.

There are also a growing number of bibliographic collections about available datasets. The biomedical and healthCAre Data Discovery Index Ecosystem (bioCADDIE) [8] is accessed via the DataMed search interface[39] and is based on a DAta Tag Suite (DATS) for datasets [9]. Other bibliographic sources of datasets include:

[27] https://www.apa.org/pubs/databases/psycinfo/
[28] http://www.healthindex.com/MANTIS.aspx
[29] https://liinwww.ira.uka.de/bibliography/
[30] https://dblp.uni-trier.de/
[31] https://dl.acm.org/dl.cfm
[32] https://www.mededportal.org/
[33] https://www.merlot.org/merlot/
[34] https://www.krugle.com/
[35] https://www.booksinprint.com/Home/Index
[36] https://www.amazon.com/
[37] https://www.barnesandnoble.com/
[38] https://www.proquest.com/products-services/pqdtglobal.html
[39] https://datamed.org/

- Google Dataset Search,[40] which provides access to online datasets [10, 11].
- Another source of research datasets is r3data.org[41]—Registry of Research Data Repositories [12].
- The (Re)usable Data Project[42] [13].

3.2.2 Web Catalogs and Feeds

While some may not consider Web catalogs to be bibliographic content, they share many features with traditional bibliographic databases. This is especially true for Web catalogs that provide other content on their sites or more exhaustive descriptions of Web sites than a traditional bibliographic database might. One of the original Web catalogs was Medical Matrix [14], which existed before the Web as a text file of medical resources on the Internet. It has since developed an exhaustive database of sites that are rated by its editorial board consisting of physicians and other healthcare professionals. For each topic area, a variety of links are provided for different types of resources. Some other early medical Web catalogs, now defunct, include Cliniweb [15] and HealthWeb [16].

Some health-oriented Web catalogs that still exist include:

- HONselect[43]—a European catalog of clinician-oriented Web content from the Health on the Net Foundation that adheres to the HONcode of trustworthy information on the Web [17]
- Translating Research into Practice (TRIP)[44]—a database of evidence-based online resources, including full-text journals, electronic textbooks, and other resources

There are also bibliographic-type Web feeds that provide short summaries of Web content and can be rendered by apps that can parse them. The original Web feed was RSS, which is claimed to stand for either Really Simple Syndication or Rich Site Summary [18]. RSS feeds provide short summaries, typically of news or other recent postings on Web sites. Many news sites, such as CNN[45] and BBC,[46] make extensive use of them. NLM also supports RSS feeds through PubMed.[47] Users receive RSS feeds by an RSS aggregator that can typically be configured for the site(s) desired and to filter based on content.

---

[40] https://datasetsearch.research.google.com/

[41] https://www.re3data.org/

[42] http://reusabledata.org/

[43] https://www.hon.ch/HONselect/

[44] http://www.tripdatabase.com

[45] https://www.cnn.com/

[46] https://www.bbc.com/

[47] https://www.nlm.nih.gov/bsd/disted/pubmedtutorial/040_060.html

There are unfortunately a number of different versions of RSS, although each has the fundamental fields and most aggregators can handle all of the different versions. The various versions can be grouped into two categories. One category (version 1.0) builds on the Resource Description Framework (RDF) and aims to allow rich metadata, while the other category (version 2.0) uses plain XML and aims to be simpler. A competing Web feed called Atom was developed but never achieved widespread use [18]. The fundamental fields of RSS include:

- Title—name of item
- Link—URL of full page
- Description—brief description of page

Here is an example of XML code from an RSS item from Wikipedia[48]:

```
<rss version="2.0">
<channel>
 <title>RSS Title</title>
 <description>This is an example of an RSS feed</description>
 <link>http://www.example.com/main.html</link>
 <lastBuildDate>Mon, 06 Sep 2010 00:01:00 +0000 </lastBuildDate>
 <pubDate>Sun, 06 Sep 2009 16:20:00 +0000</pubDate>
 <ttl>1800</ttl>

 <item>
  <title>Example entry</title>
  <description>Here is some text containing an interesting descrip-
tion.</description>
  <link>http://www.example.com/blog/post/1</link>
            <guid       isPermaLink="false">7bd204c6-1655-4c27-
aeee-53f933c5395f</guid>
  <pubDate>Sun, 06 Sep 2009 16:20:00 +0000</pubDate>
 </item>

</channel>
</rss>
```

3.2.3 Specialized Registries

A specialized registry has overlap with literature reference databases and Web catalogs but can be considered to be distinct in that it points to more diverse information resources. An example of a specialized registry is the *Catalog of US Government*

[48] https://en.wikipedia.org/wiki/RSS

Publications,[49] which provides bibliographic links to all governmental publications whether in print, online, or both.

A specialized registry specific to healthcare was the *National Guidelines Clearinghouse* (NGC). Produced by the Agency for Healthcare Research and Quality (AHRQ), it contained exhaustive information about clinical practice guidelines. In 2018, AHRQ shut down the National Guidelines Clearinghouse [19]. The original contractor developing the NGC was the nonprofit research firm, ECRI, which developed a new site, ECRI Guidelines Trust.[50] This site adheres to principles of trustworthy clinical guidelines developed by the Institute of Medicine [20] and implemented as the NGC Extent of Adherence to Trustworthy Standards (NEATS) instrument, whose items include [21]:

- Disclosure of the funding source
- Disclosure and management of conflicts of interest
- Multidisciplinary input; incorporation of patient perspectives
- Rigorous systematic review
- Recommendations accompanied by rationale, assessment of benefits and harms, clear linkage to the evidence, and assessment of strength of evidence and strength of recommendation
- Clear articulation of recommendations
- External review by diverse stakeholders and plans for updating

Another organization that has created a bibliographic resource of practice guidelines is Guidelines Central.[51]

3.3 Full-Text Content

Full-text content contains the complete text of a resource as well as associated tables, figures, images, and other graphics. If a database has a corresponding print version, then the text portions of the electronic and print versions are typically identical. The original full-text databases were online versions of journals and thus tended to be either primary literature or mixtures of primary and secondary literature. As the price of computers and CD-ROM drives fell in the early 1990s, adaptation of non-journal secondary sources such as textbooks increased. This trend has not only continued with the growth of the Internet but led to the development of vast Web sites with information aimed at a variety of audiences. Full-text products usually do not have associated human-assigned indexing terms. Instead, the indexing terms are typically the words that appear in the text, as will be described in Chap. 4.

---

[49] https://catalog.gpo.gov/

[50] https://guidelines.ecri.org/

[51] https://www.guidelinecentral.com/summaries/

3.3.1 Periodicals

The technical impediments to electronic publishing of journals have long passed, and, as was discussed in Chap. 2, the challenges now are mostly political and economic [22]. Just about all scientific journals, certainly those in health and biomedicine, are now published electronically. Commercial publishers such as Springer[52] and Elsevier[53] tend to package collections of their journals to sell to large customers, such as libraries and universities. An early publisher of online biomedical and health journals, especially those published by nonprofit publishers such as scientific and medical societies, was HighWire Press,[54] a spin-off of the Stanford University Library that provided a Web site, searching and browsing interfaces, and development tools for journals whose publishers have not moved directly into electronic publishing. Other commercial publishers now offer such services to which a number of journals have moved.

Some journals publish exclusively in electronic format, such as the journals of Biomed Central[55] and *Journal of Medical Internet Research* plus its family of sister publications.[56] Many of these journals use the open-access publishing model introduced in Sect. 2.6.1 and described more fully in Sect. 6.4.3. Biomed Central publishes dozens of peer-reviewed journals on a variety of biological and health topics, including medicine, cell biology, medical informatics, etc. and is now owned by Springer Nature. Another family of open-access journals is the Public Library of Science (PLoS).[57] One innovation from PLoS was *PLos ONE*, which aimed to break down the disciplinary walls between journals and also provide an open and innovative form of post-publication peer review (after the initial traditional peer review to deem acceptance) [23].

A number of government entities provide periodical information in full-text form. Among the best known of these are *Morbidity and Mortality Weekly Report* (MMWR)[58] from the Centers for Disease Control and Prevention (CDC) and *AHRQ WebM&M: Morbidity & Mortality Rounds on the Web*,[59] which focuses on medical errors and patient safety.

Electronic publication of journals allows additional features that were not possible in the print world. Journal Web sites can provide supplemental information, such as additional description of methods, results, images, and even raw data. A journal Web site also allows more dialogue about articles than could be published in a Letters to the Editor section of a print journal. Electronic publication also allows true bibliographic linkages, both to other full-text articles and to the MEDLINE

---

[52] https://www.springer.com/

[53] https://www.elsevier.com/

[54] http://highwire.org/

[55] https://www.biomedcentral.com/

[56] https://www.jmir.org/

[57] https://www.plos.org

[58] https://www.cdc.gov/mmwr/

[59] https://psnet.ahrq.gov/webmm/

record, typically from PubMed. Electronic journals also allow linkage to actual data from the study, with many using the Dryad system[60] for linking data to publications from which they came.

Another source for full-text journal articles is the repository PubMed Central (PMC),[61] the rationale for which is explained in Chap. 6. PMC is meant to be an archive for all literature that results from research funded in the United States by NIH. While several thousand journals deposit articles directly, researchers who publish government-funded research in other journals must deposit their final manuscripts (before typesetting by the journal) into PMC. Authors submit manuscripts directly must use the NIH Manuscript Submission System (NIHMS).[62] Most of the major biomedical and health informatics journals deposit papers reporting on NIH-funded research into PMC. Also in PMC are papers from the *AMIA Annual Symposium Proceedings*, which has been called various names over the years, dating back to the *Symposium on Computer Applications in Medical Care* (SCAMC).[63]

NLM has brought more standardization to electronic journal publishing with what was originally called the Journal Archiving and Interchange Document Type Definition (DTD) and is now called the Journal Article Tag Suite (JATS)[64] and is now an ANSI/NISO standard.[65]

Another effort of PMC is the Back Issue Digitization Project, which aims to scan back issues of participating journals.[66] The scanned pages for each article are combined into a single PDF file, with appropriate JATS metadata applied. The text has optical character recognition (OCR) applied for searching, although OCR errors are not corrected. A growing number of other journal publishers have been scanning archives back to their inception, such as BMJ to 1840 [24] and JAMA to 1883 [25].

3.3.2 Books and Reports

The most common secondary literature source is the traditional textbook, an increasing number of which are available in computer form. One of the first textbooks available electronically was *Scientific American Medicine*, later *ACP Medicine*, but now has ceased publication. Some venerable print textbooks are now available electronically include the *Physicians' Desk Reference*,[67] Micromedex,[68] and *Merck Manual*.[69]

---

[60] https://datadryad.org/

[61] https://www.ncbi.nlm.nih.gov/pmc/

[62] https://www.nihms.nih.gov/

[63] https://www.ncbi.nlm.nih.gov/pmc/journals/362/

[64] https://jats.nlm.nih.gov/

[65] https://www.niso.org/publications/z3996-2019-jats

[66] https://www.ncbi.nlm.nih.gov/pmc/about/scanning/

[67] https://www.pdr.net/

[68] https://www.ibm.com/watson-health/learn/micromedex

[69] https://www.merckmanuals.com/professional

A common approach with textbooks is to bundle them, sometimes with linkages across the aggregated texts. An early bundler of textbooks was *STAT!-Ref*,[70] which like many began as a CD-ROM product and then moved to the Web. *STAT!-Ref* now offers mostly its own content. Another early product that implemented linking early was a combination of *Harrison's Principles of Internal Medicine* and the drug reference *US Pharmacopeia*, which is now part of a large collection called *AccessMedicine*.[71] Another early online medical textbook was *MDConsult*, which was acquired by Elsevier and folded into its ClinicalKey product.[72]

Electronic textbooks offer features beyond text from the print version. While many print textbooks do feature high-quality images, electronic versions offer the ability to have more pictures and illustrations. They also have the ability to use sound and video, although few do at this time. As with full-text journals, electronic textbooks can link to other resources, including journal references and the full articles. Many Web-based textbook sites also provide access to continuing education self-assessment questions and medical news. And finally, electronic textbooks let authors and publishers provide more frequent updates of the information than is allowed by the usual cycle of print editions, where new versions come out only every 2–5 years.

Making a textbook or other tertiary literature source usable as an electronic database requires some reorganization of the text. The approach used by most vendors is to break books down into "documents" along their hierarchical structure. Since the text of most books is divided into chapters, sections, subsections, and so forth, a typical approach will be to reduce the text to the lowest level in a subsection.

Another large and growing collection of online textbooks is the NCBI Bookshelf.[73] This resource contains the full text of several thousand books as well as reports from AHRQ, the National Academy of Medicine, the National Institute for Health Research (the United Kingdom), the Canadian Agency for Drugs and Technologies in Health, and the World Health Organization. One noteworthy title in this collection is *Online Mendelian Inheritance in Man* (OMIM),[74] which is now maintained at a separate site,[75] although the version in NCBI Bookshelf is kept up to date [26]. A key feature of this reference is its linkage to references in MEDLINE as well as genomics databases, the latter of which are described in more detail in Sect. 3.4.4.

Consumer health information also has been an area of rapid growth in full-text information [27, 28]. While traditional consumer-oriented books on health topics are still plentiful in bookstores, and some have migrated online (e.g., *The Merck Manual Home Edition*[76]), the real growth has occurred with consumer-oriented Web sites, which are described in the next section.

---

[70] http://www.tetondata.com/

[71] https://accessmedicine.mhmedical.com/

[72] https://www.clinicalkey.com/

[73] https://www.ncbi.nlm.nih.gov/books

[74] https://www.ncbi.nlm.nih.gov/omim

[75] https://omim.org/

[76] https://www.merckmanuals.com/home

There have been some common trends in biomedical and health journal and textbook publishing over the years. One has been consolidation among publishers and a trend to offer large aggregations on a subscription basis. Another has been the movement to mobile devices, from smartphones to tablets.

3.3.3 *Web Collections*

As noted at the beginning of the chapter, we use the term "Web collection" for the classification of discrete collections of Web pages providing full-text information. Health-oriented Web sites are produced by everyone from individuals to nonprofit entities to companies to governments. The Web has fundamentally altered the publishing of health information. To begin with, the bar of entry has been significantly lowered. Virtually anyone can have access to a Web server, and with that access, he or she can become a "publisher" of health or any other type of information. The ease of producing and disseminating has had ramifications, e.g., the ease of copying content threatens protection of intellectual property and the ease of pasting can lead to plagiarism. The Internet, through Web sites, news groups, email lists, and chat rooms, also rapidly speeds the dissemination of information and misinformation. Nonetheless, there are a great many Web sites that empower the healthcare provider and consumer alike.

Probably the most effective user of the Web to provide health information is the US government. The bibliographic databases of the NLM, NCI, AHRQ, and others have been described. These agencies have also been innovative in providing comprehensive full-text information for healthcare providers and consumers as well. Some of these (in particular MedlinePlus) are described later as aggregations (Sect. 3.5), since they provide many different types of resources. Smaller yet still comprehensive Web sites include:

- The Diseases & Conditions[77] and Travelers' Health[78] Web sites of the Centers for Disease Control and Prevention (CDC)
- Health information from other NIH institutes besides NLM, such as the National Cancer Institute,[79] National Institute of Diabetes and Digestive and Kidney Diseases,[80] and the National Heart, Lung, and Blood Institute[81]
- Information on HIV/AIDS from NIH[82]

---

[77] https://www.cdc.gov/DiseasesConditions/

[78] https://wwwnc.cdc.gov/travel

[79] https://www.cancer.gov/

[80] https://www.niddk.nih.gov/health-information

[81] https://www.nhlbi.nih.gov/

[82] https://aidsinfo.nih.gov/

- Drug use and regulatory information from the Food and Drug Administration (FDA) for professionals[83] and consumers[84]
- Evidence reports and other information from the AHRQ Effective Health Care Program[85]

A large number of commercial consumer health Web sites have come and gone over years. Some early well-known sites that were eventually sunset included Intelihealth and NetWellness. Some sites that do remain include:

- Harvard Health Publishing[86]
- Mayoclinic.org[87]
- WebMD[88]
- Health Finder[89]

A number of medical associations and other organizations provide Web collections:

- American Academy of Dermatology[90]
- American Academy of Family Physicians[91]
- Federal Consumer Health Information Center[92]
- RxMed[93]

A number of organizations have used the Web to publish the full text of their clinical practice guidelines, including the following:

- American College of Cardiology[94]
- American College of Physicians[95]
- Institute for Clinical Systems Improvement[96]
- International Diabetes Federation[97]

---

[83] https://dailymed.nlm.nih.gov/dailymed/
[84] https://www.fda.gov/consumers
[85] https://effectivehealthcare.ahrq.gov/
[86] https://www.health.harvard.edu/
[87] https://www.mayoclinic.org/patient-care-and-health-information
[88] https://www.webmd.com/
[89] https://healthfinder.gov/
[90] https://www.aad.org/public
[91] https://familydoctor.org/
[92] https://pueblo.gpo.gov/Publications/PuebloPubs.php
[93] https://www.rxmed.com/
[94] https://www.acc.org/guidelines
[95] https://www.acponline.org/clinical-information/guidelines
[96] https://www.icsi.org/guidelines/
[97] https://www.idf.org/e-library/guidelines.html

In the computer science IR field, the ACM Special Interest Group on Information Retrieval (SIGIR)[98] maintains a repository of scanned documents of early research from the period of 1960–1991.[99] Likewise, in the space science field, the NASA Image and Video Library[100] makes available the entire collection of images, videos, sounds, and more.

A number of new types of Web content have achieved prominence over the years and found use in health and biomedicine. One of these is the wiki, or free encyclopedia. Wikis allow any individual in a community to write or edit an entry. This allows massive distributed and collaborative work to be done. For example, the prototype wiki, *Wikipedia*,[101] has millions of entries in a variety of languages. One recent commentator noted that Wikipedia has withstood the test of time and continues to be a valuable resource [29]. A number of medical wikis have been cataloged by Wikipedia,[102] including *Clinfowiki*, which is devoted to clinical informatics.[103] Wikipedia has made efforts to improve the quality of its health-related content [30], and one medical school allows fourth-year medical students to get credit for editing medical content in Wikipedia [31].

Another growing type of Web content is the weblog, or blog. A blog consists of running commentary on a topic and is usually maintained by a person or community. Some blog-like Web sites do not call themselves blogs but have characteristics of them. This author maintains a blog entitled, *The Informatics Professor*.[104]

3.4 Annotated Content

As noted above, annotated content has its metadata tightly integrated with the content (as opposed to being in a separate bibliographic database). It includes resources such as images, citation databases, and biomedical research data. Although these types of content are usually annotated with some amount of text, and searched with IR systems, their make-up is of predominantly nontextual material or nonnarrative text.

98 https://sigir.org/

99 https://sigir.org/resources/museum/

100 https://images.nasa.gov/

101 https://en.wikipedia.org/wiki/Main_Page

102 https://en.wikipedia.org/wiki/List_of_medical_wikis

103 http://www.clinfowiki.org/

104 http://informaticsprofessor.blogspot.com/

3.4.1 Images and Videos

Image and video collections have always been an important part of healthcare practice, especially in the so-called "visual" medical specialties such as radiology, pathology, and dermatology. These collections tend to come and go, and often their Web addresses change over time. Table 3.5 provides a sampling of

Table 3.5 A sampling of medical image and video databases

Name	Organization	URL
General		
Visible Human	National Library of Medicine	https://www.nlm.nih.gov/research/visible/visible_human.html
Images from the History of Medicine	National Library of Medicine	https://www.nlm.nih.gov/hmd/ihm/
Open-i	National Library of Medicine	https://openi.nlm.nih.gov/
HON Images	Health on the Net Foundation	https://www.hon.ch/Media/media.html
Bio-Image Search	Stanford University	https://lane.stanford.edu/bioimagesearch.html
Health Education Assets Library (HEAL)	University of Utah	https://library.med.utah.edu/heal/
MEDtube online medical videos	MEDtube	https://medtube.net/
Viziometrics diagrams, visualizations, and photographs from scientific publications	Viziometrics	http://www.viziometrics.org/
Dermatology		
Dermatologic Online Image Atlas	University of Heidelberg and University of Erlangen	https://www.dermis.net/
DermNet Skin Disease Image Atlas	Interactive Medical Media LLC	http://www.dermnet.com/
Interactive Dermatology Atlas		http://www.dermatlas.net/index.cfm
VisualDx—commercial decision support system	VisualDx	https://www.visualdx.com/
Pathology		
WebPath	University of Utah	https://webpath.med.utah.edu/
Pathology Education Instructional Resource (PEIR)	University of Alabama at Birmingham	http://peir.path.uab.edu/library/
Radiology		
Interactive Radiology Atlas	SUNY Downstate Medical Center	https://act.downstate.edu/courseware/rad-atlas/
MedPix Database of Teaching Cases	National Library of Medicine	https://medpix.nlm.nih.gov/home
PEIR Radiology	University of Alabama at Birmingham	http://peir.path.uab.edu/library/index.php?/category/106

current image and video databases. Several of them come from the NLM and are described in the literature:

- Visible Human Project—collection of three-dimensional representations of normal male and female bodies, consisting of cross-sectional slices of cadavers, with sections of 1 mm thickness in the male and 0.3 mm thickness in the female [32]. Also available from each cadaver are transverse computerized tomography and magnetic resonance images.
- Images from the History of Medicine—online access to images from the historical collections of the NLM.
- Open-I—collection of images from PubMed Central papers [33].

3.4.2 *Citations*

Chapter 2 described bibliometrics, the field concerned with linkage of the scientific literature. Bibliometric databases can be very useful in IR, i.e., searchers may wish to find new articles by tracing references from those they have found. The original citation databases of scientific literature were the *Science Citation Index* (SCI) and *Social Sciences Citation Index* (SSCI), which are now part of *Web of Science*.[105] A number of other Web bibliographic resources maintain cited and cited documents, in essence becoming citation databases. These include Google Scholar,[106] Microsoft Academic,[107] Semantic Scholar,[108] and Scopus.[109] An additional citation database is iCite,[110] from the NIH, which aggregates citation from a number of different sources [34].

3.4.3 *Evidence-Based Medicine Resources*

Although in some ways textbooks and in other ways aggregations, evidence-based medicine (EBM) resources deserve special mention because of their unique resources as well as importance to healthcare. As noted in Chap. 2, there has been an evolution in EBM to make it more useful for busy clinicians with the emergence of the 4S model [35] that has expanded to the 6S model [36].

Like all bodies of scientific research, the foundation of the 4S/5S/6S models consists of studies, which are typically journal articles. Of course, full articles may be long and detailed beyond what a clinician wants to read, yet just the abstract

---

[105] https://clarivate.com/webofsciencegroup/

[106] https://scholar.google.com/

[107] https://academic.microsoft.com/home

[108] https://www.semanticscholar.org/

[109] https://www.elsevier.com/solutions/scopus

[110] https://icite.od.nih.gov/

would be too short. Thus, another type of full-text information associated with EBM is summaries of journal articles. Probably the best known among these are the Massachusetts Medical Society's *Journal Watch*[111] and, from the American College of Physicians (ACP), *Journal Club*, which was originally published standalone but later folded into ACP's journal *Annals of Internal Medicine*.[112] ACP Journal Club uses a highly structured format designed to provide the reader all the important details of the study, including pertinent EBM statistics, such as patient population, intervention, and number needed to treat [37].

Another approach to annotating journal articles is *JournalWise*, which uses the McMaster Online Rating of Evidence (MORE) system,[113] where clinicians rate journal articles already filtered for scientific (i.e., evidence-based) merit [38, 39]. Several thousand clinicians rate clinically oriented journal articles on seven-point scales for relevance to practice and newsworthiness. The ratings are averaged for specific medical disciplines so that users of MORE will see ratings that have been made by physicians and nurses in their own specialties.

When the primary literature of a given topic gets large, there are likely to be syntheses about it, usually in the form of systematic reviews, which may include meta-analysis when enough studies exist and are homogeneous enough to have their results combined. Many systematic reviews are published in medical journals, although once that is done, they tend to become static documents that are not updated when new studies become available. This shortcoming has led to the development of the *Cochrane Database of Systematic Reviews*,[114] which is the largest collection (though far from covering all of medicine) of reviews of health and medical interventions. The Evidence-Based Practice Centers of AHRQ are also a source of systematic reviews (which they call evidence reports).

Of course, most systematic reviews are long and detailed, so the next level in the 4S/5S/6S models is synopses, which provide easily readable and digestible evidence-based overviews. While some EBM purists argue that *UpToDate*[115] is not completely evidence-based, e.g., not all statements are tagged with levels of evidence or support from studies of the highest-quality evidence, the resource is comprehensive and very popular among clinicians as well as those in training. Another collection of evidence-based summaries of conditions comes from *DynaMed*,[116] which tags recommendations for clinician actions such as tests and treatments with an evidence level of 1–3. DynaMed also offers an evidence overview for all topics.

Another collection of EBM content is POEMS[117] ("Patient-Oriented Evidence that Matters"), which offers short evidence-based synopses. Topics are selected

---

[111] https://www.jwatch.org/

[112] https://annals.org/aim/journal-club

[113] http://hiru.mcmaster.ca/more/

[114] https://www.cochranelibrary.com/

[115] https://www.uptodate.com/

[116] https://www.dynamed.com/

[117] https://www.essentialevidenceplus.com/content/poems

based on whether they address a question faced by physicians, measure outcomes that physicians and their patients care about (e.g., symptoms, morbidity, quality of life, and mortality), and have the potential to change the way medicine is practiced. POEMS are part of an EBM aggregation called *Essential Evidence Plus* to be discussed later in this chapter.

An additional collection of EBM resources is Epistemonikos,[118] which includes a variety of systematic reviews and bibliographic databases, accessible through a single search interface [40]. Epistemonikos allows searching in nine different languages and also features an application programming interface (API) to allow other applications to access its resources.[119]

The Family Practice Inquiries Network (FPIN)[120] is a project led by leading Departments of Family Medicine in the United States. It features several resources:

- Good Evidence Matters (GEMs)—summaries of recently published studies.
- HelpDesk Answers (HDAs)—short research articles that provide evidence-based answers to clinical questions in a structured format.
- Priority Updates from the Research Literature (PURLs)—knowledge translation that targets newly published research expected to change family medicine and primary care practice.
- Clinical Inquiries (CIs)—The goal of this resource is to develop a resource that answers 80% of primary care clinical questions in 60 s. This is being done by collecting the most common clinical questions and providing specific answers to them. In some ways this is analogous to the "Frequently Asked Questions" (FAQs) seen on many Web sites.
- *Evidence-Based Practice* (EBP)—a monthly journal focused on topics relevant to the daily practice of family medicine.

At the top of the 4S/5S/6S models are systems, which are usually provided as order sets or clinical decision support rules that can be used within electronic health records (EHRs). There is a growing market for such content, which is produced not only by EHR vendors but also by companies that produce and market them:

- Zynx[121]
- Provation[122]

A related form of structured information we may see in the future is computable knowledge that encodes the knowledge in forms that can be used by applications, including and beyond EHRs [41].

---

[118] https://www.epistemonikos.org/en/

[119] https://api.epistemonikos.org/

[120] http://www.fpin.org/

[121] https://www.zynxhealth.com/

[122] https://www.provationmedical.com/order-set-management/

3.4.4 Molecular Biology and -Omics

Another important category of annotated information is from molecular biology and the various -omics (e.g., genomics, proteomics, metabolomics, etc.). The first -omics to gain prominence was genomics, the field studying genetic material in living organisms. A milestone in genomics was reached in 2001 with the publication of a "working draft" of the human genome published simultaneously by the publicly sponsored Human Genome Project [42] and the private company Celera Genomics [43]. The final sequence of the three billion nucleotides that comprise the human genome was completed in 2003 [44].

An excellent source of information for -omics and related data is the annual Database Issue of the journal, *Nucleic Acids Research*[123] [45]. A prominent article in each year's issue is an overview of the database resources from the NLM National Center for Biotechnology Information [2]. The NLM continues to evolve and improve its genomics resources in response to new technologies, data, types, and usability concerns. A key feature is linkage across databases, from the nucleotide sequences in GenBank [46] to human clinical variation in ClinVar [47]. Some of these data sources are summarized in the Genome Data Viewer,[124] which organizes them based on the location of their activity on the chromosome, as shown in Fig. 3.2.

One unique aspect of the molecular biology research community (certainly in comparison to other biomedical sciences) has been the sharing of data among researchers. Some of this sharing has been made possible by the development of public databases from the NCBI. However, scientists themselves as well as those developing databases with genome-related content have in general made their information widely available. The myriad of genomics databases are reviewed annually in the first issue of the journal *Nucleic Acids Research*, which is now published as open access and is freely available on the Web. A related annual issue has emerged more recently devoted to Web services providing access to bioinformatics tools.

The entirety of NCBI databases, including the already-discussed PubMed and NCBI Bookshelf, is called Entrez and is available from a pan-search interface.[125] Table 3.6 shows the organization of NCBI databases as they currently stand. There are a number of other genomics-related resources maintained by NCBI:

- GenBank[126]—genetic sequence database, an annotated collection of all publicly available DNA sequences. GenBank is part of the International Nucleotide Sequence Database Collaboration, which comprises the DNA Data Bank of Japan (DDBJ), the European Nucleotide Archive (ENA), and GenBank at

[123] http://nar.oxfordjournals.org/

[124] https://www.ncbi.nlm.nih.gov/genome/gdv/

[125] https://www.ncbi.nlm.nih.gov/search/

[126] https://www.ncbi.nlm.nih.gov/genbank/

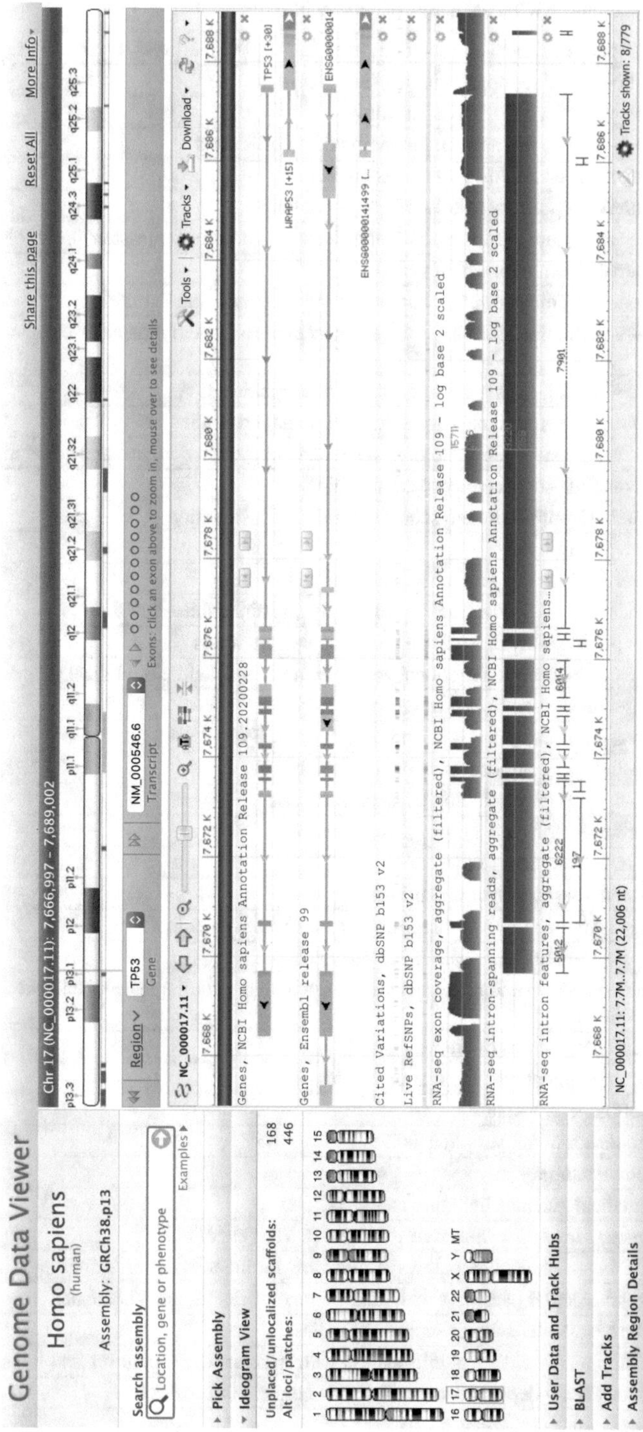

Fig. 3.2 Genome Data Viewer for the region of 7667000-7689000 on the *Homo sapiens* chromosome 17 (Courtesy of NLM)

Table 3.6 Organization of NCBI databases (Courtesy of NLM)

Literature—repository of medical and scientific abstracts, full-text articles, books, and reports
• Bookshelf—books and reports, including GeneReviews
• MeSH—vocabulary for MEDLINE indexing
• NLM Catalog—books, journals, and more in NLM collections
• PubMed—scientific and medical abstracts/citations
• PubMed Central—repository of full-text journal articles
Genes—sequences and annotations for study of orthologs structure, expression, and evolution
• Gene—collected information about gene loci
• Gene Expression Omnibus (GEO) Datasets—functional genomics studies
• Gene Expression Omnibus (GEO) Profiles—gene expression and molecular abundance profiles
• HomoloGene—homologous gene sets for selected organisms
• PopSet—sequence sets from phylogenetic and population studies
Proteins—sequences, 3D structures, and tools of functional protein domains and active sites
• Conserved Domains—conserved protein domains
• Identical Protein Groups—protein sequences grouped by identity
• Protein—protein sequences
• Protein Clusters—sequence similarity-based protein clusters
• Sparcle—functional categorization of proteins by domain architecture
• Structure—experimentally determined biomolecular structures
Genomes—sequence assemblies, functional genomics data, and source biological samples
• Assembly—genome assembly information
• BioCollections—museum, herbaria, and other biorepository collections
• BioProject—biological projects providing data to NCBI
• BioSample—descriptions of biological source materials
• Genome—genome sequencing projects by organism
• Nucleotide—DNA and RNA sequences
• Probe—sequence-based probes and primers
• Sequence Read Archive (SRA)—high-throughput sequence reads
• Taxonomy—taxonomic classification and nomenclature
Genetics—heritable DNA variations, associations with human pathologies, and clinical diagnostics and treatments
• ClinVar—human variations of clinical significance
• dbGaP—genotype/phenotype interaction studies
• dbSNP—short genetic variations
• dbVar—genome structural variation studies
• GTR—genetic testing registry
• MedGen—medical genetics literature and links
• OMIM—*Online Mendelian Inheritance in Man* (OMIM) textbook
Chemicals—information, molecular pathways, and tools for bioactivity screening
• BioSystems—molecular pathways with links to genes, proteins and chemicals
• PubChem BioAssay—bioactivity screening studies
• PubChem Compound—chemical information with structures, information, and links
• PubChem Substance—deposited substance and chemical information

https://www.ncbi.nlm.nih.gov/search/

NCBI. These three organizations exchange data on a daily basis {Sayers, 2020 #7854}.

- NCBI Reference Sequence Database (RefSeq)[127]—comprehensive, integrated, nonredundant, well-annotated set of reference sequences including genomic, transcript, and protein data [48].
- ClinGen[128]—NIH-funded resource dedicated to building a central resource that defines the clinical relevance of genes and variants for use in precision medicine and research [49].
- Genetics Home Reference[129]—consumer-friendly resource of effects of genetic variation on human health [50].
- Gene Expression Omnibus[130]—functional genomics (gene expression) data repository.
- Sequence Read Archive (SRA)[131]—raw sequencing data and alignment information from high-throughput sequencing platforms.

The various -omics databases are aggregated in different ways, especially with a focus on their content in human health and disease. There is an overview of human genome resources at NCBI.[132] Aggregated Reference Sequence (RefSeq) is viewable graphically on the different human chromosomes by the Genome Data Viewer.[133] NCBI also maintains a listing of a subset of databases related to human health on its NCBI Health page.[134]

3.4.5 Educational Resources

Another type of content that many seek on the Web is educational materials. A large amount of material is available through large repositories of what were originally called massive open online courses (MOOCs) [51]:

- Coursera[135]
- edX[136]
- Lynda.com[137]
- Khan Academy[138]

---

[127] https://www.ncbi.nlm.nih.gov/refseq/

[128] https://clinicalgenome.org/

[129] https://ghr.nlm.nih.gov/

[130] https://www.ncbi.nlm.nih.gov/geo/

[131] https://www.ncbi.nlm.nih.gov/sra/

[132] https://www.ncbi.nlm.nih.gov/projects/genome/guide/human/

[133] https://www.ncbi.nlm.nih.gov/genome/gdv/

[134] https://www.ncbi.nlm.nih.gov/home/health/

[135] https://www.coursera.org/

[136] https://www.edx.org/

[137] https://www.lynda.com/

[138] https://www.khanacademy.org/

Also available are archives of materials developed for biomedical informatics and data science, some of which this author has contributed:

- Office of the National Coordinator for Health IT Curriculum[139]
- NIH Big Data to Knowledge (BD2K) modules[140]
- Videos from the BD2K Guide to the Fundamentals of Data Science[141]
- What is Biomedical and Health Informatics?[142]

3.4.6 Linked Data

As noted in Chap. 2, many believe that a next step in data transparency and utility for biomedical research is for researchers to share their raw data. We saw in Sect. 3.1 that a number of bibliographic resources have been developed for accessing datasets. A further step is for structured data itself to be represented on the World Wide Web. This notion was originally dubbed the "Semantic Web" by Web creator Tim Berners-Lee [52]. A data structure that emerged for such data is the Resource Description Framework (RDF), which consists of subject-predicate-object triples, with each identified by URIs and queried by the SPARQL Protocol and RDF Query Language (SPARQL). RDF triples are the building blocks of ontologies, which can be expressed in the Web Ontology Language (OWL). This whole construct of annotated data across the Web is now commonly called "linked data" [53].

A number of such linked data collections exist, including:

- Springer Nature Linked Data[143]
- Wikidata[144]
- DBpedia[145] [54]
- eagle-i[146] [55]

3.4.7 Other Annotated Content

There are a variety of other databases of annotated content:

---

[139] https://www.healthit.gov/topic/health-it-resources/health-it-curriculum-resources-educators

[140] https://dmice.ohsu.edu/bd2k/topics.html

[141] https://www.youtube.com/channel/UCKIDQOa0JcUd3K9C1TS7FLQ/videos

[142] http://informatics.health

[143] https://scigraph.springernature.com/explorer

[144] https://www.wikidata.org/wiki/Wikidata:Main_Page

[145] https://wiki.dbpedia.org/

[146] https://www.eagle-i.net/

Table 3.7 Summary of information in ClinicalTrials.gov records (Courtesy of NLM)

All ClinicalTrials.gov records contain summary information about a study protocol, including:
• Disease or condition
• Intervention (e.g., medical product, behavior, or procedure being studied)
• Title, description, and design of the study
• Requirements for participation (eligibility criteria)
• Locations where the study conducted
• Contact information for study locations
• Links to relevant information on other health Web sites, MedlinePlus and PubMed
Some records also include information on the results of the study, including:
• Description of study participants—number of participants starting and completing study and their demographic data
• Outcomes of study
• Summary of adverse events experienced by study participants

https://clinicaltrials.gov/ct2/about-site/background

- *NIH RePORTER*[147]—a database of all of grants, contracts, and other projects conducted or funded by the NIH.
- HSRProj[148]—a database of ongoing projects in health services research.
- Search capabilities over the documents, emails, viewed Web pages, and so forth on one's own computer. Both the Windows and Macintosh operating systems allow searching over information in files on their disks these days.

Another annotated database of note is ClinicalTrials.gov.[149] Starting as a database of clinical trials sponsored by NIH, ClinicalTrials.gov has taken on new roles over the years. After problems were uncovered with post-inception protocol changes in clinical trials, the International Committee of Medical Journal Editors (ICMJE) adopted a policy of requiring registration at inception of study [56]. This required that clinical trials be registered in ClinicalTrials.gov [57] or other comparable databases [58] before they began in order to be later published, with the aim of preventing selective reporting or modification of study protocols after the trial had started. An additional rule expanding the legal mandate for sponsors and others responsible for clinical trials of FDA-regulated drug, biologic, and device products to register their studies and report summary results information to ClinicalTrials.gov was implemented in 2016 [59]. A next step under consideration is the inclusion of individual patient data [60]. The current contents of ClinicalTrials.gov records are listed in Table 3.7.

The US Food and Drug Administration (FDA) has improved its information availability. Two resources of note include:

[147] https://projectreporter.nih.gov/reporter.cfm

[148] https://hsrproject.nlm.nih.gov/

[149] https://clinicaltrials.gov/

- MedWatch[150]—reporting system for adverse events
- Drugs@FDA[151]—database of FDA-approved products

A comparison of results reporting for new drug approval trials from ClinicalTrials.gov and Drugs@FDA found results congruent but former with more adverse events details [61].

3.5 Aggregations

The real value of the Web, of course, is its ability to aggregate disparate information resources. This chapter so far has focused for the most part on individual resources. This section provides some examples of aggregated resources oriented toward consumers and professionals. We will also look in detail at two specific types of aggregations, the body of knowledge and model organism databases.

3.5.1 Consumer Health

One of the largest aggregated consumer information resources is MedlinePlus[152] from the NLM. MedlinePlus includes representatives of the types of resources already described, aggregated so they are easily accessed for a given topic. MedlinePlus includes nine types of information[153]:

- Health topics—pages covering wellness issues, diseases, illnesses, and health conditions
- Medical encyclopedia—articles and images related to hundreds of diseases and conditions
- External health links—links to Web pages from selected government agencies and health-related organizations
- Medical tests—articles about medical tests
- Drugs and supplements—prescription and over-the-counter medication information and information on herbs and supplements
- National Institutes of Health—links to articles and images created by the 27 Institutes and Centers at NIH
- *MedlinePlus Magazine*—articles from the online version of the NIH *MedlinePlus Magazine*
- Healthy recipes—recipes showing how to prepare tasty, healthy meals

[150] https://www.fda.gov/safety/medwatch-fda-safety-information-and-adverse-event-reporting-program

[151] https://www.accessdata.fda.gov/scripts/cder/daf/

[152] https://medlineplus.gov/

[153] https://medlineplus.gov/about/using/searchtips/

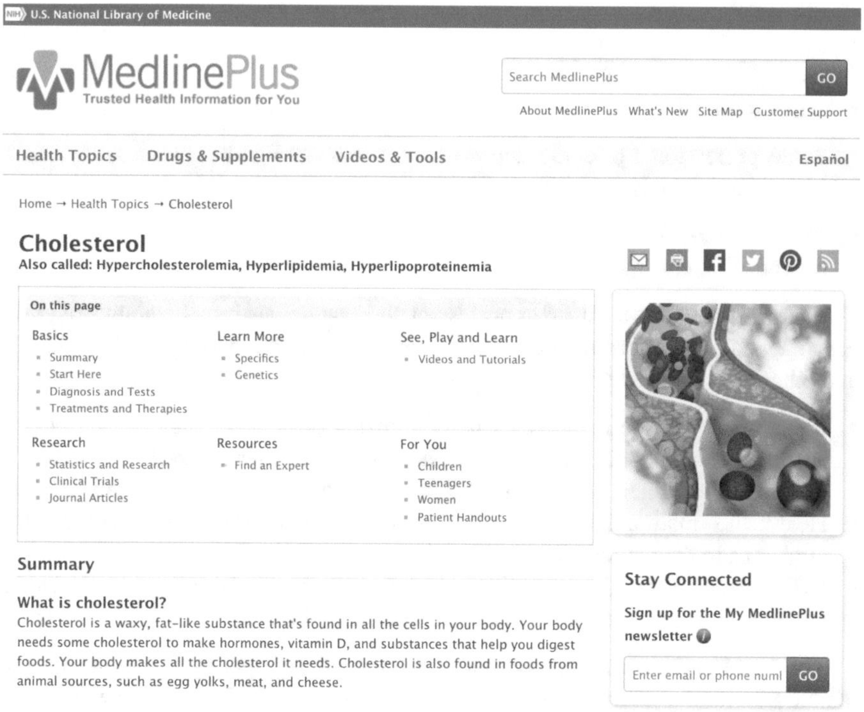

Fig. 3.3 MedlinePlus topic `Cholesterol` (Courtesy of NLM)

- Multiple languages—links to high-quality health information in languages in addition to English and Spanish

The selection of MedlinePlus topics is based on analysis of those used by consumers to search for health information on the NLM Web site [62]. Each topic contains links to health information from the NIH and other sources deemed credible by its editorial staff. There are also links to current health news, a medical encyclopedia, drug references, and directories, along with a preformed PubMed search, related to the topic. Figure 3.3 shows the top of the MedlinePlus page for `cholesterol`.

A number of consumer health Web collections mentioned in Sect. 3.3.3 are actually part of larger aggregations of content that also provide features that can be used to manage health and healthcare.

3.5.2 *Health Professionals*

Most of the large medical publishers that produce textbooks, handbooks, journals, and other resources have aggregated their content into large packages that are sold on a subscription basis:

- Elsevier[154]
- McGraw-Hill Medical[155]
- Springer Publishing[156]
- Wiley & Sons[157]

Some professional-oriented aggregations focus on EBM resources, including tools such as calculators:

- JAMAevidence[158]
- Essential Evidence Plus[159]

There are also efforts aimed at professionals to aggregate broad amounts of clinical content along with content about practice management, information technology, and other topics. These include the following:

- Medscape[160]—a site for medical news aimed at physicians, segmented to one's specialty or status (e.g., medical students, nurses, or pharmacists)
- Unbound Medicine[161]—a commercial resource for mobile device clinical content
- Health Information Online[162]—a variety of free and commercial resources for clinicians in the United Kingdom
- INFOMED[163]—the Cuban National Health Care Telecommunications Network and Portal, from a more resource-limited country [63]

The NLM organizes its content into a number of different aggregations. One is the NCBI Search system already described previously, which has an interface that allows searching over the entire collection of NCBI databases.[164] Additional pages on the NCBI site feature aggregations in more focused areas, such as:

- Literature[165]

---

[154] https://www.elsevier.com/clinical-solutions

[155] https://mhmedical.com/

[156] https://www.springerpub.com/

[157] https://www.wiley.com/en-us/

[158] https://jamaevidence.mhmedical.com/

[159] https://www.essentialevidenceplus.com/

[160] https://www.medscape.com/

[161] https://www.unboundmedicine.com/

[162] http://www.library.nhs.uk/

[163] http://www.sld.cu/

[164] https://www.ncbi.nlm.nih.gov/search/

[165] https://www.ncbi.nlm.nih.gov/home/literature/

- Health[166]
- Genomes[167]

Another NLM aggregation is its Digital Collections,[168] consisting of digitized images of documents, photographs, maps, and videos.

3.5.3 Body of Knowledge

A growing approach to aggregation in a specific domain is the body of knowledge. One of the earliest and most comprehensive was the Software Engineering Body of Knowledge (SWEBOK).[169] The goal of this resource is to map all of the knowledge of the field of software engineering [64]. The paper by Bourque et al. summarized the challenges in creating such a resource. For example, where does one draw the line between the discipline of software engineering and related ones, such as computer science, cognitive science, management science, and systems engineering? Likewise, what should be the depth of material presented? The project chose to adopt the approach of including "generally accepted" knowledge, which applies to most situations most of the time and has widespread consensus about its value and effectiveness. This type of knowledge was distinguished from "advanced and research" knowledge, which was not yet mature, and "specialized" knowledge, which was not yet generally applicable.

There is one body of knowledge project in biomedical informatics, the Health Information Management (HIM) Body of Knowledge, managed by the American Health Information Management Association (AHIMA).[170] It includes:

- Most *Journal of AHIMA* articles
- Many *AHIMA Advantage* articles
- Various AHIMA practice briefs, position statements, reports, guidelines and white papers, job descriptions, and other AHIMA information
- Government publications such as parts of the Federal Register and Department of Health and Human Services documents
- Links to other useful HIM documents
- Practice guidance reports on current e-HIM topics

---

[166] https://www.ncbi.nlm.nih.gov/home/health/

[167] https://www.ncbi.nlm.nih.gov/home/genomes/

[168] https://collections.nlm.nih.gov/

[169] https://www.computer.org/education/bodies-of-knowledge/software-engineering

[170] https://bok.ahima.org/

3.5.4 Model Organism Databases

A resource of growing importance in genomics is the model organism database, where all information (e.g., gene nomenclature, nucleotide and protein sequences, literature references, and other data) are brought together into a unified resource. Among the most-developed model organism databases are:

- Mouse Genome Informatics[171]—the house mouse, *Mus musculus*
- EcoCyc[172]—genes and metabolism from the well-studied *Escherichia coli* bacterium
- WormBase[173]—the soil-dwelling worm, *Caenorhabditis elegans*
- Saccharomyces Genome Database[174]—the yeast *Saccharomyces*, which has importance for certain types of fermented beverages
- FlyBase[175]—the ubiquitous *Drosophila melanogaster* fruit fly
- Zebrafish Information Network[176]—the zebra fish

Naturally, the development of all these model organism databases has led to the development of a toolkit to facilitate their construction, the Generic Model Organism Database[177] [65].

3.5.5 Scientific Information

Some aggregations of science-oriented Web content goes beyond health and biomedical science. The US government maintains a site called Science.gov[178] that provides access by searching or browsing to over 60 databases, 2200 scientific Web sites, and more than 200 million pages of authoritative federal science information including research and development results. Many of these are part of an even larger catalog of scientific information from around the world, WorldWideScience.org,[179] which features a federated search engine that broadcasts search to each site's search engine.

---

[171] http://www.informatics.jax.org/

[172] https://ecocyc.org/

[173] https://www.wormbase.org/

[174] https://www.yeastgenome.org/

[175] https://flybase.org/

[176] https://zfin.org/

[177] http://gmod.org/wiki/Main_Page

[178] https://www.science.gov/

[179] https://worldwidescience.org/

References

1. Riley J. Understanding metadata: what is metadata, and what is it for? Baltimore, MD: National Information Standards Organization; 2017.
2. Sayers E, Agarwala R, Bolton E, Brister J, Canese K, Clark K, et al. Database resources of the National Center for Biotechnology Information. Nucleic Acids Res. 2019;47:D23–8.
3. DeBakey M. The National Library of Medicine: evolution of a premier information center. J Am Med Assoc. 1991;266:1252–8.
4. Anonymous. Index Medicus to cease as print publication. NLM Tech Bull. 2004;2004:e2.
5. Tybaert S, Rosov J. MEDLINE data changes—2004. NLM Tech Bull. 2004;2003:e6.
6. Rickman K. Research tips: what's the difference between PubMed, Medline & Embase? Perth: King Edward Memorial Hospital; 2019.
7. Bramer W, Rethlefsen M, Kleijnen J, Franco O. Optimal database combinations for literature searches in systematic reviews: a prospective exploratory study. Syst Rev. 2016;6:245.
8. Ohno-Machado L, Sansone S, Alter G, Fore I, Grethe J, Xu H, et al. Finding useful data across multiple biomedical data repositories using DataMed. Nat Genet. 2017;49:816–9.
9. Sansone S, Gonzalez-Beltran A, Rocca-Serra P, Alter G, Grethe J, Xu H, et al. DATS: the data tag suite to enable discoverability of datasets. Sci Data. 2017;4:170059.
10. Noy N. Making it easier to discover datasets. Google. The Keyword; 2018.
11. Noy N. Discovering millions of datasets on the web. Google. The Keyword; 2020.
12. Kindling M, van de Sandt S, Rücknagel J, Schirmbacher P, Pampel H, Vierkant P, et al. The landscape of research data repositories in 2015: a re3data analysis. D-Lib Mag. 2017;23(3/4). http://www.dlib.org/dlib/march17/kindling/03kindling.html.
13. Carbon S, Champieux R, McMurry J, Winfree L, Wyatt L, Haendel M. A measure of open data: a metric and analysis of reusable data practices in biomedical data resources. BioRxiv. 2018; https://doi.org/10.1101/282830.
14. Malet G, Munoz F, Appleyard R, Hersh W. A model for enhancing Internet medical document retrieval with "medical core metadata". J Am Med Inform Assoc. 1999;6:183–208.
15. Hersh W, Brown K, Donohoe L, Campbell E, Horacek A. CliniWeb: managing clinical information on the World Wide Web. J Am Med Inform Assoc. 1996;3:273–80.
16. Redman P, Kelly J, Albright E, Anderson P, Mulder C, Schnell E. Common ground: the HealthWeb project as a model for Internet collaboration. Bull Med Libr Assoc. 1997;85:325–30.
17. Boyer C, Baujard V, Geissbuhler A. Evolution of health web certification through the HONcode experience. Stud Health Technol Inform. 2011;169:53–7.
18. Hammersley B. Developing feeds with RSS and atom. Sebastopol, CA: O'Reilly & Associates; 2005.
19. Munn Z, Qaseem A. Disappearance of the national guideline clearinghouse: a huge loss for evidence-based health care. Ann Intern Med. 2018;169:648–9.
20. Graham R, Mancher M, Wolman D, Greenfield S, Steinberg E. Clinical practice guidelines we can trust. Washington, DC: National Academies Press; 2011.
21. Jue J, Cunningham S, Lohr K, Shekelle P, Shiffman R, Robbins C, et al. Developing and testing the Agency for Healthcare Research and Quality's National Guideline Clearinghouse Extent of Adherence to Trustworthy Standards (NEATS) instrument. Ann Intern Med. 2019;170:480–7.
22. Hersh W, Rindfleisch T. Electronic publishing of scholarly communication in the biomedical sciences. J Am Med Inform Assoc. 2000;7:324–5.
23. MacCallum C. ONE for all: the next step for PLoS. PLoS Biol. 2007;4:e401.
24. Delamothe T. The new BMJ online archive. Br Med J. 2009;338:1025–6.
25. Winker M, Herron M, Jones E, Bauchner H. The JAMA Network Website: today's content on the future of medical publishing. J Am Med Assoc. 2012;307:2321.

26. Amberger J, Bocchini C, Scott A, Hamosh A. OMIM.org: leveraging knowledge across phenotype–gene relationships. Nucleic Acids Res. 2019;47:D1038–43.
27. Eysenbach G. Consumer health informatics. Br Med J. 2000;320:1713–6.
28. Slack W, Lewis D, Eysenbach G, Kukafka R, editors. Consumer health informatics: informing consumers and improving health care. New York, NY: Springer; 2005.
29. Cooke R. Wikipedia is the last best place on the Internet. Wired. 2020;17:2020.
30. Heilman J. 5 ways Wikipedia's health information is improving. London: Chartered Institute of Library and Information Professionals; 2014.
31. Azzam A, Bresler D, Leon A, Maggio L, Whitaker E, Heilman J, et al. Why medical schools should embrace Wikipedia: final-year medical student contributions to Wikipedia articles for academic credit at one school. Acad Med. 2017;92:194–200.
32. Spitzer V, Ackerman M, Scherzinger A, Whitlock D. The visible human male: a technical report. J Am Med Inform Assoc. 1996;3:118–30.
33. Demner-Fushman D, Antani S, Simpson M, Thoma G. Design and development of a multimodal biomedical information retrieval system. J Comput Sci Eng. 2012;6:168–77.
34. Hutchins B, Baker K, Davis M, Diwersy M, Haque E, Harriman R, et al. The NIH Open Citation Collection: a public access, broad coverage resource. PLoS Biol. 2019;70(10):e3000385.
35. Haynes R. Of studies, syntheses, synopses, and systems: the "4S" evolution of services for finding current best evidence. ACP J Club. 2001;134:A11–3.
36. DiCenso A, Bayley L, Haynes R. ACP Journal Club. Editorial: accessing preappraised evidence: fine-tuning the 5S model into a 6S model. Ann Intern Med. 2009;151(6):JC3–2, JC3.
37. McKibbon K, Wilczynski N, Hayward R, Walker-Dilks C, Haynes R. The medical literature as a resource for health care practice. J Am Soc Inf Sci. 1995;46:737–42.
38. Haynes R. bmjupdates+, a new free service for evidence-based clinical practice. Evid Based Nurs. 2005;8:39.
39. Haynes R, Walker-Dilks C. Having trouble deciding what's most important to read? Look to the stars. ACP J Club. 2005;143(1):A10.
40. Izcovich A, Criniti J, Popoff F, Ragusa M, Gigler C, Malla C, et al. Answering medical questions at the point of care: a cross-sectional study comparing rapid decisions based on PubMed and Epistemonikos searches with evidence-based recommendations developed with the GRADE approach. BMJ Open. 2017;7:e016113.
41. Friedman C, Flynn A. Computable knowledge: an imperative for learning health systems. Learn Health Syst. 2019;3(4):e10203.
42. Anonymous. Initial sequencing and analysis of the human genome. Nature. 2001;409:860–921.
43. Venter J, Adams M, Myers E, Li P, Mural R, Sutton G. The sequence of the human genome. Science. 2001;291:1304–51.
44. Collins F, Morgan M, Patrinos A. The Human Genome Project: lessons from large-scale biology. Science. 2003;300:286–90.
45. Rigden D, Fernández X. The 2019 Nucleic Acids Research database issue and the online molecular biology database collection. Nucleic Acids Res. 2019;47:D1–7.
46. Sayers E, Cavanaugh M, Clark K, Ostell J, Pruitt K, Karsch-Mizrachi I. Genbank. Nucleic Acids Res. 2020;48:D84–6.
47. Landrum M, Lee J, Benson M, Brown G, Chao C, Villamarin-Salomon R, et al. ClinVar: public archive of interpretations of clinically relevant variants. Nucleic Acids Res. 2016;44:D862–8.
48. Haft D, DiCuccio M, Badretdin A, Brover V, Chetvernin V, Yamashita R, et al. RefSeq: an update on prokaryotic genome annotation and curation. Nucleic Acids Res. 2018;46:D851–60.
49. Rehm H, Berg J, Brooks L, Bustamante C, Evans J, Landrum M, et al. ClinGen—the clinical genome resource. N Engl J Med. 2015;372:2235–42.
50. Collins H, Calvo S, Greenberg K, Neall L, Morrison S. Information Needs in the precision medicine era: how Genetics Home Reference can help. Interact J Med Res. 2016;5(2):e13.
51. Hollands F, Tirthali D. MOOCs: expectations and reality, vol. 2014. New York, NY: Columbia University Teacher's College; 2014.
52. Berners-Lee T, Lassila O, Hendler J. The Semantic Web. Sci Am. 2001;284(5):34–43.

53. Sakr S, Wylot M, Mutharaju R, LePhuoc D, Fundulaki I. Linked data—storing, querying, and reasoning. New York: Springer Nature; 2018.
54. Lehmann J, Isele R, Jakob M, Jentzsch A, Kontokostas D, Mendes P, et al. DBpedia—a large-scale, multilingual knowledge base extracted from Wikipedia. Semantic Web. 2015;6:167–95.
55. Torniai C, Bourges-Waldegg D, Hoffmann S. eagle-i: biomedical research resource datasets. Semantic Web. 2015;6:139–46.
56. DeAngelis C, Drazen J, Frizelle F, Haug C, Hoey J, Horton R, et al. Is this clinical trial fully registered? A statement from the International Committee of Medical Journal Editors. J Am Med Assoc. 2005;293:2927–9.
57. Zarin D, Tse T, Ide N. Trial registration at ClinicalTrials.gov between May and October 2005. N Engl J Med. 2005;353:2779–87.
58. Haug C, Gotzsche P, Schroeder T. Registries and registration of clinical trials. N Engl J Med. 2005;353:2811–2.
59. Zarin D, Tse T, Williams R, Carr S. Trial reporting in ClinicalTrials.gov—the final rule. N Engl J Med. 2016;375:1998–2004.
60. Zarin D, Tse T. Sharing individual participant data (IPD) within the context of the trial reporting system (TRS). PLoS Med. 2016;13(1):e1001946.
61. Schwartz L, Woloshin S, Zheng E, Tse T, Zarin D. ClinicalTrials.gov and Drugs@FDA: a comparison of results reporting for new drug approval trials. Ann Intern Med. 2016;165:421–30.
62. Miller N, Lacroix E, Backus J. MEDLINEplus: building and maintaining the National Library of Medicine's consumer health Web service. Bull Med Libr Assoc. 2000;88:11–7.
63. Séror A. A case analysis of INFOMED: the Cuban national health care telecommunications network and portal. J Med Internet Res. 2006;8(1):e1.
64. Bourque P, Dupuis R, Abran A. The guide to the Software Engineering Body of Knowledge. IEEE Software, 1999;16(6):35–44.
65. Stein L, Mungall C, Shu S, Caudy M, Mangone M, Day A, et al. The generic genome browser: a building block for a model organism system database. Genome Res. 2002;12:1599–610.

Chapter 4
Indexing

In the first chapter, *indexing* was defined as the process of assigning metadata, consisting of terms and attributes, to documents. This process is also called by other names, such as *annotation* or *tagging*. There are two reasons to index document collections, one cognitive and one mechanical. The cognitive reason for indexing is to represent the content of individual documents so that searchers may retrieve them accurately. The mechanical reason for indexing is to enable computer programs to more rapidly determine which documents contain content described by specific terms and attributes.

4.1 Types of Indexing

The indexing of documents for content long preceded the computer age. The most famous early cataloger of medical documents, Dr. John Shaw Billings, avidly pursued and cataloged medical reference works at the Library of the Surgeon General's Office [1]. In 1879, Billings produced the first index to the medical literature, *Index Medicus*, which classified journal articles by topic. For over a century, *Index Medicus* was the predominant method for accessing the medical literature.

By the middle of the twentieth century, however, the chore of manually cataloging and indexing of the expanding base of medical literature was becoming overwhelming. Fortunately, the beginning of the computer age was at hand. While initial efforts at automation were geared toward improving the efficiency of the indexing and publishing process, the potential value of using computers for actual retrieval became apparent as well, with the birth of MEDLINE in the 1960s. By the 1990s, MEDLINE, the electronic version of *Index Medicus*, had made the paper version obsolete and the latter was retired in 2004 [2].

W. Hersh, *Information Retrieval: A Biomedical and Health Perspective*, Health Informatics, https://doi.org/10.1007/978-3-030-47686-1_4

Even though the medium has changed, the human side of indexing the medical literature for the most part has not. The main difference in the computer age is that a second type of indexing, automated indexing, has become available. Thus, most modern commercial content is indexed in two ways:

1. Manual indexing—where human indexers, usually using standardized terminology, assign indexing terms and attributes to documents, often following a specific protocol
2. Automated indexing—where computers make the indexing assignments, usually limited to breaking out each word in the document (or part of the document) as an indexing term

Manual indexing is mostly done for bibliographic databases. In the age of proliferating electronic resources, such as online textbooks, practice guidelines, and multimedia collections, manual indexing has become either too expensive or outright infeasible for the large quantity and diversity of content now available. Thus, most content is now indexed for retrieval only by automated means.

Recall from Chap. 1 that the indexing process uses one or more *indexing languages* to represent the content of documents and queries for retrieval of documents. In the manual indexing process, the main indexing language is usually a controlled vocabulary of terminology from a field. When relationships among different terms are specified, this vocabulary is called a *thesaurus*. The indexing language for word indexing, however, consists of all the words that are used for indexing (often minus a small number of common function words, called a *stop list* or *negative dictionary*), with no control imposed.

Some authors classify indexing differently than above by distinguishing it as either *precoordinated* or *postcoordinated*. These distinctions are usually but not necessarily applied to human indexing, since they refer to whether the indexing terms are coordinated at indexing (precoordinated) or retrieval (postcoordinated) time. In precoordinated systems, the indexing terms are searchable only as a unit, thus they are "pre"-coordinated. While many early retrieval systems required precoordinated searching on full terms only, most modern systems allow searching on the individual words of indexing terms, hence are "post"-coordinated.

4.2 Factors Influencing Indexing

A variety of factors influence indexing. Usually careful consideration must be given to selecting appropriate terms that lead to the most effective retrieval by users. Two measures reflect the depth and breadth of indexing, *specificity* and *exhaustivity*, respectively. These measures can also be used as criteria for evaluating the quality of indexing for any specific purpose. Another concern with the quality of indexing is inconsistency. While not an issue with automated systems whose computer algorithms produce the same results every time, manual indexing must be consistent for users who anticipate terms being assigned to documents they expect to retrieve.

Of course, the ultimate measure of indexing quality is how well users can use the indexing to access the documents they need, which we will cover in Chap. 7.

The first measure of indexing, specificity, refers to the detail or precision of the indexing process and indicates its depth. The desired level of specificity is dependent upon both users and databases. Users with much knowledge of a subject area will likely want the highest level of specificity. Researchers, for example, may recognize distinct genes or clinical variations associated with a disease that are less known to clinicians. Thus, a researcher might find indexing geared to the clinicians to be insufficiently specific, resulting in loss of precision when searching. Likewise, a clinician who found indexing geared to the researcher too specific might experience loss of recall owing to improper use of highly specific indexing terms. In general, more indexing specificity translates into better retrieval precision, assuming that searchers understand and apply the terms in their queries properly.

Exhaustivity indicates the completeness of indexing or its breadth. In the human indexing process, terms are generally assigned to documents when they are one of the focal subjects of a document. Increasing exhaustivity of indexing will tend to increase recall, since more possible indexing terms will increase the chance of retrieving relevant documents. On the other hand, excessive exhaustivity will result in diminished precision, especially if search terms are only loosely related to documents retrieved by the searcher.

The final measure of indexing quality is *consistency*. It has been shown that indexing consistency leads to improved retrieval effectiveness [3]. Hooper's measure has been used to indicate the percentage consistency of indexing [4]:

$$\text{Consistency}(A,B) = \frac{i}{i+j+k} \tag{4.1}$$

where A and B are the two indexers, i is number of terms A and B assign in agreement, j is the number of terms assigned by A but not B, and k is the number of terms assigned by B but not A. For example, if two indexers assigned 15 and 18 terms, respectively, 11 of which were in agreement, their consistency would be 11/(11 + (1 5 − 11) + (18 − 11)) = 0.5 or 50%.

4.3 Controlled Vocabularies

Before discussing indexing processes in detail, it is important to describe controlled vocabularies. While these vocabularies are most often used in manual indexing, numerous research projects have attempted to employ them for automated indexing, as described in later chapters. This section will first discuss some general principles in thesaurus construction, followed by a description of the controlled vocabulary used most often in medical IR systems, the *Medical Subject Headings* (or MeSH) vocabulary, created by the National Library of Medicine (NLM). This will be followed by a discussion of other controlled vocabularies and the NLM's Unified Medical Language System (UMLS) project.

4.3.1 General Principles of Controlled Vocabularies

Before discussing specific vocabularies, it is useful to define some terms, since different writers attach different definitions to the various components of thesauri. A *concept* is an idea or object that occurs in the world, such as the condition under which human blood pressure is elevated. A *term* is the actual string of one or more words that represent a concept, such as `Hypertension` or `High Blood Pressure`. One of these string forms is the preferred or *canonical* form, such as `Hypertension` in the present example. When one or more terms can represent a concept, the different terms are called *synonyms*.

A controlled vocabulary usually contains a list of certified terms that are the canonical representations of the concepts. Most thesauri also contain relationships between terms, which typically fall into three categories:

1. Hierarchical—terms that are broader or narrower. The hierarchical organization not only provides an overview of the structure of a thesaurus but also can be used to enhance searching (e.g., MeSH tree explosions described in Chap. 5).
2. Synonymous—terms that are synonyms, allowing the indexer or searcher to express a concept in different words.
3. Related—terms that are not synonymous or hierarchical but are somehow otherwise related. These usually remind the searcher of different but related terms that may enhance a search.

Another term that commonly comes up when discussing controlled vocabularies is *ontology*. There are many definitions of ontologies, and the word is sometimes used to describe any type of controlled vocabulary or terminology. A commonly cited definition and general overview of ontologies comes from Arp et al. [5]: "a representational artifact, comprising a taxonomy as proper part, whose representations are intended to designate some combination of universals, defined classes, and certain relations between them." Some commonly agreed upon components of an ontology are classes of general concepts, with specific instances or instantiations that represent concepts within them. Concepts have various attributes, usually connected via relationships. Concepts also have restrictions, sometimes called facets. In a pure sense, ontologies differ from terminologies in that the former richly represent a domain, whereas the latter catalogs its formal terms. Cimino and Zhu noted that most major terminologies, while used successfully for many applications, have varying amounts to adherence to true ontological principles [6].

A repository of biomedical ontologies is the National Center for Biomedical Ontologies (NCBO)[1] and its main project, the repository of biomedical ontologies

[1] https://www.bioontology.org/

called BioPortal.[2] A key use of ontologies is mapping concepts to computer applications [7]. One important ontology is one that aims to model all human phenotypes, the Human Phenotype Ontology [8].

Another important ontology, which is aimed for use for simple manual indexing for the Web, has been developed by the major search engine companies—Google, Microsoft, and others—and is called Schema.org.[3] Schema.org is supported by the Schema.org Community Group.[4] The schemas are designed to be "microdata" that can be used to index digital content, such as Web pages. They can even be included in the Web page HTML themselves. The schemas consist of a collection of "types," each of which is associated with a set of "properties." The types are arranged in a hierarchy. The core vocabulary currently consists of nearly 600 types, over 800 properties, and over 100 enumeration values for the properties. The community has also developed a process for "extensions" to the basic schemas, which can be "hosted" as part of the Schema.org project or "external" and be maintained by outside organizations.

One important example of the latter is MedicalEntity,[5] which is related to health and the practice of medicine. The schema is not meant to be a new controlled medical vocabulary, but instead aims to complement existing vocabularies and ontologies. It provides a way to annotate entities with codes that refer to existing controlled medical vocabularies (e.g., MeSH, SNOMED, ICD, RxNorm, UMLS, etc.).

Another important extension to Schema.org is Bioschemas.org,[6] which aims to "improve the findability of data in the life sciences. It does this by encouraging people in the life sciences to use Schema.org markup in their Web sites so that they are indexable by search engines and other services." It extends the basic ontology with types, which allow for the description of life science resources (e.g., `Gene` or `Protein`), and profiles, which identify the essential properties to use in describing a resource (e.g., `DataSet` or `TrainingMaterial`).

4.3.2 The Medical Subject Headings (MeSH) Vocabulary

Created by the NLM for indexing *Index Medicus*, the MeSH vocabulary was and is now used to index most of the databases produced by the NLM [9]. The MeSH vocabulary files, their associated data, and their supporting documentation are available on the NLM's MeSH Web site.[7] MeSH consists of[8]:

---

[2] https://bioportal.bioontology.org/

[3] https://schema.org/

[4] https://www.w3.org/community/schemaorg/

[5] http://schema.org/MedicalEntity

[6] https://bioschemas.org/

[7] https://www.nlm.nih.gov/mesh/meshhome.html

[8] https://www.nlm.nih.gov/mesh/intro_record_types.html

Table 4.1 The 16 trees in MeSH, under which all headings are classified (Courtesy of NLM)

Anatomy [A]
Organisms [B]
Diseases [C]
Chemicals and Drugs [D]
Analytical, Diagnostic and Therapeutic Techniques, and Equipment [E]
Psychiatry and Psychology [F]
Phenomena and Processes [G]
Disciplines and Occupations [H]
Information Science [L]
Named Groups [M]
Health Care [N]
Publication Characteristics [V]
Geographicals [Z]

- Headings—the word MeSH uses for the canonical representation of its concepts
- Entry terms—synonyms of the MeSH headings
- Supplementary concepts—additional diseases, chemicals, protocols, and organisms

MeSH currently has over 27,000 headings, 87,000 entry terms, and 232,000 supplementary concepts.

In addition, MeSH contains three types of relationships described at the end of Sect. 4.3.1:

1. Hierarchical—MeSH is organized hierarchically into 16 *trees*, which are listed in Table 4.1.
2. Synonymous—MeSH entry terms are synonyms of headings and consist mainly of variations of the headings and entry terms in plurality, word order, hyphenation, and apostrophes. These are also called *see references* because they point the indexer or searcher back to the canonical form of the term.
3. Related—terms that may be useful for searchers to add to their searches when appropriate are suggested for many headings.

In addition to being fully available for download, MeSH can be accessed by two different search interfaces on the NLM Web site:

- MeSH Browser[9]—allows searching and browsing of the tree structure
- MeSH on Demand[10]—allows entry of larger quantities of text and uses the Medical Text Indexer (see below) to identify all MeSH terms in the entered text

[9] https://meshb.nlm.nih.gov/search

[10] https://meshb.nlm.nih.gov/MeSHonDemand

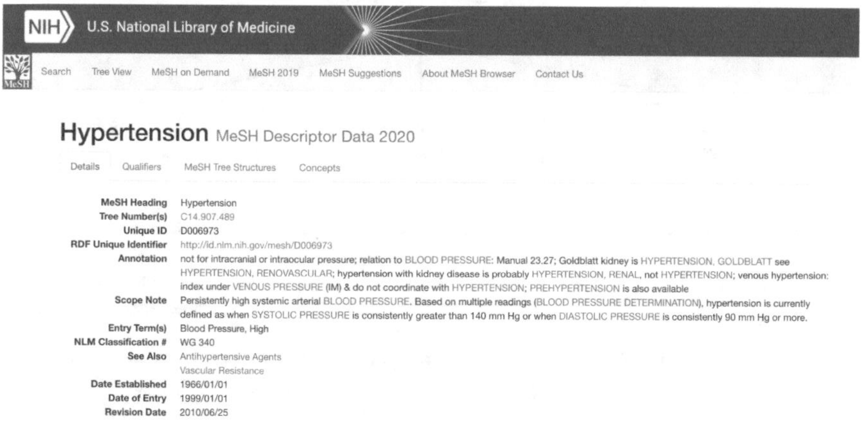

Fig. 4.1 MeSH browser page for the heading `Hypertension`. Among the components in the note are the tree number, the annotation summarizing the term usage, the scope note for searchers, an entry term (`Blood Pressure, High`), and two related terms (`Antihypertensive Agents` and `Vascular Resistance`). Other tabs include the allowable subheadings (Qualifiers) and tree structure (Courtesy of NLM)

Figure 4.1 shows the screen image from the MeSH browser containing all the data in the vocabulary for the term `Hypertension`. The page displayed by the browser also displays the location of the term in the MeSH hierarchy. Figure 4.2 shows a partially pruned version of some of the terms in hierarchical proximity to `Hypertension`.

There are additional features of MeSH designed to assist indexers in making documents more retrievable. One of these is *subheadings*, which are qualifiers to headings that can be attached to narrow the focus of a term. In `Hypertension`, for example, the focus of an article may be on the diagnosis, epidemiology, or treatment of the condition. Assigning the appropriate subheading will designate the restricted focus of the article, potentially enhancing precision for the searcher. Table 4.2 lists the subheadings of MeSH and their hierarchical organization. There are also rules for each tree restricting the attachment of certain subheadings. For example, the subheading `drug therapy` cannot be attached to an anatomic site, such as the `femur`. The allowed subheadings for a given term are shown as the *Allowable Qualifiers* in the MeSH browser (Fig. 4.1).

Another feature of MeSH that helps retrieval is *check tags*.[11] These are MeSH terms that represent certain facets of medical studies, such as age, gender, human or nonhuman, and type of grant support. They are called check tags because the indexer is required to use them when they describe an attribute of the study. For example, all studies with human subjects must have the check tag `Human` assigned. Likewise, studies about pregnancy will require the check tags `Pregnancy` and `Female`.

[11] https://www.nlm.nih.gov/bsd/indexing/training/CHK_010.html

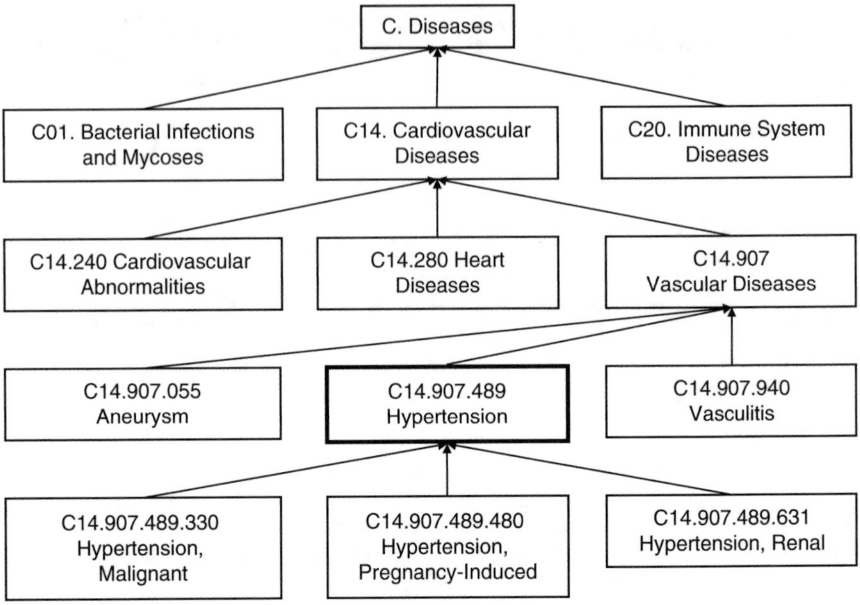

Fig. 4.2 MeSH hierarchy for the heading `Hypertension`, which is denoted by the heavy box. Other (but not all) terms at each level are shown (Courtesy of NLM)

Table 4.2 MeSH subheadings; indented terms are children terms hierarchically (Courtesy of NLM)

• Analysis
– Blood
– Cerebrospinal fluid
– Isolation & purification
– Urine
• Anatomy & histology
– Blood supply
– Cytology
Ultrastructure
– Embryology
Abnormalities
– Innervation
– Pathology
• Chemistry
– Agonists
– Analogs & derivatives
– Antagonists & inhibitors
– Chemical synthesis
• Diagnosis
– Diagnostic imaging
• Etiology
– Chemically induced

Table 4.2 (continued)

– Complications
Secondary
– Congenital
– Embryology
– Genetics
– Immunology
– Microbiology
Virology
– Parasitology
– Transmission
• Organization & administration
– Economics
– Legislation & jurisprudence
• Standards
• Supply & distribution
• Trends
• Pharmacology
– Administration & dosage
– Adverse effects
Poisoning
Toxicity
– Agonists
– Antagonists & inhibitors
– Pharmacokinetics
• Physiology
– Genetics
– Growth & development
– Immunology
– Metabolism
Biosynthesis
Blood
Cerebrospinal fluid
Deficiency
Enzymology
Pharmacokinetics
Urine
– Physiopathology
• Statistics & numerical data
– Epidemiology
Ethnology
Mortality
– Supply & distribution
• Therapeutic use
– Administration & dosage

(continued)

Table 4.2 (continued)

– Adverse effects
– Poisoning
• Therapy
– Diet therapy
– Drug therapy
– Nursing
– Prevention & control
– Radiotherapy
– Rehabilitation
– Surgery
transplantation
• Classification
• Drug effects
• Education
• Ethics
• History
• Injuries
• Instrumentation
• Methods
• Pathogenicity
• Psychology
• Radiation effects
• Veterinary

Related to check tags are the geographical locations in the Z tree. Indexers must also include these, like check tags, since the location of a study (e.g., `Oregon`) must be indicated.

Another important feature of MeSH is the *publication type*, which describes the type of publication or the type of study.[12] A searcher who wants a review of a topic will choose the publication type `Review`. Or, to find studies that provide the best evidence for a treatment, the publication type `Meta-Analysis`, `Randomized Controlled Trial`, or `Controlled Clinical Trial` would be used. MeSH features dozens of publication types. (For many years, `Systematic Review` was not a publication type but rather an entry term for the more general publication type `Review`. This belied the fact that systematic reviews are a special type of review and that some systematic reviews are not amenable to meta-analysis.)

While not necessarily helpful to a searcher using MeSH, the *tree address* is an important component of the MeSH record. The tree address shows the position of a MeSH term relative to others. At each level, a term is given a unique number that becomes part of the tree address. All children terms of a higher-level term will have the same tree address up to the address of the parent. As seen in Fig. 4.2, the tree addresses for children terms for `Hypertension` have the same tree address up

[12] https://www.nlm.nih.gov/mesh/pubtypes.html

to the last number. It should be noted that a MeSH term can have more than one tree address. `Pneumonia`, for example, is a child term of both `Lung Diseases` (C08.381) and `Respiratory Tract Infections` (C08.730). It thus has two tree addresses, C08.381.677 and C08.730.610.

Another feature of MeSH is *related concepts*. Most well-designed thesauri used for IR have related terms, and MeSH is no exception. Related concepts are grouped into three types. The first is the *see related* references. These are used when one heading is reminded of another that may be more appropriate for a particular purpose. Some examples include:

- Between a disease and its cause, e.g., `Factor XIII Deficiency` see related `Factor XIIIa`
- Between an organ and a physiological process, e.g., `Bone and Bones` see related `Osteogenesis`
- Between an organ and a drug acting on it, e.g., `Bronchi` see related `Bronchoconstrictor Agents`
- Between an organ and a procedure, e.g., `Bile Ducts` see related `Cholangiography`

Another type of related concept is the *consider also* reference, which is usually used for anatomical terms and indicates terms that are related linguistically (e.g., by having a common word stem). For example, the record for the term `Brain` suggests considering terms `Cerebr-` and `Encephal-`. A final category of related concepts consists of main heading/subheading combination notations. In these instances, unallowed heading/subheading combinations are referred to a preferred precoordinated heading. For example, instead of the combination `Accidents/Prevention & Control`, the heading `Accident Prevention` is suggested.

Figure 4.1 demonstrates two other features of MeSH terms. The first is the *Annotation*, which provides tips on the use of the term for searchers. For example, under `Congestive Heart Failure`, the searcher is instructed not to confuse the term with `Congestive Cardiomyopathy`, a related but distinctly different clinical syndrome. Likewise, under `Cryptococcus`, the searcher is reminded that this term represents the fungal organism, while the term `Cryptococcosis` should be used to designate diseases caused by *Cryptococcus*. The second feature is the *Scope Note*, which gives a description of how the term is used in indexing.

4.3.3 Other Indexing Vocabularies

MeSH is not the only thesaurus used for indexing biomedical documents. A number of other thesauri are used to index non-NLM databases. CINAHL, for example, uses the CINAHL Subject Headings,[13] which are based on MeSH but have additional domain-specific terms added. EMBASE, the so-called European MEDLINE that is

[13] https://connect.ebsco.com/s/article/CINAHL-Subject-Headings-Frequently-Asked-Questions

part of *Excerpta Medica*, has a vocabulary called EMTREE, which has many features similar to those of MeSH [10]. EMTREE is also hierarchically related, with all terms organized under 16 *facets*, which are similar but not identical to MeSH trees. Concepts can also be qualified by *link terms*, which are similar to MeSH subheadings. EMTREE includes synonyms for terms, which include the corresponding MeSH term.

The PsycINFO database[14] uses two indexing vocabularies. The first is the *Thesaurus of Psychological Index Terms*, containing over 8400 terms and constructed like a typical thesaurus. The second is a set of *Classification Categories and Codes*,[15] a set of 22 major categories and 135 subcategories that classify references into broad categories of experimental psychology, treatment, education, and others.

Another vocabulary of great importance to -omics researchers is the Gene Ontology (GO),[16] which has the goal of enabling description of aspects of molecular biology [11, 12]. GO associates gene products to GO terms using statements that describe:

- Molecular function—molecular activities of individual gene products
- Cellular component—where the gene products are active
- Biological process—pathways and larger processes to which that gene product's activity contributes

The primary use of GO is not in indexing content but rather annotating the knowledge of genes and their functions. Many of the model organism databases are devoting great resources to annotating the genes in their databases with GO codes. This work is usually done by curators who have advanced training in various fields of biology. There are over 44,000 terms in GO, which is also now included in the UMLS Metathesaurus. A GO annotation is a statement about the function of a particular gene. These annotations are created by associating a gene or gene product with a GO term and together comprise a "snapshot" of current biological knowledge.

GO also has *evidence codes* that indicate the level of evidence supporting the association of a term with a gene.[17] The current evidence codes in use are shown in Table 4.3. Some of the evidence codes represent stronger levels of evidence. For example, the weakest forms of evidence are inferred from electronic annotation (IEA), where codes have been assigned based on genes identified in a sequence similarity search which have not been manually reviewed, and non-traceable author statement (AS), where the author of a paper has made a statement about the function of a gene with a citation to a paper describing an experiment that has not been curated.

[14] https://www.apa.org/pubs/databases/psycinfo

[15] https://www.apa.org/pubs/databases/training/class-codes

[16] http://geneontology.org/

[17] http://geneontology.org/docs/guide-go-evidence-codes/

Table 4.3 Gene Ontology evidence codes

• Experimental evidence codes
– Inferred from Experiment (EXP)
– Inferred from Direct Assay (IDA)
– Inferred from Physical Interaction (IPI)
– Inferred from Mutant Phenotype (IMP)
– Inferred from Genetic Interaction (IGI)
– Inferred from Expression Pattern (IEP)
– Inferred from High Throughput Experiment (HTP)
– Inferred from High Throughput Direct Assay (HDA)
– Inferred from High Throughput Mutant Phenotype (HMP)
– Inferred from High Throughput Genetic Interaction (HGI)
– Inferred from High Throughput Expression Pattern (HEP)
• Phylogenetically inferred annotations
– Inferred from Biological aspect of Ancestor (IBA)
– Inferred from Biological aspect of Descendant (IBD)
– Inferred from Key Residues (IKR)
– Inferred from Rapid Divergence (IRD)
• Computational analysis evidence codes
– Inferred from Sequence or structural Similarity (ISS)
– Inferred from Sequence Orthology (ISO)
– Inferred from Sequence Alignment (ISA)
– Inferred from Sequence Model (ISM)
– Inferred from Genomic Context (IGC)
– Inferred from Reviewed Computational Analysis (RCA)
• Author statement evidence codes
– Traceable Author Statement (TAS)
– Non-traceable Author Statement (NAS)
• Curator statement evidence codes
– Inferred by Curator (IC)
– No biological Data available (ND)
• Electronic annotation evidence code
– Inferred from Electronic Annotation (IEA)

http://geneontology.org/docs/guide-go-evidence-codes/

The National Cancer Institute maintains two vocabulary efforts, the NCI Thesaurus and the NCI Metathesaurus. The NCI Thesaurus[18] is focused on cancer science and covers basic, preclinical, and clinical research as well as administrative terminology associated with research management. It contains over 140,000 key biomedical concepts with terms and codes, 120,000 written definitions, and more

[18] https://ncit.nci.nih.gov/

than 500,000 inter-concept relationships. The NCI Metathesaurus is described in the next section.

4.3.4 The Unified Medical Language System

One problem for the biomedical and health informatics field has been the proliferation of different controlled vocabularies. Many of these vocabularies were developed for specific applications, such as epidemiological studies, coding for billing, and medical expert systems. It was recognized by the NLM and others as early as the 1980s that a significant impediment to the development of integrated and easy-to-use applications was the proliferation of disparate vocabularies, none of which was compatible with any other. Not only did this hamper individual applications, in that the user had to learn a new vocabulary for each application, but the integration of these applications was obstructed as well. The vision of a clinician seamlessly moving among the electronic health record, literature databases, and decision support systems could not be met if those applications could not communicate with each other by means of a common underlying vocabulary.

This is not necessarily surprising, since many vocabularies were created for different purposes. For example, MeSH is used for literature indexing, while ICD-10 is used to code diagnoses for billing, SNOMED is used to represent patient-specific information, CPT-4 is used to code procedures, and so on. Many medical record systems as well as specialized decision support programs have their own vocabularies and cannot take data directly from sources other than user input. Applications designed to integrate or interact with other applications, however, cannot communicate because a common language is lacking. A number of analyses have shown that many vocabularies used in medicine for a variety of purposes do not provide comprehensive coverage of concepts [13].

The UMLS project was undertaken with the goal of providing a mechanism for linking diverse medical vocabularies as well as sources of information [14]. When the project began, it was unclear what form the final products would take, and several years of work went into defining and building experimental versions of the UMLS resources [15–17]. There are now three UMLS Knowledge Sources[19] [18, 19]:

- Metathesaurus—terms and codes from many vocabularies, along with their hierarchies, definitions, and other relationships and attributes.
- Semantic Network—broad categories (semantic types) and their relationships (semantic relations)
- SPECIALIST Lexicon—large syntactic lexicon of biomedical and general English and tools for normalizing strings, generating lexical variants, and creating indexes

[19] https://www.nlm.nih.gov/research/umls/

The most used component of the UMLS project has been the Metathesaurus, whose major focus has been to create linkages among disparate vocabularies, not only assisting inter-program communication but also providing a richer vocabulary for IR and other applications. The Metathesaurus component of the UMLS links parts or all of over 100 source vocabularies, including portions of those listed above. It is multilingual, in the sense that terms from non-English translations of its source vocabularies, mainly of MeSH, are "synonyms" of their English translations. The Metathesaurus is not a new, unified vocabulary, which some early workers advocated [15–17]. Rather, it designates conceptual linkages across existing vocabularies. Another way to conceptualize the Metathesaurus is to think of it as a "repository" of vocabularies, with the source vocabularies kept unchanged and able to be extracted from the Metathesaurus.

In the Metathesaurus, all terms that are conceptually the same are linked together as a *concept*. Each concept may have one or more *terms*, each of which represents an expression of the concept from a source vocabulary that is not just a simple lexical variant (i.e., differs only in word ending or order). Each term may consist of one or more *strings*, which represent all the lexical variants that are represented for that term in the source vocabularies. Each string has an *atom* that represents the source vocabulary from which it came. One of each concept's strings is designated as the preferred form, and the preferred string of the preferred term is known as the *canonical* form of the concept. There are rules of precedence for the canonical form, the main one being that the MeSH heading is used if one of the source vocabularies for the concept is MeSH. The "synonyms" in the Metathesaurus include not only traditional lexical and string variants but also acronyms and expressions of the concept in other languages.

Each Metathesaurus concept has a single concept unique identifier (CUI). Each term has one term unique identifier (LUI), all of which are linked to the one (or more) CUIs with which they are associated. Likewise, each string has one string unique identifier (SUI), which in turn are linked to the LUIs in which they occur. In 2004, a new Rich Release Format (RRF) was introduced that added the atomic unit identifier (AUI), which provided a unique entry for each string in its original form from its source vocabulary, in essence allowing each string of a concept to be traced back to its source vocabulary.

Table 4.4 lists the concepts and a sampling of terms, strings, and atoms for the concept `atrial fibrillation`. The English-language components are displayed graphically in Fig. 4.3. The canonical form of the concept and one of its terms is `atrial fibrillation`, with the other terms being auricular fibrillation, `AF - atrial fibrillation`, `AFib`, `AF`, and `a fib`. Within each term are several strings, which vary in word order and plurality. The Metathesaurus has a total of 191 atoms for this concept, with 81 in the English language and the remainder in 16 other languages.

Table 4.4 Concept with sampling of terms, strings, and atoms for the Metathesaurus concept `atrial fibrillation` (Courtesy of NLM)

Concept (CUI)	Term (LUI)	String (SUI)	Atom (AUI)
C0004238 Atrial Fibrillation (preferred) Atrial Fibrillations Auricular Fibrillation Auricular Fibrillations	**L0004238** Atrial Fibrillation (preferred) Atrial Fibrillations Fibrillations, Atrial	**S0016668** Atrial Fibrillation (preferred)	**A0027665** Atrial Fibrillation (from MSH) **A0027667** Atrial Fibrillation (from PSY)
		S0016669 Atrial Fibrillations (plural variant)	**A0027668** Atrial Fibrillations (from MSH)
		S0041388 Fibrillations, Atrial (word order variant)	**A0059049** Fibrillations, Atrial (from MSH)
	L0004327 Auricular Fibrillation Auricular Fibrillations (synonyms)	**S0016899** Auricular Fibrillation (preferred)	**A0027930** Auricular Fibrillation (from PSY)
		S0016900 Auricular Fibrillations (plural variant)	**A0027932** Auricular Fibrillations (from MSH)
	L0495689 AF—Atrial fibrillation (synonym)	**S0580463** AF—Atrial fibrillation (preferred)	**A2986961** AF—Atrial fibrillation (from SNMCT)
	L1217801 AFib (synonym)	**S1620090** AFib (preferred)	**A10771863** AFib (from NCI)
	L1224181 AF (synonym)	**S1620003** AF (preferred)	**A10771860** AF (from NCI)
	L6192254 a fib (synonym)	**S1459006** a fib (preferred)	**A1412324** a fib (from AB)

The current Metathesaurus contains over 3.8 million concepts from over 210 vocabularies and other sources.[20] There are over 11 million terms, 12 million strings, and 14 million atoms. A total of 25 different languages are represented. The Metathesaurus also contains a wealth of additional information. In addition to the synonym relationships between concepts, terms, and strings described earlier, there are also nonsynonym relationships between concepts. There are also a great many attributes for the concepts, terms, and strings, such as definitions, lexical types, and occurrence in various data sources. Also provided with the Metathesaurus is a word index that connects each word to all the strings it occurs in, along with its concept, term, and string identifiers.

Use of the UMLS Metathesaurus has been modest. One study surveyed about 70 users who replied [20]. The two major intended uses were access to source terminologies (75%) and mapping among source terminologies (44%). The most common

[20] https://www.nlm.nih.gov/research/umls/knowledge_sources/metathesaurus/release/statistics.html

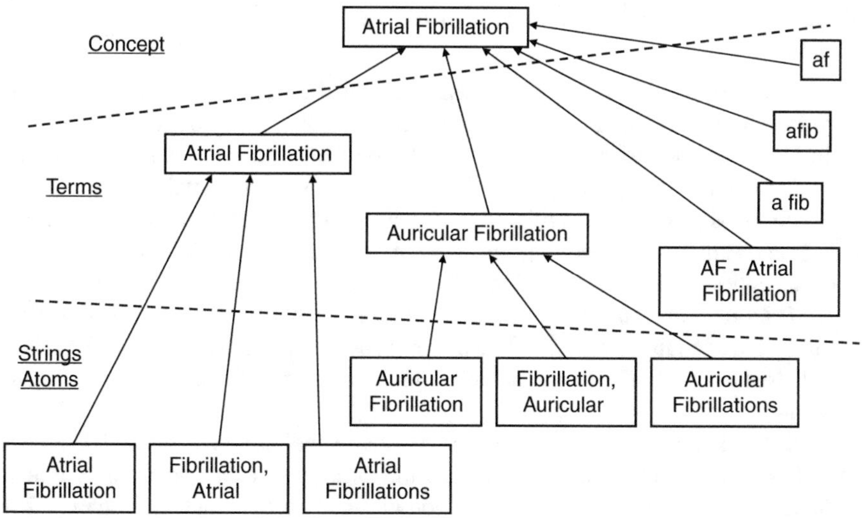

Fig. 4.3 Graphical depiction of the concept `atrial fibrillation` and its terms, strings, and atoms in the UMLS Metathesaurus (Courtesy of NLM)

reported uses were terminology research (31%), information retrieval (16%), and terminology translation (12%). Others reported UMLS was used as a terminology itself (77%) and stated they wanted NLM to develop unified hierarchy and derive a terminology (73%).

The NCI Metathesaurus[21] is based on the UMLS Metathesaurus. Sources deemed not relevant to cancer are omitted from the UMLS Metathesaurus, while those believed to be valuable to cancer science are added.[22] The NCI Metathesaurus contains about 850,000 concepts mapped to 1.5 million terms. The NCI site features a browser for many terminologies, including the NCI Thesaurus and NCI Metathesaurus.[23]

4.4 Manual Indexing

As mentioned, manual indexing was the only type of indexing possible prior to the computer age. This circumstance may have influenced much of the early work in IR systems that focused only on this aspect of indexing (along with the fact that these early machines probably also lacked the power to build large indexes of words in databases). Virtually all human indexing systems utilize a controlled vocabulary.

---

[21] https://ncim.nci.nih.gov/ncimbrowser/

[22] https://ncim.nci.nih.gov/ncimbrowser/pages/source_help_info.jsf

[23] https://ncit.nci.nih.gov/ncitbrowser/start.jsf

4.4.1 Bibliographic Manual Indexing

Manual indexing of bibliographic content is the most common and developed use of such indexing. Bibliographic manual indexing is usually done by means of a controlled vocabulary of terms and attributes, often called a thesaurus. This function has been particularly developed by the NLM through MeSH, which will be the focus of this section. Most databases utilizing human indexing usually have a detailed protocol for assignment of indexing terms from the thesaurus. The MEDLINE database is no exception. The principles of MEDLINE indexing were laid out in the two-volume *MEDLARS Indexing Manual* [21, 22]. More recent descriptions of MEDLINE indexing are available from an online training course for indexers on the NLM Web site.[24] Most MEDLINE indexers are trained in both biomedical sciences and manual indexing.

With the large volume of references constantly being added to MEDLINE, it would be impossible for indexers to read the entirety of every article they index. Rather, they follow the "read/scan" method outlined by Bachrach and Charen [23] and updated on the NLM Web site:

1. Read carefully and understand the title.
2. Read the introduction to the point where the author states the purpose of the article and correlate it with the title. Absorb but do not necessarily attempt to index the introductory material since this is usually a statement of known facts upon which the present study is based.
3. Scan the body of the article, focus on the Materials and Methods section and the Results section.
4. Note section headings and paragraph headings; italics and boldface; charts, plates, tables, and illustrations; and laboratory methods, case reports, etc. Headings supplied by the author usually herald the content of the section headed.
5. Select for indexing only those subjects actually discussed as opposed to those subjects merely mentioned (and of little or no value in retrieval).
6. Read the summary or conclusions of the author to determine whether he achieved the aims set forth in his stated purpose. Weigh conclusions based on the text but do not index implications or suggested future applications. Do not index conclusive statements not supported by discussion in the text.
7. Scan the abstract, if there, for items missed in indexing, being careful, however, to locate actual discussions within the text of the article; ignore mere implications.
8. Scan the author's own indexing if supplied or the keywords supplied by the publisher to see whether the concepts chosen are actually discussed in the text and if they have been indexed.
9. Scan the bibliographic references supplied by the author for clues and further corroboration.

[24] https://www.nlm.nih.gov/bsd/indexing/training/USE_010.html

After this process, the indexer assigns from 5 to 12 headings, depending upon the complexity and length of the article [23]. Terms are assigned if the concept is discussed and any of the following conditions is met:

- Occurs in the title, purpose, or summary
- Is significant in research generally or the results of this paper specifically
- Is a check tag
- Is covered by several sections or paragraphs
- Is in a table or figure

The major concepts of the article, usually from two to five headings, are designed as *central concept* headings and designated in the MEDLINE record by an asterisk (noncentral concepts used to be called non-*Index Medicus* terms, since they were not represented in *Index Medicus*.) The indexer is also encouraged to assign the appropriate subheadings. Finally, the indexer must also assign check tags, geographical locations, and publication types.

Tools have been developed to assist indexers in selecting MeSH terms. The NLM developed the Medical Text Indexer[25] that uses a variety of methods to suggest MeSH terms for indexers [24, 25].

The NLM also edits some of the fields of the MEDLINE record. For example, author names are formatted with the last name followed by a space and then the initials of the first and middle (if present) name. The NLM policy on the number of authors included in the MEDLINE record has varied over the years. The current policy includes all author names, though in the past years, it was limited to 10 (1984–1995) or 25 (1996–1999). When the policy changes, it applies only to new records added to the database (i.e., existing records are not changed). Author and institutional names are entered as they appear in the journal, which leads to much variation in authors' names and affiliations (e.g., some of this author's articles in MEDLINE have his name listed `Hersh WR`, while others have `Hersh W`). Starting in 2002, the NLM added full author names to MEDLINE in the FAU field, with the previous abbreviated author name with last name and first and middle initials maintained in the old AU field [26].

Another type of manual indexing used by NLM is the annotation of gene function information in the Gene Reference Into Function (GeneRIF) [27]. Assignment of GeneRIFs is now part of the MEDLINE indexing process, although others can nominate them to NCBI, and all GeneRIFs are added for a given gene to Entrez Gene [28]. GeneRIFs describe the basic biology of the gene or its protein products from the designated organism, including the isolation, structure, genetics, and function of genes/proteins in normal and disease states. They are maintained in the NLM Gene database.[26] There are presently about 1.3 million GeneRIFs from over 819,000 publications representing over 98,000 genes.

[25] https://ii.nlm.nih.gov/Interactive/MTI/mti.shtml

[26] https://www.ncbi.nlm.nih.gov/gene/about-generif

McGregor has addressed the issues of indexing with MeSH outside the NLM, i.e., those who use it to index other resources [29]. He notes that MeSH is well-tuned to indexing the biomedical literature and that the NLM devotes the resources to updating it with the terms it needs, a process that is likely to consume too much resources for most other organizations. Adding "enhanced" or "local" terminology to MeSH can be challenging. One problem is mapping terms into the proper location in the MeSH hierarchy. Another is maintaining those new terms when MeSH is revised or reorganized by the NLM. McGregor also notes that the addition of terms is sometimes political, e.g., the developer of a new surgical procedure wants to be sure his or her new procedure is in the index. A final problem he notes is the lack of use of the MeSH hierarchy. Non-NLM indexers usually do not follow the adage of indexing to the most specific level so searchers can take advantage of the explosion feature of retrieval (see Chap. 5), which leads to poorer search results.

4.4.2 Full-Text Manual Indexing

Few full-text resources are manually indexed. One type of indexing that is commonly done with traditional books is the index at the back. However, that information is rarely used in IR systems; instead, most online textbooks rely on automated indexing (see later). Some Web sites do provide the structured headings of an online book as an alphabetized index, such as the Merck Manual Professional[27] and UpToDate.[28]

4.4.3 Web Manual Indexing

The Web both is and is not a good place for manual indexing. On the one hand, with billions of pages, manual indexing of more than a fraction of it is not feasible. On the other hand, the lack of a coherent index can make searching much more difficult, especially when specific resource types are being sought. A simple form of manual indexing of the Web takes place in the development of the Web catalogs and aggregations described in Chap. 3. These catalogs make not only explicit indexing about subjects and other attributes but also implicit indexing about the quality of a given resource by the decision of whether to include it in the catalog. Some classifications are derived from well-formulated principles. The health topics selected for MedlinePlus, for example, were developed from analysis of consumers' searches on the NLM site [30].

---

[27] https://www.merckmanuals.com/professional

[28] https://www.uptodate.com/

This section focuses on more formal approaches to manual indexing of Web content. Two main approaches have been used for manual indexing of Web content. The first approach, that of applying metadata to Web pages and sites, is exemplified by the *Dublin Core Metadata Initiative* (DCMI).[29] The second approach was much more popular in the early days of the Web but has mostly faded away, which was to build directories or catalogs of content. Other approaches to manual "indexing" of Web content include user tagging, where individuals on the Web tag pages, and paid search, where bidders vie for having their results displayed for search terms entered by users.

4.4.3.1 Dublin Core Metadata Initiative

One of the first frameworks for metadata on the Web was the DCMI, which has become a standard designated by several standards bodies: IETF RFC 5013 [RFC5013], ANSI/NISO Standard Z39.85-2007 [NISOZ3985], and ISO Standard 15836:2009 [ISO15836]. The goal of the DCMI was to develop a set of standard data elements that creators of Web resources could use to apply metadata to their content. The original standard defined 15 elements,[30] as shown in Table 4.5. A number of new terms have been added to the standards that are mostly refinements of the original elements. These elements do not differ greatly from metadata elements in older paper-based resources, such as the *Dewey decimal system* for library catalogs or the MEDLINE database for medical literature. Each DCMI term has a minimal set of attributes:

- Name—token appended to the URI of a DCMI namespace to create the URI of the term
- Label—human-readable label assigned to the term
- URI—Uniform Resource Identifier used to uniquely identify a term
- Definition—statement that represents the concept and essential nature of the term
- Type of Term—as described in the DCMI Abstract Model (DCAM)

The DCMI began as more of a semantic conceptualization than a definable syntax, and as such original versions did not completely identify how to represent the metadata. One early approach, adopted by many organizations, was to put the metadata elements right in the Web page, using the HTML META tag. Figure 4.4 shows what metadata might be associated with this book if it were available on a Web site. However, this tended to imply that the metadata would reside in Web pages. It could be argued that metadata should not reside within a resource, however particularly within Web pages. First, the practice may encourage the author of the page to perform the indexing, who is not necessarily the best person to provide the metadata. He or she may be unskilled in indexing, may have an ulterior motive (such as using

[29] https://www.dublincore.org/

[30] https://www.dublincore.org/specifications/dublin-core/dcmi-terms/

Table 4.5 The Dublin Core Metadata Initiative element set

Dublin Core element	Definition
DC.title	The name given to the resource
DC.creator	The person or organization primarily responsible for creating the intellectual content of the resource
DC.subject	The topic of the resource
DC. description	A textual description of the content of the resource
DC.publisher	The entity responsible for making the resource available in its present form
DC.date	A date associated with the creation or availability of the resource
DC. contributor	A person or organization not specified in a creator element who has made a significant intellectual contribution to the resource but whose contribution is secondary to any person or organization specified in a creator element
DC.type	The category of the resource
DC.format	The data format of the resource, used to identify the software and possibly hardware that might be needed to display or operate the resource
DC.identifier	A string or number used to uniquely identify the resource
DC.source	Information about a second resource from which the present resource is derived
DC.language	The language of the intellectual content of the resource
DC.relation	An identifier of a second resource and its relationship to the present resource
DC.coverage	The spatial or temporal characteristics of the intellectual content of the resource
DC.rights	A rights management statement, an identifier that links to a rights management statement, or an identifier that links to a service providing information about rights management for the resource

```
<META NAME=“DC.title” CONTENT=”Information Retrieval: A Biomedical and Health
Perspective, Fourth Edition” >
<META NAME=“DC.creator” CONTENT=“William Hersh, M.D.”>
<META NAME=“DC.subject” CONTENT=“Information storage and retrieval”>
<META NAME=“DC.subject” CONTENT=“Biomedical Informatics”>
<META NAME=“DC.description” CONTENT=“A book describing the use of information
retrieval systems in biomedicine and health.”>
<META NAME=“DC.publisher” CONTENT=“Springer”>
<META NAME=“DC.date” CONTENT=“2020-8-1”>
<META NAME=“DC.type” CONTENT=“Book”>
<META NAME=“DC.identifier” CONTENT=“http://www.irbook.info”>
<META NAME=“DC.language” CONTENT=“en-US”>
```

Fig. 4.4 Metadata for book Web site in DCMI

excess indexing terms in an attempt to increase page hits), or may not comply with the proper format of a given standard. Just as the NLM employs trained indexers to assign MEDLINE metadata, high-quality Web catalogs should employ standards of quality control and indexing expertise.

Another problem with the implication that DCMI should reside in Web pages is the assumption that all indexed resources should be at the granularity of the individual page. Like many information resources, print or electronic, many Web sites are not mere collections of HTML pages. Rather, they have organization and structure. A simple example is the online textbook in which the content is organized hierarchically. A more complex example is an aggregation Web site with pages providing not only information but also linkages across databases and applications.

The original DCMI specification had a number of other limitations. The most obvious was the lack of a standardized syntax, i.e., no standard method for expressing the values of attributes. Dates comprise a well-known example, e.g., the date 2020-2-5 is generally interpreted as February 5, 2020, in the United States but as May 2, 2020 in European countries. As any user of MEDLINE who is searching for articles by a specific person or their institution knows, of course, the lack of a standardized syntax, of course, is not unique to the DCMI. (Names and locations in MEDLINE are complicated by inconsistent usage in source articles.) The standardized syntax problem has been partially rectified with the development of Dublin Core Qualifiers, which recommended standards for certain elements such as `DC.Format`, `DC.Language`, and `DC.Date`. These have now been replaced by the larger number of DCMI terms, a specification for using controlled vocabularies (Vocabulary Encoding Schemes), various syntax specifications (Syntax Encoding Schemes), specified attributes of resources (Classes), and enumerated types of resources (DCMI Type Vocabulary). A user guide on the DCMI site describes the process for creating DCMI metadata.[31]

There were several early medical adaptations of the DCMI, most of which are no longer operational [31–33]. Another early project still applying the DCMI to healthcare resources is the *Catalogue et Index des Sites Médicaux Francophones* (CISMeF)[32] [34, 35]. A catalog of French-language health resources on the Web, CISMeF uses DCMI to catalog tens of thousands of Web pages, including information resources (e.g., practice guidelines, consensus development conferences), organizations (e.g., hospitals, medical schools, pharmaceutical companies), and databases. The `Subject` field uses the French translation of MeSH but also includes the English translations.[33] For `Type`, a list of common Web resources was developed [36].

One early approach for moving the metadata outside of the Web page was the *Resource Description Framework* (RDF) [37]. A framework for describing and interchanging metadata, RDF is usually expressed in Extensible Markup Language (XML) or the JavaScript Object Notation (JSON), which are standards for data interchange on the Web. RDF consists of the following entities:

- A *resource* is anything that can have a URI.
- A *property* is an attribute of a resource, such as an `author` or `subject`.
- A *statement* is the combination of a resource, a property, and a value for the property.

---

[31] https://www.dublincore.org/resources/userguide/creating_metadata/

[32] http://www.chu-rouen.fr/cismef/

[33] https://www.inserm.fr/en/professional-area/scientific-and-technical-information/bilingual-mesh

```
<!DOCTYPE rdf:RDF SYSTEM "http://purl.org/dc/schemas/dcmes-xml-20000714.dtd">
<rdf:RDF xmlns:rdf="http://www.w3.org/1999/02/22-rdf-syntax-ns#"
   xmlns:dc="http://purl.org/dc/elements/1.1">
 <rdf:Description>
  <dc:title>Information Retrieval: A Biomedical and Health
                    Perspective, Fourth Edition</dc:title >
  <dc:creator>William Hersh, M.D.</dc:creator>
  <dc:subject>Information storage and retrieval</dc:subject>
  <dc:subject>Biomedical Informatics</dc:subject>
  <dc:description>A book describing the use of information retrieval
                    systems in biomedicine and health.</dc:description>
  <dc:publisher>Springer</dc:publisher>
  <dc:date>2020-8-1</dc:date>
  <dc:type>Book</dc:type>
  <dc:identifier>http://www.irbook.info<dc:identifier>
  <dc:language>en-US</dc:language>
 </rdf:Description>
</rdf:RDF>
```

Fig. 4.5 DCMI metadata for book Web site in RDF

RDF is expressed in a subject-predicate-object format. An example of an RDF statement is a book (resource) authored (property) by William Hersh (value). The object can be a literal (string) or a resource. In this example, the author can be a name (literal) or structured resource, such as an XML structure with the author's name, address, phone, email, and so on. RDF properties can be represented in XML. Figure 4.5 shows the metadata of Fig. 4.4 reformulated in RDF. The use of URIs to identify resources on the Web is the foundation of the "linked data" vision of the semantic Web [38].

Using RDF to represent DCMI moves the metadata outside the Web page, thus decoupling metadata and content. As a result of this advantage, different metadata providers can maintain different sets of metadata. Much as the metadata of MEDLINE and EMBASE cover the same content (journal articles) but with varying overlap (higher representation of non-English journals in the latter) and different metadata schemas (e.g., MeSH vs. EMTREE), RDF allows different entities to maintain their own collections of metadata. This permits different "brands" of indexing, which can compete with each other to provide the best metadata for their intended audiences. Put another way, RDF allows individuals or groups to define a common semantics expressed in a standardized syntax.

4.4.3.2 Open Directory

Another approach to cataloging content on the Web has been to create directories of content. This approach was popularized initially by the original Yahoo search engine, although Web searching on the Yahoo site is now provided by Microsoft Bing and the catalog approach is no longer used.[34] The proprietary nature of the Yahoo cata-

---

[34] https://www.yahoo.com/

log led to a more open approach with the Open Directory Project (DMOZ, which is still archived[35]). The structuring of the directory and entry of content was maintained by volunteers across the world, although this project too was not sustainable.

4.4.3.3 User Tagging

Another approach that has emerged to index various types of Web content is user tagging [39]. This approach has also been called "social bookmarking," where a community of users (sometimes anyone on the Web) indexes and/or even rates content [40]. One Web site that applies user tagging is the image sharing Web site Flickr,[36] which also uses automated methods to help users select tags. As noted in the last chapter, one resource using a form of user tagging for clinical purposes has been implemented in JournalWise, which uses the *McMaster Online Rating of Evidence* (MORE)[37] system, where clinicians rate journal articles already filtered for scientific (i.e., evidence-based) merit.

This approach is also sometimes called "collaborative filtering," where recommendations to users or customers are delivered based on measures of similarities across interests, purchases, and so forth [41]. It has probably been commercially used longest by Amazon[38] [42], although Netflix[39] is also well-known for its recommendation of movies and other content. Collaborative filtering has been employed in a variety of clinical applications, including detection of diseases [43, 44] and consumer information access [45].

4.4.3.4 Paid Search

Although we do not think of it as "indexing" in the traditional sense, the growing application of "paid search" is a form of indexing, albeit search terms paid to the highest bidder. Paid search is the assignment of indexing terms to content based on how much someone is willing to pay for them [46]. While some search engines do not distinguish between search results based on paid search, Google has developed a highly successful business model by clearly demarcating advertised pages (denoted by an AD icon) from its regular search results. Google Ads works by advertisers bidding on given words and phrases for how much they are willing to pay when a user sees the ad and clicks through to the advertiser's site. Whoever is willing to bid more for a word or phrase will rank higher in the output. Advertisers are charged only when users click-through and can set a daily maximum to not exceed a specific

[35] https://dmoz-odp.org/

[36] https://www.flickr.com/

[37] http://hiru.mcmaster.ca/more/

[38] https://www.amazon.com/

[39] https://www.netflix.com/

budget. Once the daily maximum is reached, the advertiser's ad will no longer appear until the following day. One challenge with paid search is *click fraud*, where competitors or others with malicious intent can set up robots that click-through ads just to run up the advertiser's cost to their daily maximum [47].

4.4.4 Limitations of Manual Indexing

The human indexing process is imperfect. Some of its limitations stem from the use of a thesaurus, which may not contain all the important terminology in a field or may not word the terms in a way that allows nonexpert users to readily identify and apply them. One study of 75 MEDLINE queries generated in a clinical setting contained terms that could not be found in the UMLS Metathesaurus, which is a superset of the MeSH vocabulary [48]. A thesaurus also may not be up to date. In the mid-1980s, for example, knowledge and terminology related to `AIDS` expanded and changed, with MeSH lagging several years behind.

Another problem with human indexing, described earlier, is inconsistency. Funk and Reid evaluated indexing inconsistency in MEDLINE by identifying 760 articles that had been indexed twice by the NLM [4]. The most common reasons for duplicate indexing were the accidental resending of an already-indexed article to another indexer and instances of a paper being published in more than one journal. Using Hooper's equation, Funk and Reid generated the consistency percentages for each category of MeSH term shown in Table 4.6. As can be seen, the most consistent indexing occurred with check tags and central concept headings, although even these only ranged in the level of 61–75%. The least consistent indexing occurred with subheadings, especially those assigned to non-central concept headings, which had a consistency of less than 35%. This study was replicated in the newer indexing environment of the NLM. The results showed that human indexing consistency has not changed substantially, as seen in Table 4.6 [49].

Table 4.6 Consistency of MEDLINE indexing by category of MeSH [4, 49]

Category of MeSH	Consistency (%)—Funk and Reid	Consistency (%)—Marcetich et al.
Check tags	74.7	74.5
Central concept headings	61.1	48.6
Geographics	56.6	Not measured
Central concept subheadings	54.9	46.1
Subheadings	48.7	43.4
Headings	48.2	Not measured
Central concept heading/subheading combination	43.1	28.3
Heading/subheading combination	33.8	24.3

4.5 Automated Indexing

In automated indexing, the second type of indexing that occurs in most commercial retrieval systems, the work is done by a computer. Although the mechanical running of the automated indexing process lacks cognitive input, considerable intellectual effort may have gone into development of the process, so this form of indexing still qualifies as an intellectual process. This section will focus on the automated indexing used in operational IR systems, namely, the indexing of documents by the words they contain.

4.5.1 Word Indexing

People tend not to think of extracting all the words in a document as "indexing," but from the standpoint of an IR system, words are descriptors of documents, just like human-assigned indexing terms. Most retrieval systems actually use a hybrid of human and word indexing, in that the human-assigned indexing terms become part of the document, which can then be searched by using the whole controlled vocabulary term or individual words within it. As will be seen in the next chapter, most MEDLINE implementations have always allowed the combination of searching on human indexing terms and on words in the title and abstract of the reference. With the development of full-text resources in the 1980s and 1990s, systems that allowed word indexing only began to emerge. This trend increased with the advent of the Web.

Word indexing is typically done by taking all consecutive alphanumeric sequences between "white space," which consists of spaces, punctuation, carriage returns, and other non-alphanumeric characters. Systems must take particular care to apply the same process to documents and users' queries, especially with characters such as hyphens and apostrophes. The process usually generates an inverted file, as described in Sect. 4.7. These files can store the part of the document in which the word occurs. They may also store the word's position in the document, which can use proximity searching as described in the next chapter.

4.5.2 Limitations of Word Indexing

Simple word indexing has a number of obvious limitations, as is well-known by anyone who has tried to search for information on the computer programming language Java and ended up with articles about coffee (or vice versa). The potential pitfalls include the following:

- Synonymy—different words may have the same meaning, such as high and elevated. This problem may extend to the level of phrases with no words in common, such as the synonyms hypertension and high blood pressure.
- Polysemy—the same word may have different meanings or senses. For example, the word lead can refer to an element or to a part of an electrocardiogram machine.
- Content—words in a document may not reflect its focus. For example, an article describing hypertension may make mention in passing to other concepts such as congestive heart failure that are not the focus of the article.
- Context—words take on meaning based on other words around them. For example, the relatively common words high, blood, and pressure take on added meaning when occurring together in the phrase high blood pressure.
- Morphology—words can have suffixes that do not change the underlying meaning, such as indicators of plurals, various participles, adjectival forms of nouns, and nominalized forms of adjectives.
- Granularity—queries and documents may describe concepts at different levels of a hierarchy. For example, a user might query for antibiotics in the treatment of a specific infection, but the documents might describe specific antibiotics themselves, such as penicillin.

A number of approaches to these problems have been proposed, implemented, and evaluated. For example, natural language processing techniques have been tried for recognizing synonyms, eliminating the ambiguity from polysems, recognizing the context of phrases, and overcoming morphological variation. The limited successes with these approaches have been difficult to generalize and are research problems that will be described in Chap. 8. While the MeSH vocabulary and associated features in MEDLINE (e.g., the explosion function described in the next chapter) have handled granularity well in the manual indexing approach, automated approaches to recognizing hierarchical relationships have not lent themselves to generalization.

4.5.3 Word Weighting

One limitation of word indexing that has been addressed with some success is content, or the ability to give higher weight to more important words in a document that improve retrieval output. Based on an approach developed by Salton in the 1960s [50], this approach has proven effective particularly for inexperienced searchers, who of course comprise the majority of those using Web search engines. Sadly, Salton, a true pioneer in the IR field, passed away in 1995 just as the approach he created was starting to achieve use in large-scale operational retrieval systems.

Salton's approach goes by a variety of names, such as automated indexing, natural language retrieval, statistical retrieval, and the vector-space model. A key element, no matter what the name, has been the use of techniques that do not require manual activities. Despite widespread adoption of the weighting of indexing terms and their use in natural language retrieval with relevance ranking, other techniques innovated by Salton remain research lines of investigation and will be covered in Chap. 8. The remainder of this section will focus on Salton's basic approach, sometimes called the TF*IDF approach.

Salton's work in the 1960s was influenced by work done in the 1950s by Luhn, an IBM researcher who asserted that the content of documents themselves could be used for indexing [51]. The majority of researchers until that time had assumed that human selection of indexing terms was the most appropriate method for indexing. Luhn noted that words in English followed the *law of Zipf*, where frequency of the word in a collection of text times rank of the word by frequency is a constant. He proposed, therefore, that words in a collection could be used to rate their importance as indexing terms. He asserted that words of medium frequency had the best "resolving power," that is, were best able to distinguish relevant from nonrelevant documents, and advocated that words with high and low frequency be removed as indexing terms.

The most well-known data to support the Zipfian distribution of the English language came from the *Brown Corpus*, a collection of word frequencies based on a variety of English-language texts totaling a million words [52]. Table 4.7 shows the ten most common words in English, along with the Zipfian constant. The *Brown Corpus* also showed that 20% of words in English account for 70% of usage. Zipf's law has been found to hold in other information collections, including clinical data codes in British general practice, although not in medication usage [53].

Salton extended Luhn's ideas and was the first to implement them in a functioning system [54]. Salton asserted that Luhn's proposals were probably too simplistic. One would not want to eliminate, for example, high-frequency words like `diagnosis` and `treatment`, which might be necessary to distinguish documents about these subtopics of a disease. Likewise, one would not necessarily want to eliminate very-low-frequency words like `glucagonoma`, since there might be few documents about this rare type of tumor in any medical database.

Table 4.7 The ten most common words in the million-word *Brown Corpus* with rank and frequency, adapted from [54]

Term	Rank	Frequency	(Rank × Frequency)/1000
the	1	69,971	70.0
of	2	36,411	72.8
and	3	28,852	86.6
to	4	26,149	104.6
a	5	23,237	116.2
in	6	21,341	128.0
that	7	10,595	74.2
is	8	10,099	80.8
was	9	9816	88.3
he	10	9543	95.4

Salton introduced the notion of an indexing term's *discrimination value*, which is its ability to distinguish relevant from nonrelevant documents on a given topic. In practice, a term with a high discrimination value is one that occurs frequently in a small number of documents but infrequently elsewhere. The value of this approach can be shown with a hypothetical example. Consider two databases, one focused on the topic of `AIDS` and another covering general medicine. In the former, a word like `AIDS` would be unlikely to be useful as an indexing term because it would occur in almost every document and, when it did, would be nonspecific. The words more likely to be useful in an `AIDS` database would be those associated with specific aspects of the disease, such as `Pneumocystis`, `carinii`, and `zidovudine`. In a general medicine database, on the other hand, only a small portion of documents would cover the topic of `AIDS`, and thus it would probably be a good indexing term.

The first step in word-weighted indexing is similar to all other word-based indexing approaches, which is to identify the appropriate portions of a research amenable to such indexing (e.g., the title and text of an article or its MEDLINE reference) and break out all individual words. These words are filtered to remove *stop words*, which are common words (e.g., those at the top of the *Brown Corpus* list) that always occur with high frequency and hence are always of low discrimination value. The stop word list, also called a *negative dictionary*, varies in size from the seven words of the original MEDLARS stop list (`and, an, by, from, of, the, with`) to the list of 250–500 words more typically used. Examples of the latter are the 250-word list of van Rijsbergen [55] and the 471-word list of Fox [56]. The PubMed stop list is shown in Table 4.8.

It should be noted, of course, that stop words can sometimes be detrimental. For example, most stop word lists contain the word `a`, whose elimination would be problematic in the case of documents discussing `Vitamin A` or `Hepatitis A`. In general, however, the elimination of stop words is beneficial not only for term discrimination purposes but also for making indexing and retrieval more computationally efficient. For example, their removal leads to the reduction in size of the inverted disk files that store indexing information, since stop words tend to have a large number of postings and thus consume disk space. Eliminating these words also allows faster query processing, since stop words tend to occur in many documents, adding to the computational requirement of building and ranking retrieval sets.

In the next step, words not on the stop list undergo *stemming* to reduce them to their root form. The purpose of stemming is to ensure words with plurals and common suffixes (e.g., `-ed`, `-ing`, `-er`, `-al`) are always indexed by their stem form [57]. The benefit of stemming, however, is less clear [58]. Not only are actual experimental results mixed, but simple algorithmic rules for stemming can be shown to lead to erroneous results (e.g., stemming `aids` to `aid`). Stemming does, however, tend to reduce the size of indexing files and also leads to more efficient query processing. A simple stemming algorithm to remove plurals is shown in Table 4.9.

The final step is to assign weights to document terms based on discrimination ability. A commonly used measure that typically achieves good results is TF*IDF weighting, which combines the inverse document frequency (IDF) and term

Table 4.8 The PubMed stop list (Courtesy of NLM)

A	a, about, again, all, almost, also, although, always, among, an, and, another, any, are, as, at
B	be, because, been, before, being, between, both, but, by
C	can, could
D	did, do, does, done, due, during
E	each, either, enough, especially, etc
F	for, found, from, further
H	had, has, have, having, here, how, however
I	i, if, in, into, is, it, its, itself
J	just
K	kg, km
M	made, mainly, make, may, mg, might, ml, mm, most, mostly, must
N	nearly, neither, no, nor
O	obtained, of, often, on, our, overall
P	perhaps
Q	quite
R	rather, really, regarding
S	seem, seen, several, should, show, showed, shown, shows, significantly, since, so, some, such
T	than, that, the, their, theirs, them, then, there, therefore, these, they, this, those, through, thus, to
U	upon, use, used, using
V	various, very
W	was, we, were, what, when, which, while, with, within, without, would

https://www.ncbi.nlm.nih.gov/books/NBK3827/table/pubmedhelp.T.stopwords/

Table 4.9 A simple stemming algorithm, adapted from [58]

1. If word ends in "ies" but not "eies" or "aies," then replace "ies" with "y"
2. If word ends in "es" but not "aes", "ees", or "oes," then replace "es" with "e"
3. If word ends in "s" but not "us" or "ss," then delete "s"

frequency (TF). The IDF is the logarithm of the ratio of the total number of documents to the number of documents in which the term occurs. It is assigned once for each term in the database, and it correlates inversely with the frequency of the term in the entire database. The usual formula used is:

$$\mathrm{IDF}(\text{term}) = \log \frac{\text{number of documents in database}}{\text{number of documents with term}} + 1. \tag{4.2}$$

The TF is a measure of the frequency with which a term occurs in a given document and is assigned to each term in each document, with the usual formula:

$$\mathrm{TF}(\text{term,document}) = \text{frequency of term in document}. \tag{4.3}$$

In TF*IDF weighting, the two terms are combined to form the indexing weight, WEIGHT:

$$\text{WEIGHT}(\text{term,document}) = \text{TF}(\text{term,document}) * \text{IDF}(\text{term}) \tag{4.4}$$

With this weighting approach, the highest weight is accorded to terms that occur frequently in a document but infrequently elsewhere, which corresponds to Salton's notion of discrimination value.

4.5.4 Link-Based Indexing

Another automated indexing approach generating increased interest is the use of link-based methods, fueled no doubt by the success of the Google search engine. These methods have a lineage back to bibliometrics, introduced in Chap. 2, where the notion of citation gives some idea of the quality of a publication. Extended to the Web, Google's approach goes beyond word-based indexing to also give weight to pages based on how often they are cited by other pages. A more complete description of the Google retrieval approach is presented in the next chapter, but the PageRank (PR) algorithm that gives indexing weight to pages based on linkages is presented here.

In a simple description, PR can be viewed as giving more weight to a Web page based on the number of other pages that link to it. Thus, a page from the NLM, the Mayo Clinic, or a high-profile medical journal is likely to have a very high PR, whereas a more obscure page will have a lower PR. The PR algorithm was developed by Brin and Page [59]. To calculate it for a given page *A*, it is assumed that there is a series of pages $T_1 \ldots T_n$ having links to *A*. There is another function *C*(*A*) that is the count of the number links going out of page *A*. There is also a "damping factor" *d* that is set between 0 and 1, by default at 0.85. Then PR is calculated for *A* as:

$$\text{PR}(A) = (1-d) + d\left(\frac{\text{PR}(T_1)}{C(T_1)} + \cdots + \frac{\text{PR}(T_n)}{C(T_n)}\right). \tag{4.5}$$

The algorithm begins by assigning every page a baseline value (such as the damping factor) and then iterates on a periodic basis. When implemented efficiently on a moderately powered workstation, PR can be calculated for a large collection of Web pages. Although the actual operations of Google are now highly guarded trade secrets, a number of researchers have developed and published efficient implementations to calculate it [60].

4.5.5 Web Crawling

The Web presents additional challenges for indexing. Unlike most fixed resources such as MEDLINE, online textbooks, or image collections, the Web has no central catalog that tracks all its pages and other content. The fluid and dynamic nature of the Web makes identifying pages to be indexed a challenge for search engines. While some Web site developers submit their site URLs, the search engines themselves must still identify all the pages within the sites. The usual approach to finding Web pages for indexing is to use "crawling" or "spidering" [61]. Essentially, the search engine finds a page, indexes all the words on the page, and then follows all links to additional pages. The process is repeated for all pages not already indexed. Since much Web content is dynamic, the crawling process must periodically revisit pages already crawled to update the index if the content has changed. Sites can prevent parts or all of their content from being indexed by the Robots Exclusion Protocol, whereby they place a file in their directory called robots.txt that follows a convention for allowing or disallowing crawling [62]. (The process is voluntary, although all major search engines obey the protocol.) We are also now in the era of "adversarial" IR, where an indexing or retrieval system may want to explicitly not index or retrieve some content [63].

Henzinger et al. described a number of challenges for Web-crawling search engines that are still pertinent today [64]:

- Synonymy—different words may have the same meaning, such as `high` and `elevated`. This problem may extend to the level of phrases with no words in common, such as the synonyms `hypertension` and `high blood pressure`.
- Polysemy—the same word may have different meanings or senses. For example, the word `lead` can refer to an element or to a part of an electrocardiogram machine.
- Content—words in a document may not reflect its focus. For example, an article describing `hypertension` may make mention in passing to other concepts such as `congestive heart failure` that are not the focus of the article.
- Context—words take on meaning based on other words around them. For example, the relatively common words `high`, `blood`, and `pressure` take on added meaning when occurring together in the phrase `high blood pressure`.
- Morphology—words can have suffixes that do not change the underlying meaning, such as indicators of plurals, various participles, adjectival forms of nouns, and nominalized forms of adjectives.
- Granularity—queries and documents may describe concepts at different levels of a hierarchy. For example, a user might query for `antibiotics` in the treatment of a specific infection, but the documents might describe specific antibiotics themselves, such as `penicillin`.

4.6 Indexing Annotated Content

As noted in Chap. 3, a growing category of information people seek to retrieve is either nontextual or text that is highly structured. As such, retrieval is usually done by searching over annotations. In this section, we describe the indexing of certain types of such information, such as images, identifiers, learning objects, and the increasing amount of datasets available on the Web.

4.6.1 Index Imaging

The growth of images online plus the availability of new methods for processing them, e.g., machine learning, has made the indexing and retrieval of images more important, especially in the "visual" specialties of biomedicine, such as radiology, pathology, and dermatology [65, 66]. In essence, there are two basic approaches to indexing of images. One is *semantic indexing*, also called textual indexing, which uses textual annotations of the image (or group of images). The other approach to image indexing is called *content-based indexing* or *visual indexing*. In somewhat of an analogy to document indexing, the semantic approach can be considered to be "manual" indexing, in that words usually written by humans are associated with such indexing. In contrast, the content-based approach could be called "automated" indexing, since the "indexing" is derived from automatically processing the content of images. The semantic gap is used to describe the differences between what is in the semantic and content-based indexing approaches [66].

The semantic indexing of images can be quite varied, from simple free-text descriptions (from a simple description to the detailed findings in a radiology report) to the use of more structured metadata, such as DCMI or more imaging-specific approaches, such as the Annotation and Image Markup (AIM) from the National Cancer Informatics Program (NCIP) [67]. One simple free-text approach for indexing images comes from the Google Image search tool,[40] which "indexes" images by the text of the Web pages in which they appear. A somewhat-related approach for radiology images in the medical literature is to use the text in figure legends [68]. While many systems that use controlled vocabularies for indexing images apply such standard resources as MeSH or SNOMED CT, one system has been developed specifically for radiological images called RadLex[41] [69]. The AIM approach makes use of multiple controlled vocabularies and allows specific areas of medical images to be annotated, for example, with [69]:

- Image reference—identifier and format
- Geometric shape—coordinates in image

[40] https://images.google.com/

[41] http://www.radlex.org/

- Anatomic location—body location, e.g., `liver`
- Observation—radiologic finding, e.g., `mass`
- Impression—clinical diagnosis, e.g., `hepatocellular carcinoma`

Greenes et al. noted that indexing and retrieval of images may be compromised by the fact that many clinical observations are represented along a *findings-diagnosis continuum*, where they may be expressed differently based on how much diagnostic interpretation the clinician is adding. For example, an abnormality in a chest X-ray may be described as an `increased density` by one interpreter and a `nodule` by another. The latter contains more interpretation of the finding than the former. They recommend an approach to representing findings that makes the differences along the findings-diagnosis continuum explicit. In addition to the expected fields for anatomic site, procedure type, evaluation technique, and organism observation, there are those for:

1. Elemental findings—simplest description of a finding (e.g., `increased density`)
2. Composite findings—description with some deductive information added (e.g., `nodule`)
3. Etiologic diagnosis—diagnosis based on inference from the finding, such as the `apical infiltrations` seen on a classic chest X-ray in `tuberculosis`
4. Inference procedure—procedure used to infer composite findings or etiological diagnoses from elemental findings

In content-based image indexing, computer algorithms identify *features* in the image. Although image retrieval will be discussed at greater length in the next chapter on retrieval, it should be noted here that content-based image retrieval tools typically build vectors of these features and aim to retrieve images with similar features. These features include aspects of an image that a computer algorithm can recognize, such as:

- Color, including the intensity and sets of color
- Texture, such as coarseness, contrast, directionality, linelikeness, regularity, and roughness
- Shape, including what types are present
- Segmentation, the ability to recognize boundaries

4.6.2 Indexing Learning Objects

Another type of content attracting a great deal of interest from an indexing standpoint is e-learning content. An emerging view in this area is that educational content should be developed as *learning objects*, which should be sharable, reusable, and able to be discovered by their metadata. For indexing learning objects, one clear possibility is DCMI, and in fact, they have developed a Learning Resource Metadata

Initiative (LRMI)[42] that aims to extend the terms of DCMI along with incorporating elements of the Schema.org ontology. Schema.org itself has been developed for educational content.[43] Another extension involving Schema.org and DCMI has been developed for open educational resources (OERs).[44] Schema.org has been further elaborated by Bioschemas.org for specific educational elements:

- Course[45]
- Course instance[46]
- Training material[47]

Another standard for indexing e-learning content is the IEEE 1484 Learning Object Metadata (IEEE LOM) standard.[48] The IEEE LOM consists of nine general categories:

1. General
2. LifeCycle
3. Metametadata
4. Technical
5. Educational
6. Rights
7. Relation
8. Annotation
9. Classification

A comparison between IEEE LOM and DCMI was carried out for the iLumina Digital Library Project, which covers science, technology, engineering, and mathematics content for college undergraduates [70]. The authors found that IEEE LOM was more comprehensive than DCMI (it has many more elements), but most of the elements deemed most important in IEEE LOM had correlates in DCMI. A medical-specific version of IEEE LOM, Healthcare LOM, was developed by the MedBiquitous Consortium[49] (now part of the Association of American Medical Colleges [AAMC]) and integrated with learning competencies [71]. Healthcare LOM is also used in the Health Education Assets Library (HEAL).[50] HEAL maintains a metadata standard for medical education content such as images, cases,

[42] https://www.dublincore.org/specifications/lrmi/

[43] http://schema.org/Course

[44] http://oerschema.org/

[45] https://bioschemas.org/specifications/drafts/Course/

[46] https://bioschemas.org/specifications/drafts/CourseInstance/

[47] https://bioschemas.org/specifications/TrainingMaterial/

[48] https://standards.ieee.org/project/1484_12_1.html

[49] https://www.medbiq.org/

[50] https://library.med.utah.edu/heal/

quizzes, lecture slides, and so forth so that they can be readily shared by other medical educators [72].

Another metadata schema for indexing learning content is the Harper-Lite: Simple Lesson Discovery and Aggregation,[51] which includes the following fields:

- Title
- Abstract
- Version
- Contributor
- Package—URL of learning package
- License
- Requirements—requirements for use
- Prereq—prerequisites
- Postreq—learning objectives
- Teaches—subject
- Notes

One effort for indexing educational content with a focus on data science came from the Educational Resource Discovery Index for Data Science (ERuDIte)[52] [73]. This project developed a Data Science Education Ontology (DSEO) that is housed in BioPortal and organizes concepts along six dimensions:

- Data science process—stage of data science process, e.g., `data exploration`, `data visualization`
- Domain—field of study of resource, e.g., `biology`, `medicine healthcare`
- Datatype—type(s) of data are addressed in resource, e.g., `text data`, `image data`
- Programming tool—programming tool used in or taught by resource, e.g., `R`, `Python`
- Resource format—how resource presented, e.g., `written documents`, `video`
- Resource depth—how advanced resource is, e.g., `introductory`, `advanced`

Other efforts at indexing learning content have a focus on the clinical and translational research community [74, 75]. These extend the eagle-i ontology and have been used in the following projects:

- N-Lighten[53]
- Diamond[54]

---

[51] https://github.com/gvwilson/harper

[52] https://bigdatau.ini.usc.edu/about_erudite

[53] https://github.com/NLightenGroup/nlighten-ontology

[54] https://clic-ctsa.org/index.php/diamond

4.6.3 *Indexing Biomedical and Health Data*

As noted in Chap. 2, a significant problem for science is reproducibility. This is due in part to the materials used in research not being explicitly identified. One analysis assessed recent journal articles in the fields of neuroscience, developmental biology, immunology, cell and molecular biology, and general biology, finding that 54% of resources are not uniquely identifiable in publications [76]. This has led to projects such as eagle-i,[55] which aims to explicitly catalog biological resources, such as organisms, cell lines, antibodies, reagents, and so forth [77]. A set of best practices has been proposed for the use of Web-based identifiers in biomedical research [78]. Another resource to index is the growing amount datasets that are available both from published research and also generally. The DAta Tag Suite (DATS) was developed as part of the biomedical and healthCAre Data Discovery Index Ecosystem (bioCADDIE) project [79].

A final element of importance with regard to indexing data and any other source of information is explicit identification of the author(s). Author names continue to be a challenge for bibliographic and other databases, especially as others establish linkages and metrics based on them. This is becoming even more problematic with the increasing number and productivity of Chinese authors, who tend to have short and simple names [80]. A standard for author identifiers that is achieving rapid uptake is the Open Researcher and Contributor ID (ORCID).[56] This author's ORCID is 0000-0002-4114-5148, which can be used in a URL that links to a Web page listing publications and other information.[57]

4.7 Data Structures for Efficient Retrieval

As mentioned at the beginning of the chapter, the second purpose of indexing is to build structures so that computer programs can rapidly ascertain which documents use which indexing terms. Whether indexing is by terms in a thesaurus or words, IR systems are feasible only if they can rapidly process a user's query. A timely sequential search over an indexed text database is infeasible if not impossible for any large document collection.

A computer index usually consists of a group of *inverted files*, where the terms are "inverted" to point to all the documents in which they occur. The algorithms for building and maintaining these structures are described well by Frakes and Baeza-Yates [81]. An inverted file group for a sample document collection as it would be stored on a computer disk is shown in Fig. 4.6. The first file is the *dictionary* file,

---

[55] https://www.eagle-i.net/

[56] http://orcid.org

[57] http://orcid.org/0000-0002-4114-5148

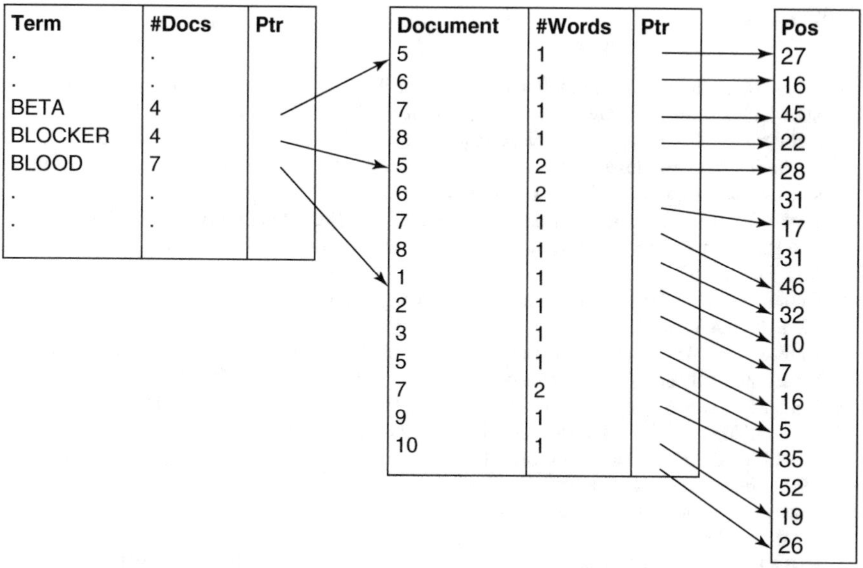

Fig. 4.6 Inverted file for a group documents and their indexing terms BETA, BLOCKER, and BLOOD. The dictionary file contains the indexing terms, the number of documents in which they occur, and a pointer to the list of documents containing each term in the postings file. The postings file contains the document number for each indexing term, the number of words in the document, and a pointer to the list of word positions in the position file. The position file contains the word positions for the document. The pointers represent file addresses on the disk and are given by arrows rather than numbers to enhance readability

which contains each indexing term along with a number representing how many documents contain the term and a pointer to the *postings* file. The postings file consists of a sequential list of all the documents that contain the indexing term. If it is desired to keep positional information for the indexing term (to allow proximity searching), then the postings file will also contain a pointer to the *position* file, which sequentially lists the positions of each indexing term in the document. The structure of the position file depends on what positional information is actually kept. The simplest position file contains just the word position within the document, while more complex files may contain not only the word number but also the sentence and paragraph number within the document.

The final component of inverted files is a mechanism for rapid lookup of terms in the dictionary file, which is typically done with methods developed in computer science, such as the B-tree or hashing [82]. Of course, with the need to process millions of queries each minute, just having an efficient file and lookup structure is not enough. Systems must be distributed across many servers in disparate geographic locations. Although the details of its approach are proprietary, Google has published some on how it maintains its sub-second response time to queries from around the globe [83, 84].

References

1. Miles W. A history of the National Library of Medicine: the nation's treasury of medical knowledge. Bethesda, MD: U.S. Department of Health and Human Services; 1982.
2. Anonymous. Index Medicus to cease as print publication. NLM Tech Bull. 2004;2004:e2.
3. Leonard L. Inter-indexer consistency and retrieval effectiveness: measurement of relationships. Champaign, IL: University of Illinois; 1975.
4. Funk M, Reid C. Indexing consistency in MEDLINE. Bull Med Libr Assoc. 1983;71:176–83.
5. Arp R, Smith B, Spear A. Building ontologies with basic formal ontology. Cambridge, MA: MIT Press; 2015.
6. Cimino J, Zhu X. The practical impact of ontologies on biomedical informatics. Methods Inf Med. 2006;45(Supp 1):124–35.
7. Harrow I, Balakrishnan R, Jimenez-Ruiz E, Jupp S, Lomax J, Reed J, et al. Ontology mapping for semantically enabled applications. Drug Discov Today. 2019;24:2068–75.
8. Köhler S, Vasilevsky N, Engelstad M, Foster E, McMurry J, Groza T, et al. The human phenotype ontology in 2017. Nucleic Acids Res. 2017;45:D865–76.
9. Coletti M, Bleich H. Medical subject headings used to search the biomedical literature. J Am Med Inform Assoc. 2001;8:317–23.
10. Anonymous. A comparison of Emtree® and MeSH®. Amsterdam: Elsevier R&D Solutions; 2015.
11. Blake J. Ten quick tips for using the Gene Ontology. PLoS Comput Biol. 2013;9(11):e1003343.
12. Dessimoz C, Škunca N, editors. The Gene Ontology handbook, Methods in molecular biology. New York: Springer Nature; 2017.
13. Cimino J. Desiderata for controlled medical vocabularies in the twenty-first century. Methods Inf Med. 1998;37:394–403.
14. Lindberg D, Humphreys B, McCray A. The Unified Medical Language System project. Methods Inf Med. 1993;32:281–91.
15. Evans D, editor. Pragmatically-structured, lexical-semantic knowledge bases for unified medical language systems. Proceedings of the 12th Annual Symposium on Computer Applications in Medical Care; 1988; Washington, DC: IEEE.
16. Masarie F, Miller R, Bouhaddou O, Giuse N, Warner H. An interlingua for electronic exchange of medical information: using frames to map between clinical vocabularies. Comput Biomed Res. 1991;24:379–400.
17. Barr C, Komorowski H, Pattison-Gordon E, Greenes R, editors. Conceptual modeling for the Unified Medical Language System. Proceedings of the 12th Annual Symposium on Computer Applications in Medical Care; 1988; Washington, DC: IEEE.
18. Humphreys B, Lindberg D, Schoolman H, Barnett G. The Unified Medical Language System: an informatics research collaboration. J Am Med Inform Assoc. 1998;5:1–11.
19. Bodenreider O. The Unified Medical Language System (UMLS): integrating biomedical terminology. Nucleic Acids Res. 2004;32:D267–70.
20. Chen Y, Perl Y, Geller J, Cimino J. Analysis of a study of the users, uses, and future agenda of the UMLS. J Am Med Inform Assoc. 2007;14:221–31.
21. Charen T. MEDLARS indexing manual, part I: bibliographic principles and descriptive indexing, 1977. Springfield, VA: National Technical Information Service; 1976.
22. Charen T. MEDLARS indexing manual, part II. Springfield, VA: National Technical Information Service; 1983.
23. Bachrach C, Charen T. Selection of MEDLINE contents, the development of its thesaurus, and the indexing process. Med Inform. 1978;3:237–54.
24. Mork J, Jimeno-Yepes A, Aronson A, editors. The NLM medical text indexer system for indexing biomedical literature. BioASQ Workshop; 2013, Valencia.
25. Mork J, Aronson A, Demner-Fushman D. 12 years on—is the NLM medical text indexer still useful and relevant? J Biomed Semant. 2017;2017(8):8.
26. Nahin A. Full author searching comes to PubMed. NLM Tech Bull. 2003;2003:e4.

27. Mitchell J, Aronson A, Mork J, Folk L, Humphrey S, Ward J, editors. Gene indexing: characterization and analysis of NLM's GeneRIFs. Proceedings of the AMIA 2003 Annual Symposium; 2003; Washington, DC: Hanley & Belfus.
28. Maglott D, Ostell J, Pruitt K, Tatusova T. Entrez Gene: gene-centered information at NCBI. Nucleic Acids Res. 2007;35:D26–31.
29. McGregor B. Medical indexing outside the National Library of Medicine. J Med Libr Assoc. 2003;90:339–41.
30. Miller N, Lacroix E, Backus J. MEDLINEplus: building and maintaining the National Library of Medicine's consumer health Web service. Bull Med Libr Assoc. 2000;88:11–7.
31. Malet G, Munoz F, Appleyard R, Hersh W. A model for enhancing Internet medical document retrieval with "medical core metadata". J Am Med Inform Assoc. 1999;6:183–208.
32. Dolin R, Boles M, Dolin R, Green S, Hanifin S, Hochhalter B, et al., editors. Kaiser Permanente's "metadata-driven" national clinical intranet. MEDINFO 2001—Proceedings of the Tenth World Congress on Medical Informatics; 2001; London: IOS Press.
33. Robertson W, Leadem E, Dube J, Greenberg J, editors. Design and implementation of the National Institute of Environmental Health Sciences Dublin Core Metadata schema. Proceedings of the International Conference on Dublin Core and Metadata Applications 2001; 2001; Tokyo: National Institute of Informatics (NII).
34. Soualmia L, Darmoni S. Combining different standards and different approaches for health information retrieval in a quality-controlled gateway. Int J Med Inform. 2005;74:141–50.
35. Merabti T, Lelong R, Darmoni S. InfoRoute: the CISMeF context-specific search algorithm. Stud Health Tech Inform. 2015;216:544–8.
36. Darmoni S, Thirion B. A standard metadata scheme for health resources. J Am Med Inform Assoc. 2000;7:108–9.
37. Manola F, Miller E. RDF primer. Cambridge, MA: World Wide Web Consortium; 2004.
38. Sakr S, Wylot M, Mutharaju R, LePhuoc D, Fundulaki I. Linked data—storing, querying, and reasoning. Cham: Springer Nature; 2018.
39. Morrison P. Why are they tagging, and why do we want them to? Bull Am Soc Inf Sci Technol. 2007;34(1):12–5.
40. Hammond T, Hannay T, Lund B, Scott J. Social bookmarking tools (I)—a general review. D-Lib Mag. 2005;11(4). http://www.dlib.org/dlib/april05/hammond/04hammond.html.
41. Nandi M. Recommender systems through collaborative filtering. Domino Data Lab; 2017.
42. Smith B, Linden G. Two decades of recommender systems at Amazon.com. IEEE Internet Comput. 2017;2017:12–8.
43. Caplan E, Rosenthal N. Collaborative filtering: an interim approach to identifying clinical doppelgängers. Health Affairs Blog; 2013.
44. Shen F, Liu S, Wang Y, Wen A, Wang L, Liu H. Utilization of electronic medical records and biomedical literature to support the diagnosis of rare diseases using data fusion and collaborative filtering approaches. JMIR Med Inform. 2018;6(4):e11301.
45. Wiesner M, Pfeifer D. Health recommender systems: concepts, requirements, technical basics and challenges. Int J Environ Res Public Health. 2014;11:2580–607.
46. Scott D. The new rules of marketing and PR: how to use social media, online video, mobile applications, blogs, newsjacking, and viral marketing to reach buyers directly. Hoboken, NJ: Wiley; 2017.
47. Soubusta S. On click fraud. Informationswissenschaft. 2008;59(2):136–41.
48. Hersh W, Hickam D, Haynes R, McKibbon K. A performance and failure analysis of SAPHIRE with a MEDLINE test collection. J Am Med Inform Assoc. 1994;1:51–60.
49. Marcetich J, Rappaport M, Kotzin S, editors. Indexing consistency in MEDLINE. MLA 04 Abstracts; 2004; Washington, DC: Medical Library Association.
50. Salton G. Developments in automatic text retrieval. Science. 1991;253:974–80.
51. Luhn H. A statistical approach to mechanized encoding and searching of literary information. IBM J Res Dev. 1957;1:309–17.
52. Kucera H, Francis W. Computational analysis of present-day American English. Providence, RI: Brown University Press; 1967.

53. Kalankesh L, New J, Baker P, Brass A. The languages of health in general practice electronic patient records: a Zipf's law analysis. J Biomed Semant. 2014;5:2.
54. Salton G, McGill M. Introduction to modern information retrieval. New York: McGraw-Hill; 1983.
55. van Rijsbergen C. Information retrieval. London: Butterworth; 1979.
56. Fox C. Lexical analysis and stop lists. In: Frakes W, Baeza-Yates R, editors. Information retrieval: data structures and algorithms. Englewood Cliffs, NJ: Prentice-Hall; 1992. p. 102–30.
57. Frakes W. Stemming algorithms. In: Frankes W, Baeza-Yates R, editors. Information retrieval: data structures and algorithms. Englewood Cliffs, NJ: Prentice-Hall; 1992. p. 131–60.
58. Harman D. How effective is suffixing? J Am Soc Inf Sci. 1991;42:7–15.
59. Brin S, Page L. The anatomy of a large-scale hypertextual Web search engine. Comput Netw ISDN Syst. 1998;30:107–17.
60. Yates E, Dixon L. PageRank as a method to rank biomedical literature by importance. Source Code Biol Med. 2015;10:16.
61. Cambazoglu B, Baeza-Yates R. Scalability challenges in web search engines. Synthesis lectures on information concepts, retrieval, and services. San Rafael, CA: Morgan & Claypool Publishers; 2015.
62. Koster M. A method for web robots control. San Francisco: America Online; 1996.
63. Castillo C, Davison B. Adversarial web search. foundations and trends in information retrieval. Delft: Now Publishers; 2011.
64. Henzinger M, Motwani R, Silverstein C. Challenges to Web search engines. SIGIR Forum. 2002;36:11–22.
65. Müller H, Unay D. Retrieval from and understanding of large-scale multi-modal medical datasets: a review. IEEE Trans Multimedia. 2017;19(9):17099710.
66. Li Z, Zhang X, Müller H, Zhang S. Large-scale retrieval for medical image analytics: a comprehensive review. Med Image Anal. 2018;43:66–84.
67. Mongkolwat P, Kleper V, Talbot S, Rubin D. The National Cancer Informatics Program (NCIP) Annotation and Image Markup (AIM) foundation model. J Digit Imaging. 2014;27:692–701.
68. Kahn C, Thao C. GoldMiner: a radiology image search engine. Am J Roentgenol. 2007;188:1475–8.
69. Wang K. Standard lexicons, coding systems and ontologies for interoperability and semantic computation in imaging. J Digit Imaging. 2018;31:353–60.
70. Heath B, McArthur D, McClelland M, Vetter R. Metadata lessons from the iLumina digital library. Commun ACM. 2005;48(7):68–74.
71. Hersh W, Bhupatiraju R, Greene P, Smothers V, Cohen C, editors. Adopting e-learning standards in health care: competency-based learning in the medical informatics domain. Proceedings of the AMIA 2006 Annual Symposium; 2006; Washington, DC: American Medical Informatics Association.
72. Candler C, Uijtdehaage S, Dennis S. Introducing HEAL: the Health Education Assets Library. Acad Med. 2003;78:249–53.
73. Ambite J, Fierro L, Geigl F, Gordon J, Burns G, Lerman K, et al., editors. BD2K ERuDIte: the educational resource discovery index for data science. Proceedings of the 26th International Conference on World Wide Web Companion; 2017; Perth.
74. Calvin-Naylor N, Jones C, Wartak M, Blackwell K, Davis J, Unsworth K, et al. Education and training of clinical and translational study investigators and research coordinators: a competency-based approach. J Clin Trans Sci. 2017;1:16–25.
75. Hornung C, Jones C, Calvin-Naylor N, Kerr J, Sonstein S, Hinkley T, et al. Competency indices to assess the knowledge, skills and abilities of clinical research professionals. Int J Clin Trials. 2018;5:46–53.
76. Vasilevsky N, Brush M, Paddock H, Ponting L, Tripathy S, Larocca G, et al. On the reproducibility of science: unique identification of research resources in the biomedical literature. PeerJ. 2013;5(1):e148.

77. Vasilevsky N, Johnson T, Corday K, Torniai C, Brush M, Segerdell E, et al. Research resources: curating the new eagle-i discovery system. Database. 2012;2012:bar067.
78. McMurry J, Juty N, Blomberg N, Burdett T, Conlin T, Goble C, et al. Identifiers for the 21st century: how to design, provision, and reuse persistent identifiers to maximize utility and impact of life science data. PLoS Biol. 2017;15(6):e2001414.
79. Sansone S, Gonzalez-Beltran A, Rocca-Serra P, Alter G, Grethe J, Xu H, et al. DATS: the data tag suite to enable discoverability of datasets. Sci Data. 2017;4:170059.
80. Qiu J. Scientific publishing: identity crisis. Nature. 2008;451:766–7.
81. Frakes W, Baeza-Yates R, editors. Information retrieval: data structures and algorithms. Englewood Cliffs, NJ: Prentice-Hall; 1992.
82. Wartik S, Fox E, Heath L, Chen Q. Hashing algorithms. In: Frakes W, Baeza-Yates R, editors. Information retrieval: data structures and algorithms. Englewood Cliffs, NJ: Prentice-Hall; 1992. p. 293–362.
83. Barroso L, Dean J, Hölzle U. Web search for a planet: the Google Cluster Architecture. IEEE Micro. 2003;23(2):22–8.
84. Dean J, Ghemawat S. MapReduce: simplified data processing on large clusters. Commun ACM. 2008;51(1):107–13.

Chapter 5
Retrieval

The last two chapters discussed the content and organization of textual databases. Chapter 3 covered the different types of databases available, while Chap. 4 showed how they are indexed for optimal retrieval. This chapter, which explores the interaction of the IR system with the user, the person whom it is intended to serve, covers the entire retrieval process, from search formulation to system interaction to content delivery.

The relationship between the information retrieval (IR) system and its users has changed considerably over the years. In the 1960s, users of the only database available, MEDLINE, had to undergo formal training at the National Library of Medicine (NLM) before being provided access. Searching itself was done by filling out a form that had to be mailed to the NLM, with a "turnaround" time of 2–3 weeks for the results to be mailed back. In the 1970s, NLM databases could be directly accessed by trained searchers over time-sharing computer networks, though clinicians, researchers, and others wanting searches done still had to go through trained intermediaries, typically librarians. The user typically had to make an appointment with the intermediary and wait for him or her to perform the search and return the results, but this did reduce the turnaround time from weeks to days. In the 1980s, online databases first became available to "early adopter" end users. Connecting to networks, then information providers, and then databases was still somewhat laborious. The 1990s saw the explosion of end user searching on the Web. The ease of use provided by powerful servers and graphical user interfaces as well as the general ubiquity of the Internet made searching a mainstream task performed by millions, with a turnaround time now down to 2–3 s. Well into the twenty-first century, what advances will speed or improve searching next?

The original version of this chapter was revised and updated. The correction to this chapter can be found at https://doi.org/10.1007/978-3-030-47686-1_9

W. Hersh, *Information Retrieval: A Biomedical and Health Perspective*,
Health Informatics, https://doi.org/10.1007/978-3-030-47686-1_5

5.1 Search Process

Chapter 2 discussed the three general reasons for consulting IR systems [1]: a need for information to solve a certain problem, a need for background information, or a need to keep up with a subject. Furthermore, within each information need, there was a spectrum of possible amounts of information needed, from a single fact to a few documents to an exhaustive collection of literature. The variation in these needs results in different strategies for interacting with the IR system.

Pao described four stages a searcher might go through before actually using an IR system [2]:

1. Information problem—user determines that an information deficiency exists
2. Information need—user decides what must be known to solve the information problem
3. Question—user determines what motivates the interaction with the IR system
4. Request—user submits the search statement to the IR system

Based on the results of any stage, the user may return to earlier stages and modify them.

While any type of user can have any type of information need, the needs of certain groups of users are likely to differ from those of other groups. In the biomedicine and health field, one can readily discern the different needs of clinicians and researchers [3]. Clinicians, including physicians, nurses, dentists, and other allied healthcare providers, are likely to have specific needs in solving problems [4]. In general, they want a search to be more precise and to include the most relevant documents to their specific need. Researchers, on the other hand, are more likely to have broader needs on a given topic. For example, someone writing a paper will want a definitive overview of the topic, whereas a researcher exploring a new topic will want a great deal of background information. Researchers are likely to be more tolerant of retrieving nonrelevant references to make sure they find all the relevant ones and in fact may benefit from the "serendipity" of off-focus retrievals [5].

5.2 General Principles of Searching

Whereas each of the four stages identified by Pao is important in helping users to meet their information needs, the step of going from question to request is most important for IR system designers [2]. After all, this is the step that will allow users to actually find documents that will meet their needs and ultimately solve their information problems. This section describes the general principles for retrieval in most currently available IR systems. It initially compares the two most common approaches to searching, exact-match (or Boolean or set-based) searching and partial-match (or natural language, ranked, or automated) searching. Then the selection of search terms and attributes, to prepare for the description of specific searching interfaces, is discussed in Sect. 5.3.

5.2.1 Exact-Match Searching

In *exact-match searching*, the IR system gives the user all documents that exactly match the criteria specified in the search statement(s). Since the Boolean operators AND, OR, and NOT are usually required to create a manageable set of documents, this type of searching is often called *Boolean searching*. Furthermore, since the user typically builds sets of documents that are manipulated with the Boolean operators, this approach is also called *set-based searching*. Most of the early operational IR systems in the 1950s through 1970s used the exact-match approach, even though Salton was developing the partial-match approach in research systems during that time [6]. In modern times, exact-match searching tends to be employed by more expert searchers, while the partial-match approach tends to be used by novices or those having simple information needs.

Typically, the first step in exact-match retrieval is to select terms to build sets. Other attributes, such as the author name, publication type, or gene identifier (in the secondary source identifier field of MEDLINE), may be selected to build sets as well. Since the user typically has an information need less broad than "all documents on a particular disease or treatment," the Boolean operators are used to focus the search output on all the elements in the information need. These operators also serve to create a document set that can be realistically analyzed. Blair spoke of the "futility point" of search results, the number of documents beyond which a searcher would stop looking at the results [7]. He speculated that the value of this point was 50 documents, although modern search systems typically have 10 (Google) or 20 (PubMed) documents per screen of output.

Once the search term(s) and attribute(s) have been selected, they are combined with the Boolean operators. The use of Boolean operators derives from *Boolean algebra*, which is based on *set theory*, the branch of mathematics dealing with sets and their algebraic manipulation. In set theory, a set is defined as a collection of elements. Examples of sets include all documents with the indexing term `Hypertension` or all students in a class. There are three common operations that are performed on sets, which correspond to the three common Boolean operators used in IR systems: intersection, union, and complement. These operations are depicted by Venn diagrams in Fig. 5.1.

The *intersection* of two sets is the set that contains only the elements that are common to both sets. This is equivalent to the Boolean AND operator. This operator is typically used to narrow a retrieval set to contain only documents about two or more concepts. For example, if one desired documents on the use of the drug `propranolol` in the disease `Hypertension`, a typical search statement might be `propranolol` AND `Hypertension`. Using the AND would most likely eliminate articles, for example, on the use of `propranolol` in `migraine headaches` and the `diagnosis` of `hypertension`.

The *union* of two sets is the set that contains all the elements that occur in either set, equivalent to the Boolean OR operator. This operator is usually used when there is more than one way to express a concept. For example, the name of the virus that causes `AIDS` has carried a number of names and acronyms over the years. When

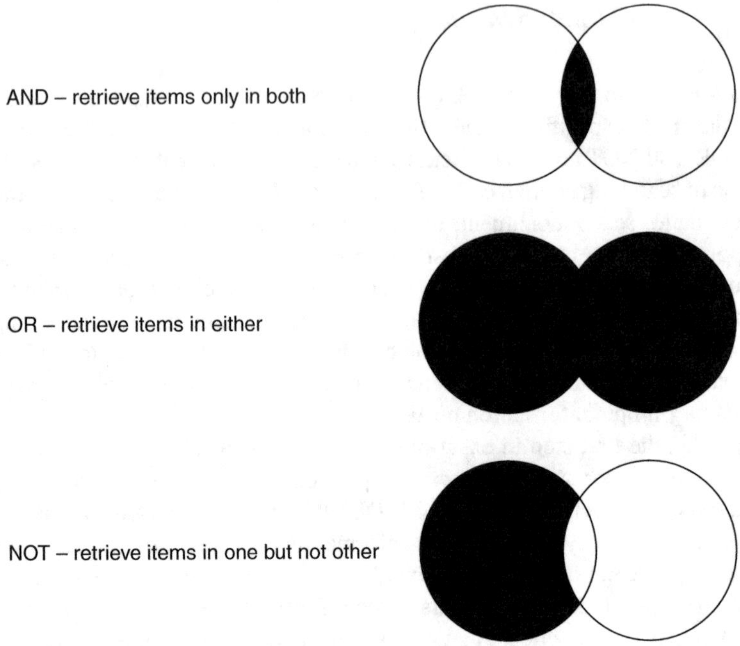

Fig. 5.1 Boolean operators AND, OR, and NOT

simultaneously discovered by French and American scientists, it was assigned the names `Lymphadenopathy Associated Virus` (LAV) and `Human T-Cell Leukemia Virus 3` (`HTLV-3`), respectively. It was later renamed `Human Immunodeficiency Virus` (`HIV`). Likewise, one of the early treatments for `AIDS` was originally called `azidothymidine` or `AZT` but was later called `zidovudine`.

The *complement* of a set is the set with all the elements of some universal set that are not contained in the complemented set, equivalent to the Boolean NOT operator. However, for practical reasons, most IR systems use the NOT operator as a complement. In a large database such as MEDLINE, with its many millions of documents, the set of all documents that do not, for example, contain the term `Hypertension`, could be very large. As a result, most IR systems use NOT as a subtraction operator that must be applied to another set. Some systems more accurately call this the ANDNOT operator.

Boolean operations can be demonstrated by looking at Table 5.1, which shows a small five-document, five-term database. The query A AND B will only retrieve document 5, since that is the only term common to both documents. The query A OR B, on the other hand, will retrieve documents 1, 2, 4, and 5, since one of the query terms is present in these four documents. The query A NOT B will retrieve documents 1 and 4, since they contain term A but not B.

Table 5.1 Five-document by five-term database

	Documents						
Terms	1	2	3	4	5	Documents with term	IDF
A	1	0	0	3	1	3	1.22
B	0	2	0	0	1	2	1.40
C	1	0	0	2	3	3	1.22
D	0	1	1	0	0	2	1.40
E	1	0	0	0	0	1	1.70

5.2.2 Partial-Match Searching

Although *partial-match searching* was conceptualized by Salton and others in the 1960s, it did not achieve widespread use in IR systems until the advent of Web search engines in the 1990s. This is most likely because exact-match searching tends to be preferred by "power users," whereas partial-match searching is preferred by novice searchers. Whereas exact-match searching requires an understanding of Boolean operators and (often) the underlying structure of databases (e.g., the many fields in MEDLINE), partial-match searching allows a user to simply enter a few terms and start retrieving documents. Despite the surface simplicity of partial-match searching, however, its effectiveness can be comparable to that of exact-match searching (see Chap. 7), and new research approaches using it (see Chap. 8) can be quite complex.

The development of partial-match searching is usually attributed to Salton [8], who pioneered the approach in the 1960s. Although partial-match searching does not exclude the use of nonterm attributes of documents and for that matter does not even exclude the use of Boolean operators (e.g., see [9]), the most common use of this type of searching is with a query of a small number of words, also known as a *natural language query*. Because Salton's approach was based on vector mathematics, it is also referred to as the *vector-space model* of IR. In the partial-match approach, documents are typically ranked by their closeness of fit to the query. That is, documents containing more query terms will likely be ranked higher, since those with more query terms will in general be more likely to be relevant to the user. As a result, this process is called *relevance ranking*. The entire approach has also been called *statistical retrieval*, *lexical-statistical retrieval*, and *ranked retrieval*.

The most common approach to document ranking in partial-match searching is to give each a score based on the sum of the weights of terms common to the document and query. Terms in documents typically derive their weight from the TF*IDF calculation described in Chap. 4. Terms in queries are typically given a weight of one if the term is present and zero if it is absent. The following formula can then be used to calculate the document weight across all query terms:

Table 5.2 TF*IDF weighting for the terms and documents in Table 5.1

	Documents					
Terms	1 (NR)	2 (R)	3	4 (R)	5 (NR)	Relevance feedback query
A	1.22	0	0	3.67	1.22	1.61
B	0	2.80	0	0	1.40	1.70
C	1.22	0	0	2.44	3.67	−0.22
D	0	1.40	1.40	0	0	0.70
E	1.70	0	0	0	0	0

$$\text{Document weight} = \Sigma_{\text{all query terms}} (\text{Weight of term in query} * \text{Weight of term in document}) \quad (5.1)$$

This may be thought of as a giant OR of all query terms, with sorting of the matching documents by weight. The usual approach is for the system to then perform the same stop word removal and stemming of the query that was done in the indexing process. (The equivalent stemming operations must be performed on documents and queries so that complementary word stems will match.)

The sample database in Table 5.1 can demonstrate partial-match searching. To simplify calculations, Table 5.1 shows the IDF for each term, and Table 5.2 shows the TF*IDF weighting for each term in each document. A query using the terms "A B C" will retrieve four documents with the following ranking:

1. Document 5 (1.22 + 1.40 + 3.67 = 6.29)
2. Document 4 (3.67 + 2.44 = 6.11)
3. Document 2 (2.80)
4. Document 1 (1.22 + 1.22 = 2.44)

In general, documents that contain more of the query terms will be ranked higher. As seen in the sample query, document 5 contains three terms in the query, while document 4 contains two. However, document 2 only has one query term while document 1 has two. But it achieves its higher ranking because the term present in document 2 has a higher weight than the two terms in document 1 combined. These results often occur when a term has a higher IDF, which is consistent with the rationale of IDF in that terms which occur with less frequency across the entire database are more "discriminating" than those which are more common.

One problem with TF*IDF weighting is that longer documents accumulate more weight in queries simply because they have more words. As such, some approaches "normalize" the weight of a document. The most common approach is cosine normalization:

$$\text{Document weight} = \frac{\sum_{\text{all query terms}} (\text{Weight of term in query} * \text{Weight of term in document})}{\sqrt{\left(\sum_{\text{all query terms}} \text{Weight of term in query}^2\right) * \left(\sum_{\text{all document terms}} \text{Weight of term in document}^2\right)}} \quad (5.2)$$

A variety of other variations to the basic partial-matching retrieval approach have been developed. All are considered to be research approaches and are covered in more detail in Chap. 8. Some apply different weighting than the simple TF*IDF, while others add more weight to certain parts of documents, such as the title or the anchor text in a Web link. Some apply different approaches to normalization.

Relevance feedback, a feature allowed by the partial-match approach, permits new documents to be added to the output based on their similarity to those deemed relevant by the user. This approach also allows reweighting of relevant documents already retrieved to higher positions on the output list. The most common approach is the modified Rocchio equation [10]. In this equation, each term in the query is reweighted by adding value for the term occurring in relevant documents and subtracting value for the term occurring in nonrelevant documents. There are three parameters, α, β, and γ, which add relative value to the original weight, the added weight from relevant documents, and the subtracted weight from nonrelevant documents, respectively. In this approach, the query is usually expanded by adding a specified number of query terms (from none to several thousand) from relevant documents to the query. Each query term takes on a new value based on the following formula:

$$\begin{aligned}
&\text{New query weight} = \\
&\alpha * \text{Original query weight} \\
&+\beta * \frac{1}{\text{number of relevant documents}} * \sum_{\text{all relevant documents}} \text{weight in document} \\
&-\gamma * \frac{1}{\text{number of nonrelevant documents}} * \sum_{\text{all nonrelevant documents}} \text{weight in document}
\end{aligned} \tag{5.3}$$

When the parameters, α, β, and γ, are set to one, this formula simplifies to:

$$\begin{aligned}
&\text{New query weight} = \\
&\text{Original query weight} \\
&+\text{Average term weight in relevant documents} \\
&-\text{Average term weight in nonrelevant documents}
\end{aligned} \tag{5.4}$$

In its rightmost column, Table 5.2 shows the new weight for each query term when documents 2 and 4 are relevant, documents 1 and 5 are not relevant, and term D is added to the query (since it occurs in document 2, which is relevant). As can be seen, none of the query terms maintains its original weight of 1.0. The weights of terms in query are now:

1. A = 1 + (3.67/2) – (2.44/2) = 1.61
2. B = 1 + (2.8/2) – (1.4/2) = 1.70
3. C = 1 + (2.44/2) – (4.89/2) = -0.22
4. D = 0 + (1.7/2) – 0 = 0.70
5. E = 0 (no relevant docs so none added)

Table 5.3 Weighting of terms in documents after Rocchio relevance feedback process

	Documents				
Terms	1	2	3	4	5
A	1.97	0	0	5.90	1.97
B	0	4.75	0	0	2.38
C	−0.27	0	0	−0.54	−0.81
D	0	0.98	0.98	0	0
E	0	0	0	0	0

By applying these new query weights to Eq. 5.1 above, the weight of terms in document can be recalculated, as shown in Table 5.3. These weights can then be used with Eq. 5.1 above to reweight the documents after the relevance feedback process:

1. Document 2 = 4.75 + 0.98 = 5.73
2. Document 4 = 5.90 − 0.54 = 5.36
3. Document 5 = 1.97 + 2.38 − 0.81 = 3.54
4. Document 1 = 1.97 − 0.27 = 1.70
5. Document 3 = 0.98

As can be seen, document 2 has moved to the top of the list, while document 5 has fallen, and document 3 has been added. These phenomena typically occur with relevance feedback, in general (but not always) achieving the goal of moving existing relevant documents higher in the output list, adding new relevant ones, and moving existing nonrelevant documents lower.

A number of IR systems offer a variant of relevance feedback that finds similar documents to a specified one. PubMed allows the user to obtain "similar articles" from any given one in an approach similar to relevance feedback but which uses a different algorithm [11, 12]. A number of Web search engines allow users to similarly obtain related articles from a specified Web page.

5.2.3 *Term Selection*

As noted in Chap. 5, search terms are generally either terms from a controlled vocabulary assigned by a manual indexing process or words extracted from the documents themselves by means of an automated process. While either type of term can be used in either type of searching approach, controlled vocabulary terms are most commonly employed in exact-match systems. Typically, when appropriate controlled terms are not available, document words are applied. Partial-match systems almost always use document words as indexing terms, though they may be qualified by where they occur, such as in the title or anchor text.

5.2.3.1 Term Lookup

Whereas early IR systems required users to enter search terms with minimal assistance (i.e., terms had to be found in telephone-book-sized catalogs and typed in exactly), most modern systems provide assistance with term lookup.

PubMed, for example, provides a MeSH lookup function that allows users to type in one or more words from a term, select the appropriate term, and build a search with it. The Ovid system[1] also allows user lookup of MeSH terms but uses a somewhat different approach, displaying a ranked list of MeSH terms that most commonly appear in MEDLINE references when the word(s) entered also occurs.

5.2.3.2 Term Expansion

Some systems allow terms in searches to be expanded by using the *wildcard character*, which adds all words to the search that begin with the letters up until the wildcard character. This approach is also called *truncation*. Unfortunately, there is no standard approach to using wildcard characters, so syntax for them varies from system to system. PubMed, for example, allows a single asterisk at the end of a word to signify a wildcard character. Thus, the query entry `can*` will lead to the words `cancer` and `Candida`, among others, being added to the search (although PubMed warns when more than 600 citations are retrieved.). Ovid allows the use of four different wildcard characters. In its basic mode interface, the asterisk character can be used, and it functions similarly to the asterisk in PubMed. In the advanced mode, however, there are three different wildcard characters:

- Limited truncation allows all terms with the root and the specified number of digits to be added to the query. It is specified by the dollar sign followed by a digit. For example, dog$1 retrieves documents containing `dog` and `dogs` but not `dogma`.
- Mandated wild card allows single characters to be substituted within or at the end of a word. It is specified by the pound sign (#). For example, `wom#n` will lead to retrieval of documents containing `woman` or `women`. There must be a character present; that is, `dog#` will not retrieve `dog`.
- Optional wild card allows zero or more characters to be substituted within or at the end of a word. It is specified by the question mark. For example, `colo?r` will lead to retrieval of documents containing `color` or `colour`. This character cannot be used after the first letter of a word.

5.2.3.3 Other Word-Related Operators

Some IR systems have operators that require more than just the term being present. The proximity operator, for example, specifies not only that two words be present but also that they occur within a certain distance of each other in the document. It is essentially an AND with the additional restriction that the words be within a specified proximity. These operators can help control for the context of words in a concept. For example, a user looking for documents on `colon cancer` might specify

[1] https://www.ovid.com/

that the words colon and cancer appear within five words of each other. This would capture documents with phrases like colon cancer and cancer of the colon but would avoid documents that discuss cancer in one part and mention colon in another (e.g., description of the effect of a type of cancer that somehow affects colon motility).

As with other features, different systems implement and have varying syntax for proximity operators. PubMed does not provide proximity searching although it does, as will be described shortly, allow searching against a list of common multiword phrases, such as health planning. Ovid, on the other hand, does provide this capability. Its ADJ operator requires words to be adjacent and in the order specified. For example, the query blood ADJ pressure will retrieve only documents that have the phrase blood pressure. The operator ADJn, where n is a digit, requires words to be within *n* characters of each other. For example, colon ADJ5 cancer will retrieve documents with both colon cancer and cancer of the colon. The Web search engine AltaVista has a proximity operator NEAR, which requires target words to be within ten words of each other.

Another word-related term specification feature in Ovid is the FREQ=n command, which will not retrieve a document unless a word or phrase is present n or more of times. One word-related feature no longer found in most systems is synonym specification. The long-retired STAIRS system from IBM had a SYN operator that allowed a user to designate two words as synonymous. For example, entering cancer SYN carcinoma would cause the two words to be used interchangeably (i.e., connected to the other with OR whenever either is used).

5.2.3.4 Subheadings

Recall from Chap. 4 that some thesauri, including MeSH, contain *subheadings*, which are modifiers that can be attached to terms. For example, one can restrict the retrieval of documents on the subject of Hypertension to just those covering diagnosis or treatment. Many MEDLINE systems also allow searching with the so-called floating subheadings, which allow the searcher to specify just the subheading itself, as if it were a solitary, unattached indexing term.

Subheadings have the effect of increasing the precision of a search, since documents on other aspects of the search term should be eliminated from the retrieval set. They should have no effect on recall, since the documents not retrieved should be focused on other aspects of the term. However, it is possible that the indexers may not assign a subheading where one is warranted; thus, the use of the subheading will preclude that document from being retrieved. Since subheading assignment is the least consistent area of indexing term assignment (see Chap. 4), most expert searchers advise care in the use of subheadings.

5.2.3.5 Explosions

Like the subheading, the *explosion* operation requires a controlled vocabulary. It further requires that the vocabulary have a hierarchical organization. The explosion operation is an OR of the term exploded with all the narrower terms below it in the hierarchy. It is typically used when a user wants to retrieve documents about a whole class of topics. For example, a user might want to obtain documents on all types of `anemia`. There are many types of `anemia`, due to deficiencies of nutrients (`iron, vitamin B12, folate`), disease processes (`hemolytic anemia, anemia of chronic disease`), and genetic disorders (`sickle cell anemia` and other `hemoglobinopathies`). If a searcher wanted to obtain information on all those anemias in the MEDLINE database, the general MeSH term `Anemia` would be exploded which would have the effect of combining the general and specific terms together with the OR operator. Another common reason for using explosions is to search on a category of drugs. For example, most drugs in the `ACE Inhibitors` category (e.g., `captopril, enalapril, lisinopril`) function similarly, so the user interested in the category would want to explore the general MeSH term `ACE Inhibitors`.

PubMed automatically explodes all terms that are not *terminal terms* or *leaf nodes* in the hierarchy (i.e., do not have a more specific term below them). Ovid, on the other hand, gives the user the choice of exploding or not. While autoexplosion is in general effective (especially for the examples just given), it can be detrimental when the MeSH hierarchy is not a true "is-a" or "part-of" hierarchy, that is, the more general term is not a generalization of the more specific terms. This occurs with the MeSH term `Hypertension`, which is autoexploded. The terms underneath it in the hierarchy represent elevated blood pressure in specific body locations, such as the portal vein of the liver (`Portal Hypertension`) or the arteries of the lung (`Pulmonary Hypertension`). These terms are included in the autoexplosion even though most searches on `essential hypertension` (designated by the MesH term `Hypertension`) would not want to search on them.

As with subheadings, explosions require quality, consistent indexing. One of the principles taught to MEDLINE indexers to make explosions work well is that documents should be indexed to the "deepest" level of a hierarchy. Thus, if a document deals with a specific type of `anemia`, such as `iron-deficiency anemia`, it will be indexed on that specific term. This allows searchers to home in on documents specifically about the disease with the MeSH term `Iron-deficiency anemia` or still capture it more broadly by exploding the MeSH term, `Anemia`.

Explosions have the effect of increasing recall, since additional documents indexed on related but more specific terms are brought into the retrieval set. The effect on precision is variable, since the exploded topics may be relevant to the more general search term or they may be too specific for the needs of the searcher.

5.2.3.6 Spelling Correction

A common feature of modern search engines, such as Google and PubMed, is detection of likely spelling errors and the offering of words for their correction. In PubMed, when a word entered in the search has few or no matches, the user is presented with an alternative spelling and the number of citations that would be retrieved if that option was selected [13, 14]. The spelling option is deactivated when the user enters a search tag, e.g., [mh]. An example of how the spelling correction of Google or PubMed works can be seen by entering `breast cancerr` into either.

5.2.4 Other Attribute Selection

As noted already, indexing not only consists of terms but also entails other attributes about documents against which the user might desire to search. In MEDLINE, for example, the user might wish to search for papers by a specific author, in a specific journal, or represent a certain type of publication, such as a review article or a randomized controlled trial. On the Web, one might wish to search against only certain parts of Web pages, such as the text in a title or the anchor text in links. One might also wish to restrict Web searches to specific domains or hosts. The syntax for specifying these attributes is explained in the discussion of the different searching interfaces in the next section.

5.3 Searching Interfaces

In describing interfaces to various IR systems, the goal is not to exhaustively cover all features of all systems but rather to demonstrate how features are implemented within various systems. Precedence is given to displaying systems of historical or market importance. The organization of this section follows the classification of content that was used to describe in Chap. 3.

Before we begin describing actual interfaces, let us make a few general comments. First, searching interfaces are constantly changing, so what is seen in this book reflects what they looked like when the book was written. Second, most systems do things somewhat differently, sometimes minimally and sometimes substantially. There is no standard approach to searching that has been adopted by all interfaces. Finally, many systems provide both "simple" and "advanced" interfaces, with the former allowing quick searches and the latter giving more control over refinement of the results.

5.3.1 *Bibliographic*

As noted in Chap. 3, bibliographic content includes literature reference databases, Web catalogs, and specialized registries. Literature reference databases, or bibliographic databases, continue to be the flagship IR application in healthcare. Even though most users want to obtain the full text of biomedical articles online, PubMed still provides an entry point to finding them.

5.3.1.1 Literature Reference Databases

Until the mid-1990s, MEDLINE was most commonly accessed using a command-line interface on a system called ELHILL over time-sharing networks accessed either by a dedicated line or telephone modem connection. ELHILL was mostly unforgiving, requiring users to enter MeSH terms exactly or get a "No postings" message. Its command-line interface also required users to remember set numbers for their Boolean combination.

One early innovative system from the 1980s was PaperChase, which was also the first MEDLINE system geared to clinicians [15]. PaperChase provided features taken for granted in modern systems, such as input of word fragments (instead of requiring the whole MeSH term), assistance with MeSH term lookup, intuitive description of the Boolean operators, and ability to handle American and British spelling variants.

Another innovative approach to MEDLINE came from the NLM in the 1980s. Grateful Med was the first MEDLINE system to run on a personal computer and feature a "full-screen" interface that provided text boxes for specific fields (such as author, title, and subject), check boxes for tags such as English language and review articles, and expression of subject terms both as MeSH terms and text words [16]. Grateful Med eventually moved to the Web in Internet Grateful Med, sporting an expert assistant called COACH that helped users diagnose problematic searches but was discontinued by NLM with the advent of PubMed [17].

While there are still other interfaces for accessing MEDLINE, such as Ovid described above, the majority of searching MEDLINE in modern times is done via PubMed, which can be accessed through most Web browsers by simply entering `pubmed.gov`. PubMed has been constantly improved by NLM, both to respond to the needs of users and to take advantage of new technology. A new version of its interface was launched in early 2020 [18]. PubMed is also well-documented on a page[2] linked from every search page. Technical information about PubMed and other NLM services is available from the *NLM Technical Bulletin*.[3]

---

[2] https://pubmed.ncbi.nlm.nih.gov/help/

[3] https://www.nlm.nih.gov/pubs/techbull/

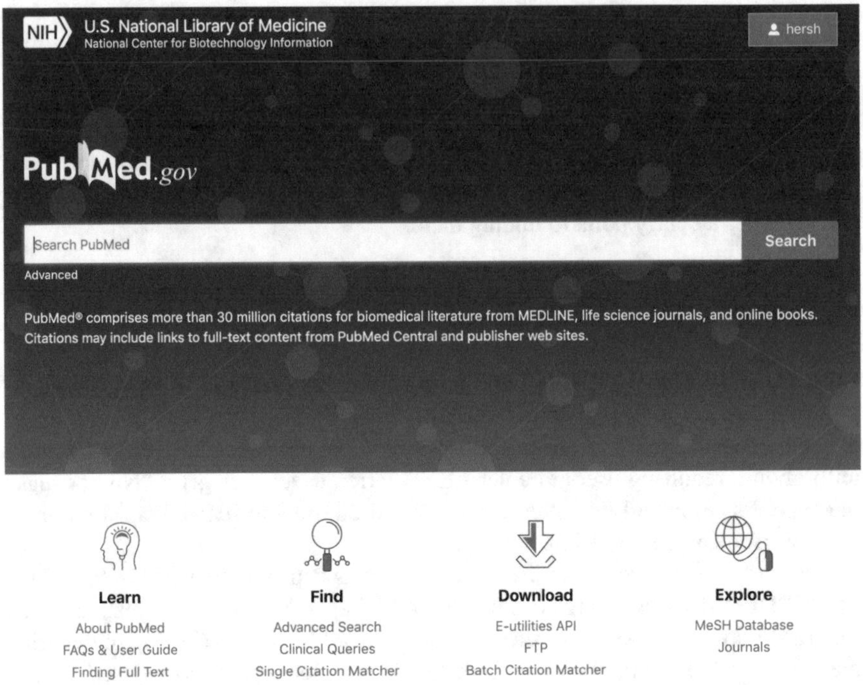

Fig. 5.2 PubMed search screen (Courtesy of NLM)

Fig. 5.3 PubMed search autocomplete (Courtesy of NLM)

The initial searching screen for PubMed is shown in Fig. 5.2. As with most modern search engines, the user begins by entering search text. A drop-down list provides suggested autocompletions of terms as the user types, as shown in Fig. 5.3. Further down the page are links for learning about PubMed, using more specialized user interfaces, accessing an application programming interface (API) and downloadable files, and exploring MeSH or available journals in the database. Still

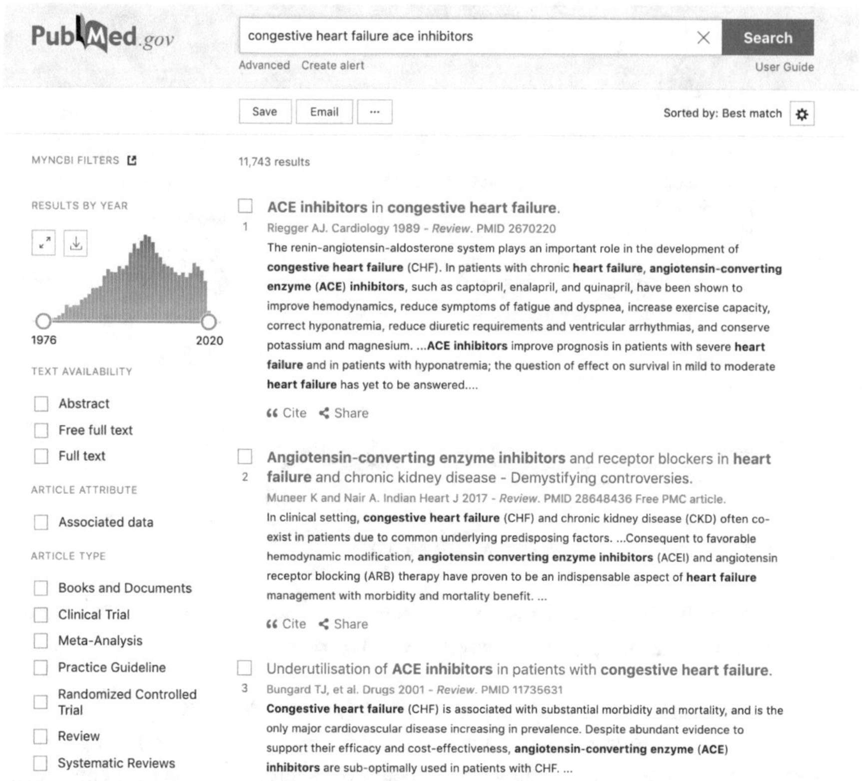

Fig. 5.4 PubMed search results (Courtesy of NLM)

further down the page is a list of "trending" articles and new articles from highly accessed journals.

After entering an appropriate query and either clicking the Search button or hitting return on their computer keyboard, the user is shown the first page of results, as shown in Fig. 5.4. In a break from long-standing historical practice, results in the most recent version of PubMed are sorted by "best match," which uses a relevance ranking approach tailored for PubMed [19]. A user can select, however, to have results sorted by the previously used reverse-chronological order, which some prefer so they can access the most recently published articles first. Although the user can choose between these sorting methods, behind the scenes, a "field sensor" algorithm determines if the query is "informational" [20] and will be triggered if the query returns less than 20 results or if other results are displayed, such as those of the spell checker.

Also by default, the results page starts by displaying ten references but that can be expanded by clicking on the Show more button. Each record in the results shows the title of the article, followed by a new line with the author(s), journal name, year published, and some additional identifier information. This is followed by a

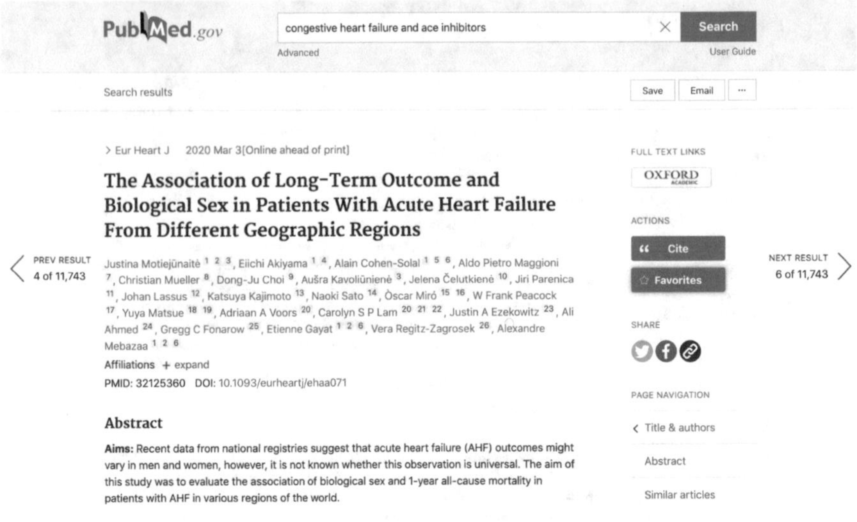

Fig. 5.5 PubMed record displayed (Courtesy of NLM)

summary of the beginning of the article abstract, if an abstract is present. The default Summary presentation can be changed to Abstract, where more information is shown.

The results page provides a number of other features. At the very top right, the user can log in (or see their login name) to their MyNCBI account, which provides additional features described below. Underneath the search box, the user can access an advanced search interface that allows set-based Boolean searching (see below), create an "alert" to send new articles added to the database that match this search, or access the user guide for documentation on PubMed features.[4] Down the left side of the results page are various filters that can be applied to the results related to text availability, article type, and years back of publication date. Additional filters can be accessed and set from the bottom of this area.

To select a PubMed record to view, the user clicks on the title of the article, which takes them to a display of the full record, as shown in Fig. 5.5. Further down the page is a list of Similar Articles based on similarity to other records [12]. On the right of PubMed record are links to (when available) the publisher's site with the full text of the article and/or the full text in PubMed Central. Also on the right side are links for (a) downloading the citation text of the article and (b) adding the article to one's Favorites. Below these links are the ability to share the article to various social media sites.

The front page of PubMed offers access to two advanced searching methods (under the Find heading). The advanced search interface[5] allows set-based

[4] https://pubmed.ncbi.nlm.nih.gov/help/

[5] https://pubmed.ncbi.nlm.nih.gov/advanced/

searching, which some prefer to maintain more control over their search results and sets. Sets can search over all fields in the record or just specific ones, such as Author, Title, or Title/Abstract. The results of different sets can be combined with the Boolean AND, OR, or NOT. A history of the user's search sets is maintained, with a given set accessed by clicking on the hyperlinked number under Results. The user can download the results to a spreadsheet or clear them from the search history.

Let us explore in more detail a user searching for studies assessing the reduction of mortality in patients with `congestive heart failure` through the use of medications from the `angiotensin-converting (ACE) inhibitors` class of drugs. A simple approach might be to combine the terms `congestive heart failure` and `ACE Inhibitors` with an AND, as shown in Fig. 5.4. It turns out that entering the operator `AND` is not required, as the PubMed mapping process does that automatically (i.e., the same results are obtained whether `AND` is used or not).

A more advanced searcher might make use of filters to reduce the 11,743 articles obtained by the basic search. If the searcher is a clinician, he or she might make use of Publication Type filters to narrow the search and limit it to the best evidence for patient care. The searcher could set filters for `Randomized Controlled Trial`, `Systematic Review`, or `Practice Guideline` to successively reduce the retrieval output size. It is important to note that these filters must be used one at a time since no articles are likely to be, for example, both a randomized controlled trial and a systematic review. All of this successive searching can also be done from the Advanced Search interface, as shown in Fig. 5.6.

Another advanced searching approach used in PubMed and focused toward evidence-based medicine is the Clinical Queries interface. This work began with the development of queries where the subject terms were limited by filters designed to retrieve the best evidence based on principles of EBM for the four common types of clinical questions as shown in Table 5.4: therapy, diagnosis, harm, and prognosis [21]. A recent fifth type of question has been added for clinical prediction guides. For each of these question types, there are two strategies, one Broad, emphasizing sensitivity (leading to higher recall, i.e., including as many relevant articles as possible) and the other Narrow, emphasizing specificity (leading to higher precision, i.e., excluding as many nonrelevant articles as possible). Further clinical queries include the ability to find systematic reviews and perform genetics-related searches. When the clinical queries interface is used, the search statement is processed by the usual automatic term mapping and the resulting output limited (via AND) with the appropriate statement. Figure 5.7 shows the choices for clinical query questions.

The very top of the PubMed window offers a link to the older "legacy" version of PubMed, which offers some features not available from the newer and simpler version. In the legacy version, a drop-down menu to the left of the search box lets the user select other resources for searching beside PubMed, such as PubMed Central, Books, MeSH, and the myriad of -omics databases. A link just below the text box takes the user to an advanced set-based searching interface. Below the

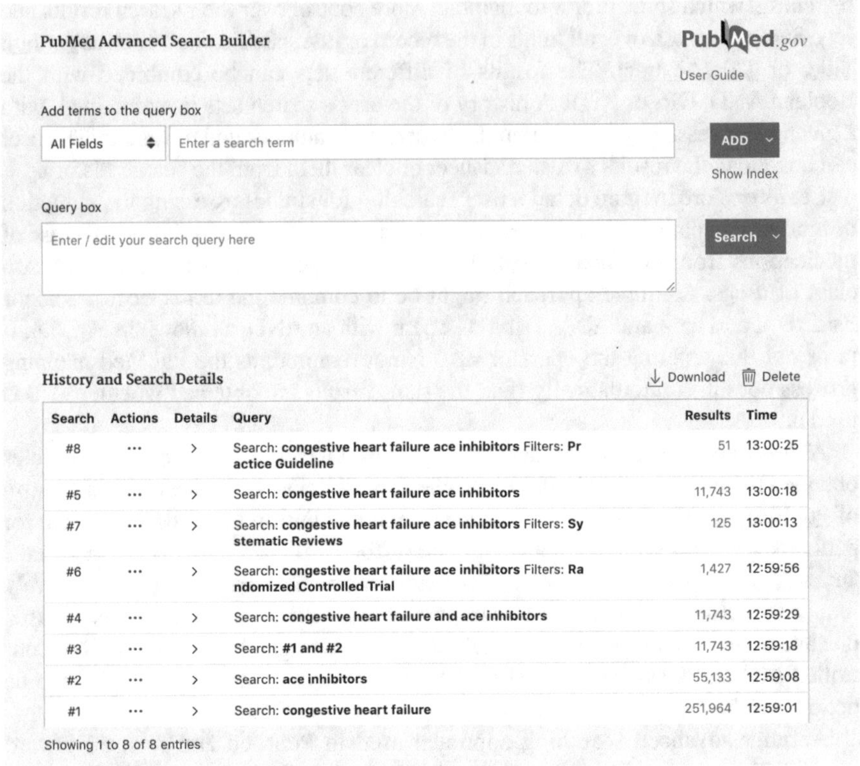

Fig. 5.6 PubMed Advanced Search interface (Courtesy of NLM)

PubMed banner are sets of links for learning to use PubMed, accessing various tools, and providing linkage to additional resources.

In the upper right corner is to log into an NCBI account (MyNCBI) that any user can establish, which provides the ability to establish a personal bibliography (if they have publications in PubMed or associated with their name through other means such as being a training grant principal investigator), view recent search activity, set up "saved" searches that can send periodic updates when new records match the search criteria, establish default filters and collections, and help build a curriculum vitae (CV).

Although presenting the user with a simple text box, PubMed does a great deal of processing of the user's input to identify MeSH and other subject terms, author names, and journal names. PubMed also translates a number of characters into specific functions (other non-alphanumeric characters are converted into spaces, with the exception of single quotes and hyphens due to their use in the naming of substances):

- Parentheses ( )—used to create Boolean nesting
- Square brackets [ ]—search field tag qualification

Table 5.4 PubMed Clinical Queries (Courtesy of NLM)

Category	Optimized for	Sensitivity/ specificity	PubMed search
Therapy	Sensitive/ broad	99%/70%	((clinical[Title/Abstract] AND trial[Title/Abstract]) OR clinical trials[MeSH Terms] OR clinical trial[Publication Type] OR random*[Title/Abstract] OR random allocation[MeSH Terms] OR therapeutic use[MeSH Subheading])
	Specific/ narrow	93%/97%	(randomized controlled trial[Publication Type] OR (randomized[Title/Abstract] AND controlled[Title/ Abstract] AND trial[Title/Abstract]))
Diagnosis	Sensitive/ broad	98%/74%	(sensitiv*[Title/Abstract] OR sensitivity and specificity[MeSH Terms] OR diagnos*[Title/Abstract] OR diagnosis[MeSH:noexp] OR diagnostic * [MeSH:noexp] OR diagnosis,differential[MeSH:noexp] OR diagnosis[Subheading:noexp])
	Specific/ narrow	64%/98%	(specificity[Title/Abstract])
Harm	Sensitive/ broad	93%/63%	(risk*[Title/Abstract] OR risk*[MeSH:noexp] OR risk *[MeSH:noexp] OR cohort studies[MeSH Terms] OR group*[Text Word])
	Specific/ narrow	51%/95%	((relative[Title/Abstract] AND risk*[Title/Abstract]) OR (relative risk[Text Word]) OR risks[Text Word] OR cohort studies[MeSH:noexp] OR (cohort[Title/Abstract] AND stud*[Title/Abstract]))
Prognosis	Sensitive/ broad	90%/80%	(incidence[MeSH:noexp] OR mortality[MeSH Terms] OR follow up studies[MeSH:noexp] OR prognos*[Text Word] OR predict*[Text Word] OR course*[Text Word])
	Specific/ narrow	52%/94%	(prognos*[Title/Abstract] OR (first[Title/Abstract] AND episode[Title/Abstract]) OR cohort[Title/Abstract])
Clinical prediction guide	Sensitive/ broad	96%/79%	(predict*[tiab] OR predictive value of tests[mh] OR scor*[tiab] OR observ*[tiab] OR observer variation[mh])
	Specific/ narrow	54%/99%	(validation[tiab] OR validate[tiab])

https://www.ncbi.nlm.nih.gov/books/NBK3827/#pubmedhelp.Clinical_Queries_Filters

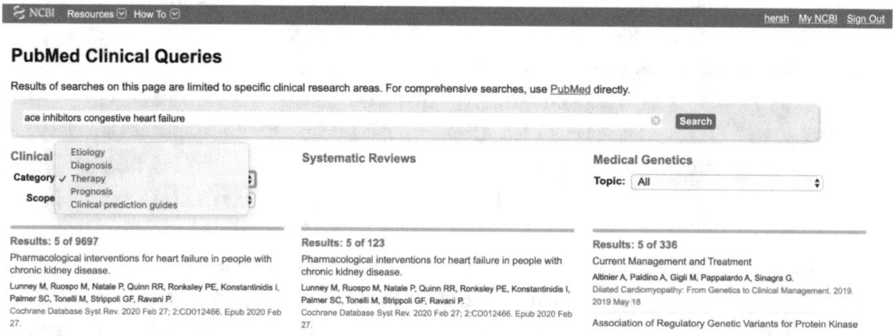

Fig. 5.7 PubMed Clinical Queries interface (Courtesy of NLM)

- Ampersand &—Boolean operator AND
- Pipe |—Boolean operator OR
- Forward slash /—MeSH/subheading combinations
- Comma ,—typically forces a space, e.g., a,b is translated to a, b
- Colon :—designates a range operation
- Double quotes "—used to force a phrase search
- Pound sign #—designates an advanced search statement when immediately followed by a number, e.g., #1 AND cat
- Asterisk *—wildcard symbol for search term truncation, e.g., toxicol*

As noted in the PubMed User Guide, unless tagged by the user, terms entered into PubMed are matched (in order entered) against:

- Subjects using the MeSH translation table
- Journals using the Journals translation table
- Authors and investigators, using the Full Author translation table, Author index, Full Investigator translation table, and Investigator index

If a match is found in any of translation tables, the mapping process stops. When subject or journal matches are found, the query and individual terms are also searched in all fields of MEDLINE records. If no match is found in any tables, terms are searched in All Fields and connected by the AND operator.

In automatic term mapping, the following steps are taken after removal of stop words:

1. MeSH translation—PubMed first tries to map input text to MeSH headings and entry terms. If this is unsuccessful, it then tries to map the text into subheadings, terms from publication types, phrases (from UMLS and elsewhere), pharmaceutical action terms, and supplementary concepts. When a term is found, it is searched as both the MeSH term and its text words. For example, the query `congestive health failure and ace inhibitors` is translated to this search:
   `(((("heart failure"[MeSH Terms] OR ("heart"[All Fields] AND "failure"[All Fields])) OR "heart failure"[All Fields]) OR (("congestive"[All Fields] AND "heart"[All Fields]) AND "failure"[All Fields])) OR "congestive heart failure"[All Fields]) AND ((((("angiotensin converting enzyme inhibitors"[Pharmacological Action] OR "angiotensin-converting enzyme inhibitors"[MeSH Terms]) OR (("angiotensin converting"[All Fields] AND "enzyme"[All Fields]) AND "inhibitors"[All Fields])) OR "angiotensin converting enzyme inhibitors"[All Fields]) OR ("ace"[All Fields] AND "inhibitors"[All Fields])) OR "ace inhibitors"[All Fields])`
2. Journal name translation—For all remaining words that do not map to MeSH (which could be all words if no MeSH terms are found), an attempt is made to map them to the journal abbreviation used in PubMed, although this is avoided for some journals whose names are common searches, such as `heart fail-`

ure [22]. An example of journal name translation is the string ann intern med mapping to the journal Annals of Internal Medicine.
3. Author mapping—If the remaining words contain at least two words, one of which has only one or two letters, word pairs are matched against the MEDLINE full and abbreviated author fields. For example, the strings William Hersh or hersh wr map to an author search by this author.

Remaining text that PubMed cannot map is searched as text words (i.e., words that occur in any of the MEDLINE fields). As noted already, PubMed allows the use of wildcard characters. It also allows phrase searching in that two or more words can be enclosed in quotation marks to indicate they must occur adjacent to each other. If the specified phrase is in PubMed's phrase index, then it will be searched as a phrase. Otherwise, the individual words will be searched. Both wildcard characters and specification of phrases turn off the automatic term mapping.

PubMed allows specification of other indexing attributes by two means. First, the user may type the attribute and its value directly into the text box. (This can also be done to directly enter MeSH terms.) For example, a search of asthma/therapy [mh] AND review [pt] will find review articles indexed on the MeSH term Asthma and its subheading Therapy. The use of field tags turns off automatic term mapping.

PubMed also has a mobile Web interface that is detected when the URL is accessed from a smartphone. Figure 5.8 shows the main search page, while Fig. 5.9 shows the same congestive heart failure and ACE Inhibitors from above.

NLM also makes available other interfaces and apps for accessing PubMed and other databases on mobile devices:

- PubMed for Handhelds (PubMed4Hh)[6] mobile app and also available by the Web, with multiple features:
  - PICO Search—oriented to patient, intervention, comparison, and outcome clinical study searching
  - askMEDLINE—natural language searching interface
  - Journal Browser—searching by journal name
  - Clinical Queries—applying the search approaches of clinical queries
- Wireless Information System for Emergency Responders (WISER)[7]—system designed to assist first responders in hazardous material incidents, providing information on hazardous substances, including its identification, physical characteristics, human health information, and advice about containment and suppression

[6] https://pubmedhh.nlm.nih.gov/

[7] https://wiser.nlm.nih.gov/

Fig. 5.8 PubMed mobile Web interface (Courtesy of NLM)

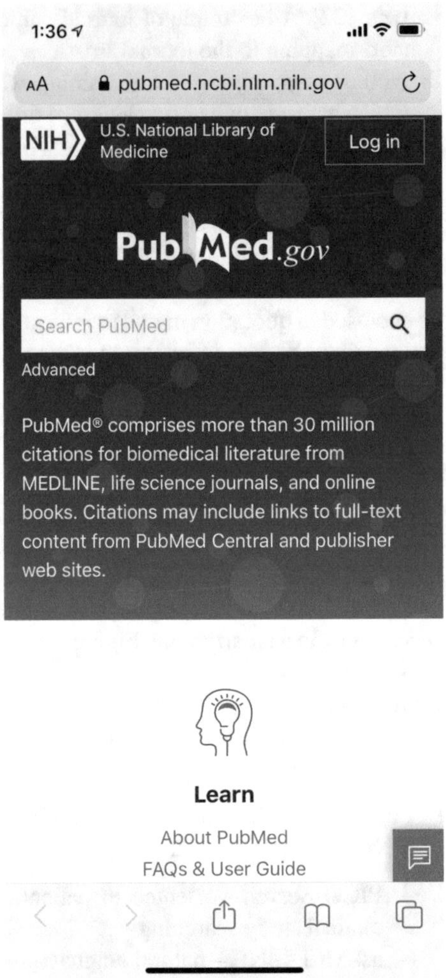

The NLM supports a number of other ways to access data in PubMed and other databases. The PubMed E-Utilities offer application programming interface (API) access to nine utility functions[8]:

- ESearch—search a text query in a single Entrez database
- ESummary—retrieve document summaries
- EFetch—retrieve full records
- EPost—upload a list for later use
- ELink—retrieve related or linked records or LinkOut URLs
- EInfo—retrieve information and statistics about a single database
- ESpell—retrieve spelling suggestions for a text query

[8] https://dataguide.nlm.nih.gov/

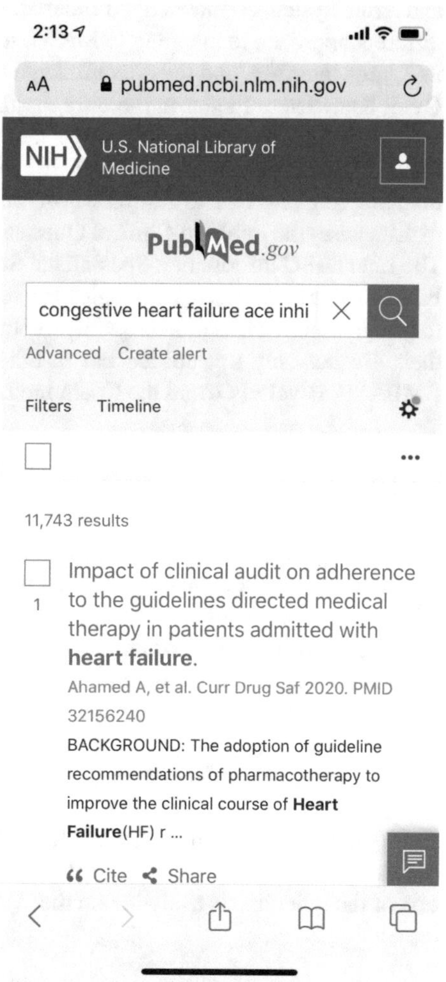

Fig. 5.9 PubMed mobile search results (Courtesy of NLM)

- ECitMatch—search PubMed for a series of citation strings
- EGQuery—search a text query in all Entrez databases and return the number of results for the query in each database

Many programming packages have been developed for accessing the PubMed E-Utilities, including those using R[9] and Python.[10]

PubMed is, of course, not the only interface for searching MEDLINE. Two well-known commercial interfaces used at many medical centers are produced by Ovid

[9] https://cran.r-project.org/package=rentrez

[10] https://biopython.org/DIST/docs/api/Bio.Entrez-module.html

and Aries Systems (Knowledge Finder[11]). The most notable features of Ovid are its different approach to mapping to MeSH, the availability of virtually all features via its Limits interface, and the direct linkage to full text of the articles also licensed by Ovid. Knowledge Finder is the only major MEDLINE interface to offer a partial-match approach to retrieval (though many exact-match features are available as well). It also provides linkages to EBM resources along with automated synonym mapping (e.g., `Advil` to `Ibuprofen`) and British/American spelling equivalents.

Likewise, the PubMed Clinical Queries is not the only approach search filtering. The InterTASC Information Specialists' Sub-Group (ISSG) has developed a Search Filter Resource that gives strategies for search filtering on about 20 study designs (e.g., economic evaluations, quality of life, and quasi-experimental studies) and their use not only in PubMed but in other well-known search resources such as EMBASE, PsycINFO, and the Cochrane Library.[12]

5.3.1.2 Web Catalogs

Web catalogs take a variety of approaches to searching. Some of them allow searching directly over their catalog and then provide links to the items referenced, while others take more of a browsing approach. HON Select[13] allows both browsing of a hierarchy and searching for terms. Translating Research into Practice (TRIP),[14] on the other hand, has only a searching interface over its catalog.

5.3.1.3 Specialized Registries

Both the ECRI Guidelines Trust[15] and Guidelines Central[16] offer searching and browsing interfaces to their clinical practice guidelines collections. When the full text of the guideline is available on the Web, a link is provided directly to it.

5.3.2 *Full Text*

In general, full-text searching interfaces offer fewer features than their bibliographic counterparts. This is in part because the amount of metadata available for full-text resources is usually smaller. Unlike the rich metadata provided in bibliographic

[11] https://kfinder.com/kfinder/

[12] https://sites.google.com/a/york.ac.uk/issg-search-filters-resource/

[13] https://www.hon.ch/HONselect/

[14] http://www.tripdatabase.com

[15] https://guidelines.ecri.org/

[16] https://www.guidelinecentral.com/summaries/

databases, most full-text “documents” consist of just a title and body of text. One advantage of full text is its complete body of text, which provides more words to search against; but when those words do not represent the focus of the content of the document, this feature can be a disadvantage.

5.3.2.1 Periodicals

As noted in Chap. 3, many journals have become available in full text on the Web. Journal articles are often accessed through bibliographic databases such as PubMed described above. Most journal Web sites also have full-text searching capabilities and also have articles retrieved via direct linkage as described further in Chap. 6. Another source for full-text articles is PubMed Central (PMC),[17] an archive for all literature that results from research funded in the United States by NIH. PMC can be searched via the PubMed interface (selecting the PMC option from the drop-down list to the left of the search box) or directly on the PMC site, which has comparable functionality to PubMed on its results and retrieved records pages. The latter allows viewing in several different formats:

- PubReader[18]—screen-friendly format
- ePub ebook standard format
- PDF—either the article itself deposited by the publisher or a version of the last manuscript prior to typesetting by the author
- Citation—in several common formats, such as APA and NLM

Once a full-text article has been found on a publisher site, a wealth of additional features may be available. Most full-text articles are typically presented both in HTML and PDF form, with the latter providing a more readable and printable version. Links are also usually provided to related articles from the journal as well as the PubMed reference and its related articles. Also may be linked are all articles in the journal that cited this one, and the site can be configured to set up a notification email when new articles cite the item selected. There may also be comments allowed by the publisher.

5.3.2.2 Textbooks

Most electronic textbook searching interfaces offer variations on the basic theme of entering words to search and allowing browsing along the book’s organizational structure. As many textbooks are now part of aggregations, the interface may allow selection of some or all of the books. This and autocompletion of searches are demonstrated in the freely available *Merck Manual*.[19]

---

[17] https://www.ncbi.nlm.nih.gov/pmc/

[18] https://www.ncbi.nlm.nih.gov/pmc/about/pubreader/

[19] https://www.merckmanuals.com/professional

5.3.2.3 Web Search Engines

Web search engines have become ubiquitous, and they are even difficult to avoid since the URL/address bar of most Web browsers will send the text entered by the user to a search engine if it is not a correctly formatted URL. Therefore, essentially everyone who uses a Web browser has used a search engine. While there are a number of niche search engines, most general search engine use goes to three systems. comScore provides an up-to-date ranking of major Web search engine usage, showing the consistent lead of Google (62%), Microsoft Bing (25%), and Verizon (formerly Yahoo) (11%), with no other search engines above 1%.[20] Wikipedia maintains a list of the features of the major search engines.[21]

The major Web search engines use a basic variant of partial-match searching. The pages have generally been discovered by "crawling" the Web, and their words are typically indexed by means of a word-based approach. Because most search engines have indexed billions of Web pages, the default operation between words entered is AND. The general approach to retrieval is that users enter a natural language query statement and the search engine responds with a ranked list of matching Web pages. Most search engines show ten matching Web pages per screen of output, but usually it is possible to configure the page to allow a different number to be displayed.

Google's Web site has a portion devoted to *How Google Search Works*.[22] The site notes that Google crawls every site that it knows about, with the exception of those that it instructs it not to crawl with a robots.txt file. The words on each page, along with a number of other attributes such as "freshness" of the Web site, are indexed. The site claims Google has indexed "hundreds of billions" of Web pages and that the index is 100 petabytes in size. A Knowledge Graph identifies other information about the page for the index. Although a proprietary secret, Google uses machine learning to identify other clues of what users are searching for to present what it considers to be the best results. Google continually updates its entire search system, for example, with the recent addition of a machine learning approach called Bidirectional Encoder Representations from Transformers (BERT) [23], which leverages richer language in queries, aiming to provide more relevant results [24].

Google offers a variety of features beyond basic word-based searching:

- Require inclusion of words—put + in front of a word to be included, e.g., `+heart` (comparable to a Boolean AND)
- Search for an exact match—put a word or phrase inside quotes, e.g., `"heart failure"` (comparable to an AND with required proximity when there is more than one term)
- Exclude words from a search—put – in front of a word to be left out, e.g., `information -retrieval` (comparable to a Boolean NOT)

---

[20] https://www.comscore.com/Insights/Rankings#tab_search_share/

[21] https://en.wikipedia.org/wiki/Comparison_of_web_search_engines

[22] https://www.google.com/search/howsearchworks/

- Combine searches—put OR between each search query, e.g., `hypertension OR HTN`
- Search for a specific site—put site: in front of a site or domain, e.g., `site:www.ohsu.edu` or `site:.gov`
- Search for related sites—put related: in front of a Web address already known, e.g., `related:cnn.com`
- Search social media—put @ in front of a word to search social media, e.g., @twitter
- Search for a price—put $ in front of a number, e.g., `camera $400`
- Search within a range of numbers—put .. between two numbers, e.g., `camera $50..$100`
- Search hashtags—put # in front of a word, e.g., `#throwbackthursday`
- See Google's cached version of a site—put cache: in front of site address

Google has many other features. One is an "autocomplete" function that provides suggestions to the user as they type in a query.[23] Google can search across everything or limit output to news, books, images, videos, maps, shopping, flights, and finance. Google attempts (usually successfully) to offer spelling corrections. It also has some medical features, e.g., entering the name of a disease will lead to a disease "card" to be shown in the output. The Google search box can also determine when something entered is a question or other non-search information need, such as:

- Time, e.g., `what time is it in Singapore?`
- Flight status, e.g., `united 250`
- Definitions, e.g., `define: informatics`
- Weather forecasts, e.g., `weather portland oregon`

In addition, Google provides an advanced search page that allows setting of various features.[24] It also has a library of application programming interface (API) functions that allow computer programs to call those functions.[25]

Since the use of Web search engines is free, they are supported by revenues mainly from advertising. Google Ads is its highly lucrative advertising platform for "paid search".[26] In Google Ads, advertisers bid for their results to be placed in the sponsored links portion of the results, with those paying more ranking higher. A related program is AdSense pays Web sites to put context-specific advertisements on their pages.[27]

---

[23] https://www.blog.google/products/search/how-google-autocomplete-works-search/

[24] https://www.google.com/advanced_search

[25] https://developers.google.com/apis-explorer

[26] https://ads.google.com/home/

[27] https://www.google.com/adsense/start/

5.3.3 *Annotated*

As noted in Chap. 3, a number of health resources on the Web consist of collections of annotated content. This section describes the searching approaches to these resources.

5.3.3.1 Images

As explained in Chap. 4, image collections are generally indexed by textual descriptions of individual images, although with the increased capabilities of machine learning more systems are making use of content-based image retrieval (CBIR) [25, 26]. Most image retrieval systems have relatively simple text-searching interfaces, usually consisting of simple word matching between query and image description terms. One early system for CBIR was the GNU Image-Finding Tool (GIFT).[28] As shown in Fig. 5.10, "searching" on one or more images tends to find others that "look like" it.

Most of the major Web search engines also feature some form of image retrieval. Their output usually displays images associated with the text of the Web pages on which they are located. Google allows imaging from its main search page or has a separate image retrieval page.[29] Some of the features of Google are particularly useful in image retrieval, such as filetype (e.g., limit to GIF). When an image is retrieved, Google displays both a thumbnail of the image and the page from which it came. Google also allows "reverse image search," where a user can drag an image into the search box and retrieve similar images, Web sites that contain the image, and other sizes of the picture with which the user searched.

A number of biomedical and health image retrieval systems are available. UpToDate allows one to select a Graphics facet for search results that shows images related to the query term(s).[30] The NLM Open-I system provides both text and reverse image searching.[31]

5.3.3.2 Citations

While the main use of citation databases is to identify linkages in the scientific literature, there is sometimes the need to search them in a conventional manner. If nothing else, the user may need to identify the specific works of an author or a particular citation. Google Scholar allows searching by topic initially but then features ability to navigate citations in the results by clicking on the following:

[28] https://www.gnu.org/software/gift/

[29] https://support.google.com/websearch/answer/1325808

[30] https://www.uptodate.com/contents/search

[31] https://openi.nlm.nih.gov/

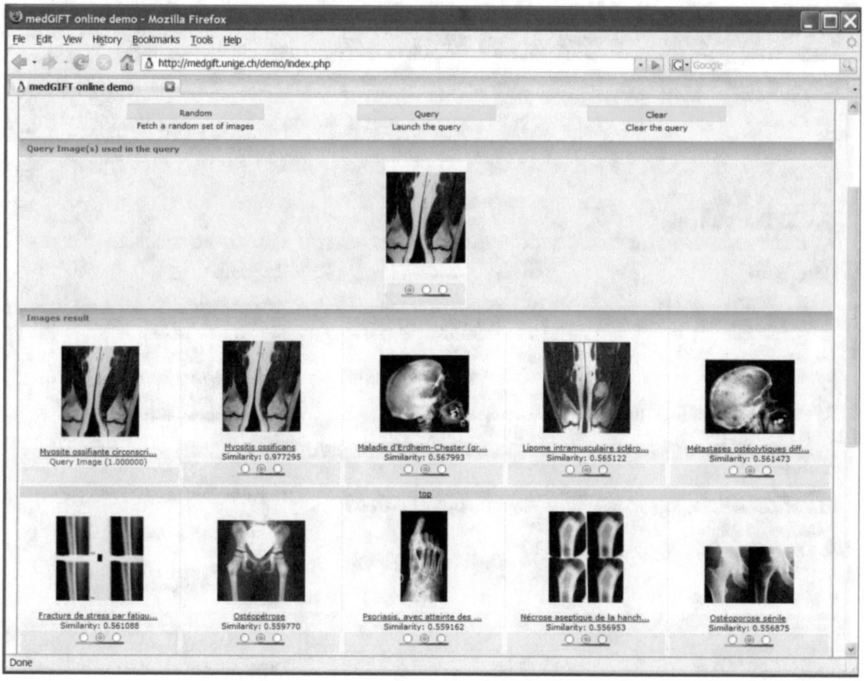

Fig. 5.10 GIFT image retrieval results screen (Courtesy of VIPER Project)

- Author name—view their Google Scholar profile (if they have created one)
- Cited by—shows all results citing this particular one

An author's Google Scholar profile shows their publications sorted by number of citations along with research productivity in number of citations and h-index. For a given publication, one can click on CITED BY: to retrieval all citations of that publication. Microsoft Academic shows similar information but also includes top co-authors, institutions, journals, conferences, and publication types for all of the retrieval results.

5.3.3.3 Molecular Biology and -Omics

Another type of annotated content is molecular biology and -omics databases. Searching in these resources may involve text strings such as disease and drug names but may also involve codes such as gene identifiers or numbers such as chromosome locations. NLM resources can be searched in a number of ways. All of the individual resources have search interfaces for the resource. One can search across resources by changing the drop-down selection from the legacy PubMed menu or

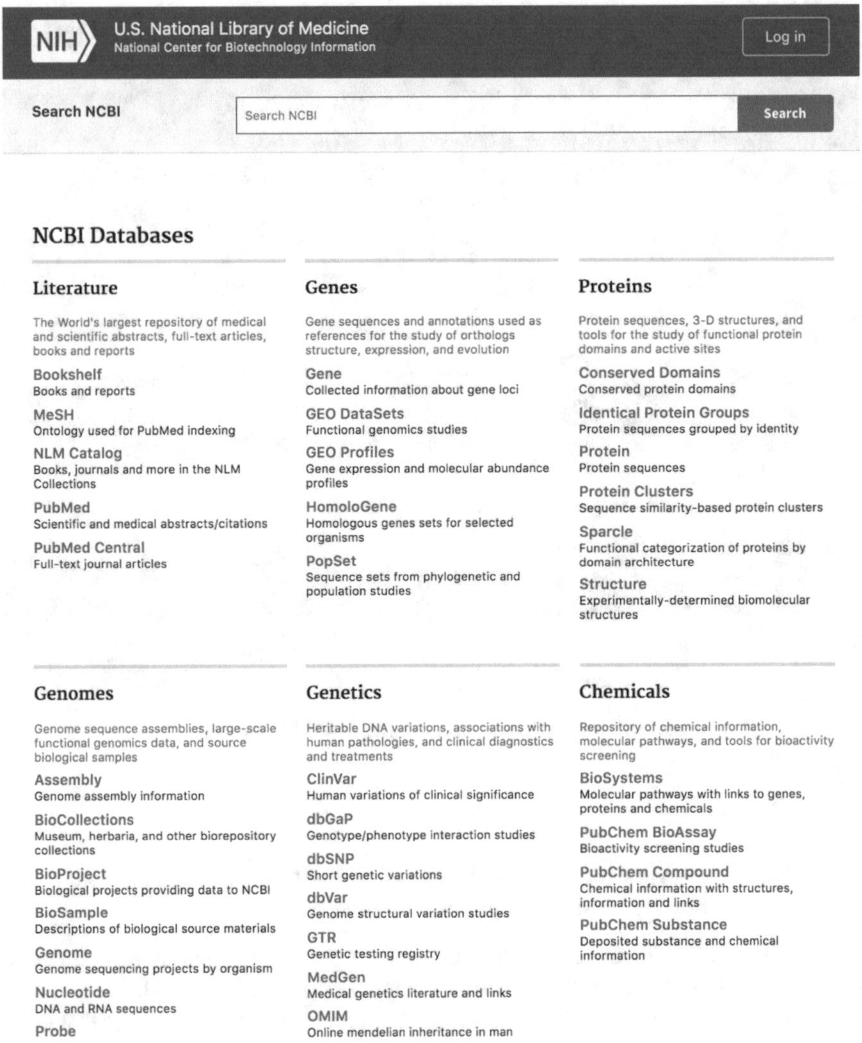

Fig. 5.11 NCBI search interface (Courtesy of NLM)

by using NCBI Search[32] as shown in Fig. 5.11. In a similar vein, the Mouse Genome Informatics resource[33] allows search over the entire collection of information or specific aspects, such as genes, gene expression, and human-mouse disease connection.

---

[32] https://www.ncbi.nlm.nih.gov/search

[33] http://www.informatics.jax.org/

5.3.3.4 Other Databases

Chapter 3 listed a variety of annotated content in the "other" category. Many of these employ simple text-word searching. The ClinicalTrials.gov site has a simple interface that allows entry of trial status, condition or disease, other terms, and country.[34] One can also browse by topic or geographic location on a map. An advanced search interface allows finer-grained searching for clinical trials. The results page shows studies listed with columns for study status, title, conditions, interventions, and locations (Fig. 5.12). Tabs of the search results allow them to be viewed by topic, on a map, and with additional details about the search. On the left side of the results window is a set of filters to narrow the number of studies by status, eligibility criteria, study type, study phase, funder, and more. Clicking on a study retrieves details for that study.

5.3.4 Aggregations

The final group of information resources described in Chap. 3 consisted of aggregations of content. The MedlinePlus system of aggregated consumer health resources provides a simple searching interface but then offers more complexity with presentation of the results.[35] The retrieval interface shows a simple text box but, like PubMed, uses a thesaurus to expand search terms and spelling correction suggestions for unrecognized terms. Searching can be restricted to certain Web sites with the site: operator, e.g., `site: cancer.gov`. Other features of the interface include:

- + or – to require a word to be present or not, e.g., `+heart` or `-heart`
- Quotation marks to require phrases, e.g., `"congestive heart failure"`
- OR operator to allow Boolean OR
- Wildcard character for terms three letters or longer, e.g., `can*`

The output of MedlinePlus, shown in Fig. 5.13, provides the definition of a disease when one is detected in the search and also categorizes results by source and format.

Another aggregated resource from NCBI mentioned in Sect. 5.3.3.3 is NCBI Search,[36] which allows searching across all of the NLM databases. Most of the other professionally oriented aggregations described in Chap. 3 have searching functionality with various advanced features and segregation by resources (e.g., journals, books, educational resources, images, etc.).

[34] https://clinicaltrials.gov/

[35] https://medlineplus.gov/about/using/searchtips/

[36] https://www.ncbi.nlm.nih.gov/search/

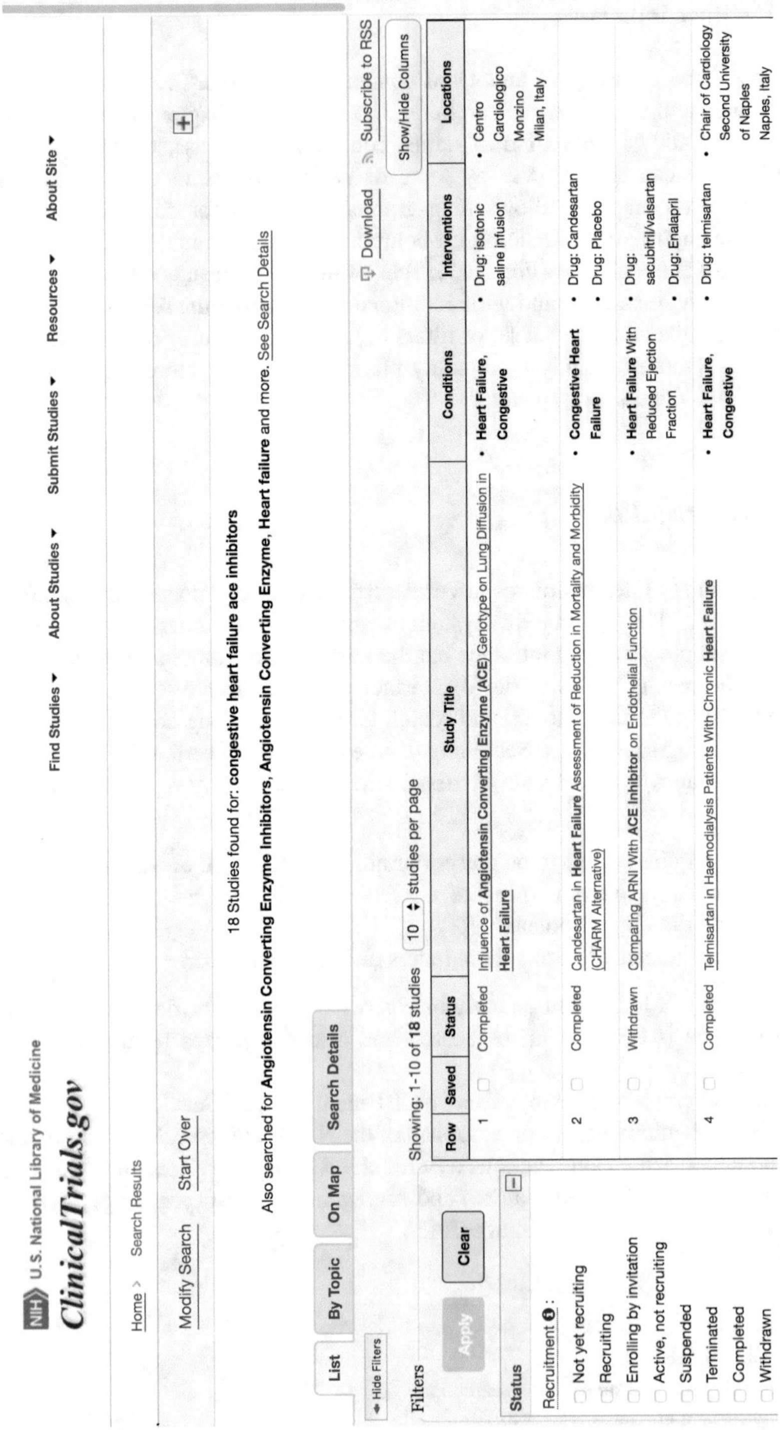

Fig. 5.12 ClinicalTrials.gov search results (Courtesy of NLM)

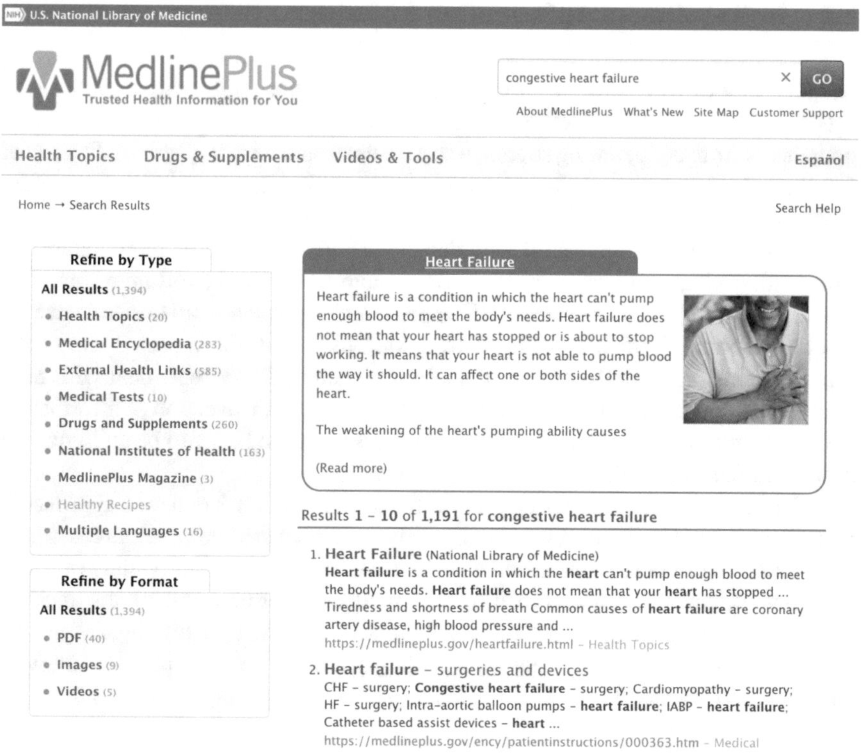
U.S. National Library of Medicine
MedlinePlus
Trusted Health Information for You
congestive heart failure
GO
About MedlinePlus
What's New
Site Map
Customer Support
Health Topics
Drugs & Supplements
Videos & Tools
Español
Home → Search Results
Search Help
Refine by Type
All Results (1,394)
Health Topics (20)
Medical Encyclopedia (283)
External Health Links (585)
Medical Tests (10)
Drugs and Supplements (260)
National Institutes of Health (163)
MedlinePlus Magazine (3)
Healthy Recipes
Multiple Languages (16)
Refine by Format
All Results (1,394)
PDF (40)
Images (9)
Videos (5)
Heart Failure
Heart failure is a condition in which the heart can't pump enough blood to meet the body's needs. Heart failure does not mean that your heart has stopped or is about to stop working. It means that your heart is not able to pump blood the way it should. It can affect one or both sides of the heart.
The weakening of the heart's pumping ability causes
(Read more)
Results 1 - 10 of 1,191 for congestive heart failure
1. Heart Failure (National Library of Medicine)
Heart failure is a condition in which the heart can't pump enough blood to meet the body's needs. Heart failure does not mean that your heart has stopped ... Tiredness and shortness of breath Common causes of heart failure are coronary artery disease, high blood pressure and ...
https://medlineplus.gov/heartfailure.html - Health Topics
2. Heart failure - surgeries and devices
CHF - surgery; Congestive heart failure - surgery; Cardiomyopathy - surgery; HF - surgery; Intra-aortic balloon pumps - heart failure; IABP - heart failure; Catheter based assist devices - heart ...
https://medlineplus.gov/ency/patientinstructions/000363.htm - Medical

Fig. 5.13 MedlinePlus results screen for search on `heart failure` (Courtesy of NLM)

5.4 Document Delivery

A historical function of libraries has been *document delivery*, also called *interlibrary loan (ILL)*, when expanded to include loan of items such as paper books. Before IR systems, libraries would provide, usually by email, photocopies of journal articles or physical books or other resources. In the early days of IR systems, before the advent of widespread full-text journal availability, the IR systems might be used to request fax or mailing of copies of journal articles. Now, of course, with essentially all journal articles available electronically, the major use of ILL is to distribute articles that may only be available behind a paywall.

Many libraries of academic medical centers provide ILL services, e.g., Oregon Health & Science University.[37] The NLM has an ILL service called DOCLINE[38] that delivers documents through the National Network of Libraries of Medicine (NNLM).[39] Fees are typically charged for these services, including copyright fees charged by the publisher.

[37] https://www.ohsu.edu/library/get-it-for-me-service

[38] https://docline.gov/docline/

[39] https://nnlm.gov/

5.5 Notification or Information Filtering

Another way of accessing information is via *notification*, *information filtering*, or *selective dissemination of information*. Information filtering is the retrieval of new documents from an incoming stream, a sort of electronic clipping system. It is suited for user who is perpetually interested in a topic, wanting to gather all new documents that are generated. The filtering system is used to set up a profile, which is a search statement run against all new documents added to one or more databases. Information filtering is very similar to IR, though Belkin and Croft note some distinct differences [27]. For example, IR systems are oriented toward one-time use for distinct information needs, while filtering systems imply the repeated use of the same system for the same query. In addition, whereas IR systems deal with relatively static databases, filtering systems are concerned with selection of information from dynamic streams of data. Finally, timeliness is more likely to be an important aspect of the functionality of filtering systems.

Information filtering has been around for decades, but some newer approaches make it easier and integrate it more effectively with other searching resources. Many systems make use of RSS feeds and allow users to receive them in a variety of ways, including directly through Web browsers such as Firefox. Most of the modern MEDLINE search systems offer some variant of information filtering. MyNCBI allows users to create a list of Saved Searches that can be run at specified intervals and delivered via email.

References

1. Lancaster F, Warner A. Information retrieval today. Arlington, VA: Information Resources Press; 1993.
2. Pao M. Concepts of information retrieval. Englewood, CO: Libraries Unlimited; 1989.
3. Wallingford K, Humphreys B, Selinger N, Siegel E. Bibliographic retrieval: a survey of individual users of MEDLINE. MD Comput. 1990;7:166–71.
4. DelFiol G, Workman T, Gorman P. Clinical questions raised by clinicians at the point of care: a systematic review. JAMA Intern Med. 2014;174:710–8.
5. Belkin N, Vickery A. Interaction in the information system: a review of research from document retrieval to knowledge-based system. London: The British Library; 1985.
6. Salton G, Lesk M. The SMART automatic document retrieval system: an illustration. Commun ACM. 1965;8:391–8.
7. Blair D. Searching biases in large interactive document retrieval systems. J Am Soc Inf Sci. 1980;31:271–7.
8. Salton G. Developments in automatic text retrieval. Science. 1991;253:974–80.
9. Salton G, Fox E, Wu H. Extended Boolean information retrieval. Commun ACM. 1983;26:1022–36.
10. Buckley C, Salton G, Allan J, editors. The effect of adding relevance information in a relevance feedback environment. Proceedings of the 17th Annual International ACM SIGIR Conference on Research and Development in Information Retrieval; 1994; Dublin: Springer-Verlag.

11. Wilbur W, Yang Y. An analysis of statistical term strength and its use in the indexing and retrieval of molecular biology texts. Comput Biol Med. 1996;26:209–22.
12. Lin J, Wilbur W. PubMed related articles: a probabilistic topic-based model for content similarity. BMC Bioinform. 2007;8:423.
13. Canese K. New PubMed spell checking feature. NLM Tech Bull. 2004;2004:e12.
14. Wilbur W, Kim W, Xie N. Spelling correction in the PubMed search engine. Inf Retr. 2006;9:543–64.
15. Horowitz G, Jackson J, Bleich H. PaperChase: self-service bibliographic retrieval. JAMA. 1983;328:2495–500.
16. Haynes R, McKibbon K. Grateful Med. MD Comput. 1987;4:47–57.
17. Kingsland L, Syed E, Lindberg D, editors. COACH: an expert searcher program to assist Grateful Med users searching MEDLINE. MEDINFO 92; 1992; Geneva: North-Holland.
18. Collins M. The new PubMed is here. NLM Tech Bull. 2019;2019:e3.
19. Fiorini N, Canese K, Starchenko G, Kireev E, Kim W, Miller V, et al. Best match: new relevance search for PubMed. PLoS Biol. 2018;16(8):e2005343.
20. Yeganova L, Kim W, Comeau D, Wilbur W, Lu Z. A field sensor: computing the composition and intent of PubMed queries. Database. 2018;2018:bay052.
21. Haynes R, Wilczynski N, McKibbon K, Walker C, Sinclair J. Developing optimal search strategies for detecting clinically sound studies in MEDLINE. J Am Med Inform Assoc. 1994;1:447–58.
22. McGhee M. PubMed subject searching avoids conflicts with journal titles. NLM Tech Bull. 2005;2005:e3.
23. Devlin J, Chang M, Lee K, Toutanova K, editors. BERT: pre-training of deep bidirectional transformers for language understanding. Proceedings of the 2019 Conference of the North American Chapter of the Association for Computational Linguistics: Human Language Technologies; 2019; Minneapolis, MN.
24. Nayak P. Understanding searches better than ever before. Google; 2019.
25. Müller H, Unay D. Retrieval from and understanding of large-scale multi-modal medical datasets: a review. IEEE Trans Multimedia. 2017;19(9):17099710.
26. Zhou W, Li H, Tian Q. Recent advance in content-based image retrieval: a literature survey. arXivorg. 2017:arXiv:1706.06064.
27. Belkin N, Croft W. Information filtering and information retrieval: two sides of the same coin? Commun ACM. 1992;35:29–38.

Chapter 6
Access

The ubiquitous Internet and World Wide Web provide literally planetwide access to knowledge-based information, although there are a variety of impediments for accessing it. There are challenges with finding it, being allowed to access it, and protecting and preserving it. This chapter covers some of the barriers and how they may be overcome to create a scientific "commons" of data and information that can be used to apply knowledge to better health while protecting those who produce and make available data and information for this. We begin with discussion of the historical locations of knowledge, namely, libraries, and then address other issues of access, openness, and protection of intellectual property as well as the data and information themselves.

6.1 Libraries

Historically, the entity associated with managing and providing access to scientific information was the library. While libraries continue to play critical roles in the scientific information ecosystem, the Internet and Web have changed the role of the library. In earlier editions of this book, there was prominent discussion of the emerging *digital library* (DL). But like many information-related activities, the distinction between traditional "brick and mortar" libraries and DLs has blurred. Just as healthcare systems, merchants, banks, and others have had to unify their physical and digital presence, libraries have had to do the same. As such, essentially all libraries are now DLs.

Libraries have traditionally performed a variety of functions, including:

- Acquisition and maintenance of collections
- Cataloging and classification of items in collections

W. Hersh, *Information Retrieval: A Biomedical and Health Perspective*, Health Informatics, https://doi.org/10.1007/978-3-030-47686-1_6

- Serving as a place where individuals can go to seek information with assistance, including information on computers
- Providing work or studying space (particularly in universities)

There are a number of organizations concerned with libraries. The American Library Association (ALA)[1] focuses on libraries in general, while the Special Library Association (SLA)[2] takes a narrower view on scientific and technical libraries. As noted in Chap. 1, the Medical Library Association (MLA)[3] addresses the issue of health science libraries.

Probably the main function of libraries is to maintain and facilitate access to collections of published literature. They may also store nonpublished literature, such as letters, notes, and other documents, in archives. But the general focus on published literature has implications. One of these is that, for the most part, quality control can be taken for granted. At least until the recent past, most published literature came from commercial publishers and specialty societies that had processes such as peer review that, although imperfect, allowed the library to devote minimal resources to assessing their quality. While libraries can still cede the judgment of quality to those information providers in the Internet era, they cannot ignore the myriad of information published only on the Internet, for which the quality cannot be presumed.

The historical nature of paper-based traditional libraries also carried other implications. For example, paper-based items are produced in multiple copies. This frees the individual library from excessive worry that an item cannot be replaced. In addition, items are fairly static, simplifying their cataloging. In modern times, these implications are challenged. As noted in Chap. 2 and as described further shortly, there is a great deal of concern about archiving of content and managing its change when fewer "copies" of it exist on the file servers of publishers and other organizations. A related problem is that libraries may not own the "artifact" of the paper journal, book, or other item. This is exacerbated by the fact that when a subscription to an electronic journal is terminated, access to the entire journal is lost; that is, the subscriber does not retain accumulated back issues, as was taken for granted with paper journals.

Another major function of libraries has been to facilitate access to their collections. The traditional means for accessing collections was the *card catalog*: users picked a subject or author name and flipped through cards representing items in the library. Card catalogs have been replaced by online public access catalogs (OPACs), which are similar to but have differences from document retrieval systems [1]. The main difference emanates from the general differences between books and "documents." That books tend to be larger and to cover more subject material is exemplified by envisioning the difference between a medical journal article on a specific disease and its treatment and a book on internal medicine. As such, catalogers of books tend to use much broader indexing terms.

---

[1] http://www.ala.org/

[2] https://www.sla.org/

[3] https://www.mlanet.org/

Some challenges for libraries from the twentieth century have changed in the twenty-first century. One traditional concern, for example, was managing the physical size of collections [2]. With the exponential growth curve of scientific literature [3], libraries had to determine where to store the ever-increasing number of volumes. However, with the modern transition to electronic publishing of journals, shelf space has become less critical of an issue.

Of course, libraries provide value beyond physical or digital access to journals. As most journals are still published under the subscription model, libraries typically must pay fees to subscribe and provide access. Even in modern times, selecting which journals to maintain subscriptions is a major task of libraries. Furthermore, libraries have had limited budgets, requiring hard decisions about which resources to maintain free availability for their institutions. As such, another major activity of libraries has been sharing of collections. Few libraries can maintain complete collections, so most participate collaboratively with other libraries to attaining materials via *interlibrary loan* (ILL). This of course potentially sets up conflict, as the needs of publishers to maintain revenues to continue being in business must be weighed against the desire of libraries to reduce costs by sharing. Aspects of copyright and intellectual property protection are covered in Sect. 6.4.

Another important historical goal of libraries has been the preservation of their collections. For paper-based materials, the aim has always been for survival of the physical object. There were a number of impediments to preservation:

- Loss, theft, and general deterioration from use
- "Perfect binding" or the use of glue in binding instead of sewing, which reduces the longevity of books
- Acid paper, that is, materials printed of paper produced by means of an acid process, used mainly between 1850 and 1950, which has led to a better understanding for preserving paper-based resources [4]

Digital materials have their own set of preservation issues, which are described in Sect. 6.5.

6.1.1 Definitions and Functions of DLs

Borgman reviewed the various definitions of DLs and concluded that there were two competing views: a researcher-oriented view of DLs defined to represent specific collections of content and/or technologies and a service-oriented view, with DLs thought to represent a set of services provided to a specific community, such as a university or a company [5]. Even in the emerging DL era, many noted that the library was still a physical place and that there was virtue to that place [6]. However, Monastersky has noted that the modern library has had to "reboot" to handle changes in the scientific publishing arena, such as managing much larger types and quantities of content, including publishing and archiving of raw data from research [7]. Still, most who work in academic institutions expect that the content from their library is available both at the library and probably more importantly over computer networks.

A number of overviews of DLs have been written. These include books, with earlier general overviews [8, 9, 2] now giving way to those that focus on how to develop and maintain digital collections [10, 11]. Perhaps in an indication that DL functions have become subsumed into the roles of all libraries, a well-known DL journal, *Digital Library Magazine*,[4] suspended publication in 2017. But important work still goes on with regard to DLs, as evidenced by a conference focused on the scientific aspects of DLs, the Joint Conference on Digital Libraries (JCDL).[5]

A report by the US National Commission on Libraries and Information Science (NCLIS) addressed information policy issues in the face of "mass digitization" of information, identifying identified nine areas with potential impact on information policy [12]:

1. Copyright—how should it be handled in digitization projects?
2. Quality—what is the quality of optical character recognition (OCR), content, and authentication?
3. Libraries—what are their roles and priorities for the digital age?
4. Ownership and preservation—who will assume long-term ownership of books, journals, and other media as well as preserve the public record?
5. Standardization and interoperability—how can systems and their content communicate with each other?
6. Publishers—what are the roles of publishers in this era?
7. Business models—what business models are needed, and what will be the impact of the open access movement?
8. Information literacy—what should be done about information illiteracy?
9. Assessment—what assessment is being undertaken, and how will we know if content and systems are meeting people's needs?

Fox et al. developed the 5S model to describe the foundational aspects of DLs [13]:

- Streams—sequences of elements of arbitrary types that can be static or dynamic
- Structures—structures of the parts that comprise content in the digital library, usually defined via markup languages (e.g., XML, HTML)
- Spaces—objects and operations on them that provide constraint yet meaning
- Scenarios—the situation that describes how digital libraries are used by real people
- Societies—the entities and their relationships, from the people to the technology systems

Fox et al. also described a taxonomy that defined the facets of a DL based on the above five elements [13]:

---

[4] http://www.dlib.org/

[5] http://www.jcdl.org/

- Actors—who interacts with or within DLs?
- Activities—what happens in DLs?
- Components—what constitutes DLs?
- Social, economic, and legal aspects—what surrounds DLs?
- Environments—in what contexts are DLs embedded?

Despite the changes in libraries, librarians still provide important services, especially in academic health science centers, as documented in a systematic review [14]. For those in training (e.g., students and residents), librarians facilitated improvement in skills for searching the literature and in integrating research evidence into clinical decision-making. For clinicians, librarians were effective in helping to save time and provide relevant information for decision-making.

6.2 Access to Content

Despite the nearly complete digitization of the world's scientific information, there are still challenges to its access. The IR systems described in the previous chapters help find the information, but even if we know its (virtual) location, that is no guarantee of access. This section focuses on access to individual items, collections of items, and the metadata that describes them. Many have advocated that knowledge-based information and underlying data should be available based on the FAIR (Findability, Accessibility, Interoperability, and Reusability) principles [15]. The FAIR principles have been further extended to data being TLC (Traceable, Licensed, and Connected) [16]. The FairSharing.org Web site[6] provides a curated and educational resource on data and metadata standards, interrelated to databases and data policies.

6.2.1 Access to Individual Items

Probably every Web user is familiar with clicking on a Web link and receiving an error message that the page is not found. In the early days of the Web, this was the dreaded message: `HTTP 404 - File not found`. DLs and commercial publishing ventures need mechanisms to ensure that documents have persistent identifiers so that when the document itself physically moves, it is still obtainable. The original architecture for the Web envisioned by the Internet Engineering Task Force was to have every Uniform Resource Locator (URL), the address entered into a Web browser or used in a Web hyperlink, linked to a uniform resource name (URN) that would be persistent [17]. The combination of a URN and URL, a uniform resource

[6] https://fairsharing.org/

identifier (URI), would provide persistent access to digital objects. The resource for resolving URNs and URIs was never implemented on a large scale.

The lack of widespread implementation of URIs did not stop advocacy for persistent identifiers of digital scholarly works. One approach that has achieved widespread adoption by publishers, especially scientific journal publishers, is the Digital Object Identifier (DOI).[7] The DOI standard (ISO 26324) is maintained by the International DOI Foundation (IDF), a membership organization that assigns a portion of the DOI to make it unique. An overview of the DOI system is described in the DOI Handbook.[8] The DOI system consists of four components:

1. Enumeration—location of the identifier, the DOI
2. Description—metadata of the entity association with the DOI
3. Resolution—means to resolve the identifier to actually locate the object
4. Policies—rules that govern the operation of the system

The DOI consists of a prefix that is assigned by the IDF to the publishing entity and a suffix that is assigned and maintained by the entity. For example, the DOI for articles from the *Journal of the American Medical Informatics Association* (*JAMIA*) have the prefix `10.1197` and the suffix `jamia.M####`, where `####` is a number assigned by the journal editors. For example, a publication in *JAMIA* by this author on image retrieval [18] has the DOI https://doi.org/10.1197/jamia.M2082. Likewise, the previous edition of this book has a DOI of https://doi.org/10.1007/978-0-387-78,703-9 based on the publisher (Springer) DOI prefix of `10.1007`.

The DOI can also be encoded into a URL and resolved by the DOI Web site in a standardized fashion. For example, the JAMIA article cited above [18] is accessed by the URL https://doi.org/10.1197/jamia.M2082, which is resolved to the URL on the JAMIA Web site.[9] Similarly, the DOI for the previous edition of this book is resolved to the URL on the Springer Web.[10]

Evidence that the DOI has become the de facto universal identifier for scientific information is the fact that it is included in MEDLINE records. MEDLINE allows designation of the DOI in its Article Identifier (AID) field, which is populated by the publisher. AID values may include the controlled Publisher Item Identifier (PII), which is any internal reference identifier used in the publishing process, or the DOI that is assigned in accordance with the publisher's use of the DOI system. The AID field may also contain Bookshelf accession numbers for citations for books and book chapters from the *NCBI Books* Database.

An outgrowth of the standardization on the DOI is the CrossRef project, which aims to create an infrastructure for linking citations across publishers.[11] Publishers

[7] https://www.doi.org/

[8] https://www.doi.org/hb.html

[9] https://academic.oup.com/jamia/article/13/5/488/733702

[10] https://link.springer.com/book/10.1007/978-0-387-78703-9

[11] https://www.crossref.org/

who are members of CrossRef can insure that the DOIs for the content items they publish will resolve to a valid URL. They can also be assured that outbound links to other content adhering to the CrossRef standard will resolve to a valid URL.

Another important identifier related to scientific publications is linkage to their published data, which authors or publishers might also want to have in citable form. DataCite[12] provides a metadata record that includes a DOI to digital datasets so they are persistent and findable. FORCE11, a group devoted to research communications and e-scholarship, has developed a set of principles for data citation.[13] The Web site Zenodo allows anyone to assign a DOI to research artifacts, such as datasets or a GitHub repository.[14]

6.2.2 Access to Collections

With myriad resources online, there has always been a desire to provide seamless access to collections of them. In the pre-Web Internet era, a standard was developed to provide a standard means for IR clients and servers to interact with each other. Called Z39.50, it aimed to enable any server to allow searching on its collection (with appropriate restriction based on access rights) and at the same time to allow any client (with the proper access rights) to search on any server [19]. This separation of the user interface from the back-end IR system allowed users on different platforms and with different clients to access the same collections. A limitation of this approach was that it limited the amount of retrieval capabilities, since each of the disparate components, client and server, needed to understand the functionality of the other. Early versions of the protocol, for example, did not provide for natural language searching capabilities. The momentum for Z39.50 was also hampered by the early search engines of the Web, which developed their own mechanisms for sending queries from Web page forms to IR servers.

Another early effort to provide access to collections was a component of the original Unified Medical Language System (UMLS) project called the Information Sources Map (ISM) [20]. The two major goals of the ISM were to describe electronically available information sources in machine-readable format, so that computer programs could determine which sources are appropriate to a given query, and to provide information on how to connect to those sources automatically. The ISM was essentially a database about databases, indexed by terms in the Metathesaurus. The ISM was ultimately abandoned, mainly because of the sheer increase in volume of information sources. In addition, effective systems for using it were never able to be constructed [21, 22].

---

[12] https://www.datacite.org/

[13] https://www.force11.org/datacitationprinciples

[14] https://zenodo.org/

Although many organizations provide catalogs to collections that they license or otherwise want to highlight availability of their clientele, there is probably no way to keep track of all of the different collections available on the Web. In addition, the ability of search engines to link to or index multiple sites makes the need for ISM-like systems less compelling.

6.2.3 Access to Metadata

As noted throughout this book, metadata is a key component for accessing content in IR systems. It takes on additional value in the DL, where there is a desire to allow access to diverse but selected resources. Most Web sites exist as silos that cannot be accessed in this manner, whereas we might want access the metadata for content in the visible and/or invisible Web. Arms et al. noted that three levels of agreement must be achieved to attain the desired interoperability for metadata [23]:

1. Technical agreements over formats, protocols, and security procedures
2. Content agreement over the data and the semantic interpretation of its metadata
3. Organizational agreements over ground rules for access, preservation, payment, authentication, and so forth

The most prominent early approach to metadata interoperability was the Open Archives Initiative (OAI)[15] [24]. While the OAI effort was rooted in access to scholarly communications, its methods could be applicable to a broader range of content. Its fundamental activity was to promote the "exposure" of archives' metadata such that DL systems could learn what content is available and how it could be obtained. The OAI recognized two classes of participants, both of whom agreed to adhere to the OAI protocol that provided a low-cost, low-barrier approach to interoperability:

1. Data providers that expose metadata about their content
2. Service providers that harvest metadata to provide value-added services

Each record in the OAI system had an XML-encoded record and contained three parts:

1. Header—a unique identifier and a date stamp indicating creation or latest modification
2. Metadata—a set of unqualified Dublin Core Metadata Initiative (DCMI) tags describing the resource
3. About—an optional container for information about the metadata, such as its schema

The OAI also had a process of harvesting metadata called the OAI Protocol for Metadata Harvesting (OAI-PMH), based on a set of six allowable actions [25]

[15] http://www.openarchives.org/

Table 6.1 Allowable actions in Open Archives Initiative Protocol for Metadata Harvesting (Adapted from [24])

Action	Description
GetRecord	Retrieve a single record
Identify	Retrieve information about a repository including, at a minimum, the name, base URL, version of OAI protocol, and email address of the administrator of the resource
ListIdentifier	Retrieve list of identifiers that can be harvested from a repository
ListMetadataFormats	Retrieve metadata formats from a repository
ListRecords	Harvests records from a repository, with optional argument for filtering based on attributes of records, either date-based or set-based
ListSets	Retrieve set structure in a repository

(Table 6.1). Further developments for OAI included the Open Archives Initiative Object Reuse and Exchange (OAI-ORE), which aimed to define standards for the description and exchange of complex aggregations of Web resources, and ResourceSync,[16] which provided tools for maintaining synchronization of resources on servers. Some biomedical publishers adopted OAI, but the only active access at this time is provided by PubMed Central (PMC).[17]

Another important aspect of access to metadata is its standardization. As in other areas of biomedical and health informatics, standards for describing all artifacts of the research process allow better understanding and reproducibility of the research. One project that maintains standardized identifier and descriptions of research artifacts is eagle-I[18] [26, 27].

An additional important metadata item to maintain for research is authors. As names are ambiguous (even rare names such as William Hersh [28]), it is important for proper identification and attribution for authors to be explicitly identified. This notion gave rise to the Open Researcher and Contributor ID (ORCID) system, which allows any research to obtain a unique identifier, which can be associated with a URL, e.g., this author.[19] Growing numbers of journals and other publishing entities encourage or require the use of ORCIDs.

6.2.4 Integration with Other Applications

The early researchers whose work was described in Sect. 10.1.1 recognized the importance of linkage of information, even if the technology at the time did not permit optimal solutions. Work continues in the area of linking various aspects of

[16] http://www.openarchives.org/rs/resourcesync

[17] https://www.ncbi.nlm.nih.gov/pmc/tools/oai/

[18] https://www.eagle-i.net/

[19] http://orcid.org/0000-0002-4114-5148

content, some of which was described in state-of-the-art systems described earlier in the book. For example, the genomics databases described in Sect. 3.4.4 demonstrated how information from gene sequences (GenBank) and their variants (ClinVar) to scientific papers describing them (MEDLINE) to textbook descriptions of diseases they occur in (Online Mendelian Inheritance in Man) can be integrated. This section focuses on linkage of knowledge-based content to the electronic health record (EHR).

Most IR applications are stand-alone applications; that is, the user explicitly launches an application or goes to a Web page. A number of researchers have hypothesized that the use of IR systems can be made more efficient in the clinical setting by embedding them in the EHR. Not only would this allow their quicker launching (i.e., the user would not have to "switch" applications), but the context of the patient could provide a starting point for a query. Cimino [29] reviewed the literature on this topic and noted that embedding had been a desirable feature since the advent on the EHR. More recently, however, the ability to link systems and their resources via the Internet, particularly using Web browsers, has made such applications easier to develop and disseminate. Cimino noted that the process of linking patient information systems to IR resources consisted of three steps:

1. Identifying the user's question
2. Identifying the appropriate information resource
3. Composing the retrieval strategy

Although IR systems typically provide a simple query box for identifying the user's question, the EHR contains context about the patient, such as diagnoses, treatments, test results, and demographic data, which might be leveraged to create a context-specific query. Some early approaches looked at extracting information from dictated reports [30, 31] but were limited by the nonspecificity of much of the data in those reports. Cimino et al. developed *generic queries* that were based on analyses of real queries posed to medical librarians [32]. They subsequently developed *infobuttons* that allowed the user to retrieve specific information. For example, an infobutton next to an ICD-9 code translated the code into a Medical Subject Headings (MeSH) term using the Unified Medical Language System (UMLS) Metathesaurus and sent a query to MEDLINE [33]. Likewise, an infobutton next to a laboratory result generated a MEDLINE search with the appropriate term based on whether the result was abnormal or not [34].

Additional work by Cimino and colleagues included development of an *Infobutton Manager*, which kept track of the various information resources, generic questions that could be asked of them, and contexts in which those questions and resources might be used. The specific context of the patient is derived from the EHR or clinical information system (CIS), e.g., demographic information, diagnoses, test results, and so forth. The system then creates specific infobuttons that provide linkage to available resources with queries to find knowledge-based information appropriate to that context [35]. The Infobutton Manager matches a group of context parameters to information needs and then matches those needs to actual resources. The context parameters include:

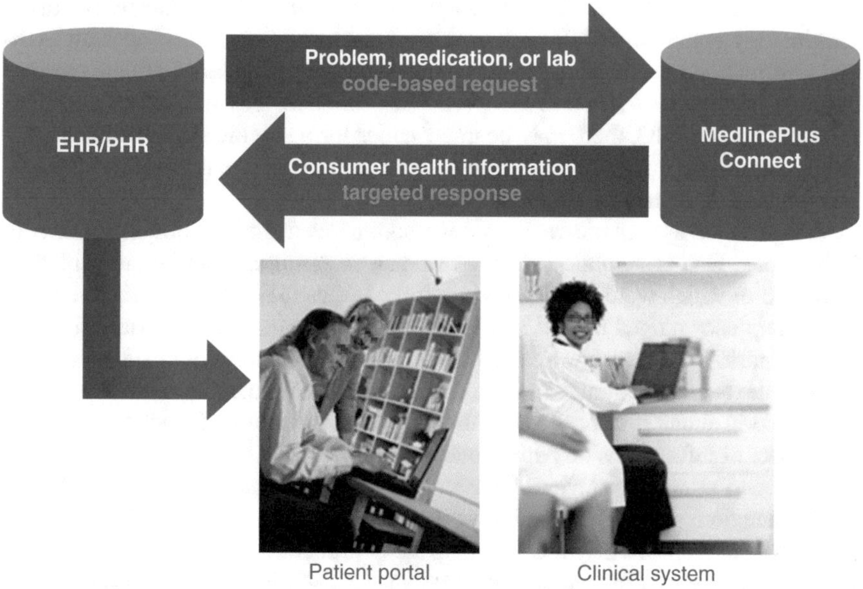

Fig. 6.1 Infobutton operations for Medline PLUS Connect. (Courtesy of NLM)

- User type—nurse, physician, patient
- Patient age—newborn, infant, child, adolescent, young adult, middle aged, and elderly
- Patient gender—male, female
- Concept of interest—e.g., diagnosis, medication, test result, organism
- Institution—used to determine which resources are available/preferred at a given institution

There has been widespread adoption of infobuttons in EHR systems. The standards organization HL7 developed the *Context-Aware Knowledge Retrieval (Infobutton)* specification,[20] which provided a standard mechanism for clinical information systems to request context-specific clinical knowledge from online resources. EHR vendors now must provide its functionality to achieve certification for systems to be eligible in US government healthcare quality programs.[21] Likewise, many information providers provide explicit mechanisms for infobuttons to access their content, such as Medline Plus Connect,[22] as shown in Fig. 6.1. They have also been expanded to provide access to genomics resources in the context of the EHR [36].

[20] https://wiki.hl7.org/Infobutton

[21] https://www.healthit.gov/test-method/patient-specific-education-resources

[22] https://medlineplus.gov/connect/overview.html

There are still some challenges to implementing infobuttons, mostly related to terminology granularity [37]. With the use of diagnosis (e.g., ICD) codes by EHRs and information resources, there can be mismatches in granularity of terms as well as in coding in the EHR and/or information resource. For vocabularies such as RxNorm and LOINC, there may be many codes for a specific drug or test, respectively. For matching of other attributes, such as user type, e.g., physician, nurse, patient, etc., there may be mismatches as well.

A couple of systematic reviews have summarized the use and evaluation of infobuttons. One systematic review of studies assessing infobuttons identified 17 studies, 3 of which were randomized controlled trials [38]. The analysis found that usage frequency ranged from 0.3 to 7.4 uses per month per user and was influenced by EHR task. Infobuttons were used about one-fifth to one-third as often as direct (non-context-sensitive) links. In three studies, users were found to answer their clinical question about 70% of the time that they used infobutton. No studies assessed the impact of infobuttons on patient outcomes.

A second systematic review focused on approaches that improved the design, implementation, and functionality of infobuttons [39]. These studies assessed infobutton interoperability, tools to help tailor infobutton functionality, interventions to improve user experience, and interventions to improve content retrieval by improving prediction of relevant knowledge resources and information needs. One study found the HL7 Infobutton standard was easy to implement. Another study demonstrated the value of a tool to help medical librarians tailor functionality of infobuttons. User studies found that access to resources with which users were familiar increased user satisfaction ratings and that links to subsections of drug monographs increased information-seeking efficiency. In one instance, improved content indexing was found to improve content retrieval across three healthcare organizations.

6.3 Copyright and Intellectual Property

As with other DL-related concerns, IP issues have already been described at various places in this book. IP is difficult to protect in the digital environment because although the cost of production is not insubstantial the cost of replication is near nothing. Furthermore, in circumstances such as academic publishing, the desire for protection is situational. For example, individual researchers may want the widest dissemination of their research papers, but each one may want to protect revenues realized from synthesis works or educational products that are developed. The global reach of the Internet has required IP issues to be considered on a global scale. The World Intellectual Property Organization (WIPO)[23] is an agency of the United Nations attempting to develop worldwide policies, although understandably there is considerable variation in opinion about what such policies should be.

[23] https://www.wipo.int/portal/en/

6.3.1 Copyright and Fair Use

The right to protection of IP is enshrined in the US Constitution (Article I, Section 8, Clause 8), which states that Congress has the power to "promote the progress of science and useful arts, by securing for limited times to authors and inventors the exclusive right to their respective writings and discoveries." Copyright law for the United States is detailed in Title 17 of the United States Code.[24] Within this law, however, is a provision for *fair use*,[25] which allows copyrighted work to be reproduced for purposes of "criticism, comment, news reporting, teaching (including multiple copies for classroom use), scholarship, or research." In particular, there are four factors to be considered whether an activity constitutes fair use:

1. Purpose of use—educational vs. commercial
2. Nature of work—photos and music more protected than text
3. Amount of copying—should be for use by individuals
4. Effect of copying—out-of-print materials easier to justify than in-print

Fair use guidelines vary among libraries. A Web site that provides pointers to a wide range of material on the topic has been developed by Stanford University Libraries,[26] while the Association of Research Libraries has created a code for best practices in fair use [40]. The actual interpretation of fair use varies from library to library [2]. Some typical copying guidelines might limit users to 1000 words or 10% of book, a single journal article, or 1 illustration or image per book or journal. Publishers responded to fair use guidelines by creating the Copyright Clearance Center (CCC),[27] which provides a succinct overview of what is and is not subject to copyright [41] (Table 6.2). The CCC standardizes the process of royalty payments for use of journal articles that are reproduced. Royalty payment amounts are usually listed at the bottom of the first page of journal articles. They apply to individual use and not reproduction in other published works. The CCC acts as a clearinghouse, with libraries and copy shops forwarding royalties to CCC, which distributes them to publishers.

Copyright laws impact access by not only the user but also the creator of the content, who might wish for a middle ground between complete and no copyright protection. The notion gave rise to the Creative Commons (CC),[28] which formalizes a group of licenses based on the premise that some people do not necessarily want full copyright protection (which is the default under law) to apply to their works. Instead, they desire to attach certain restrictions to their use. In essence, the CC License allows a creator of IP to retain some rights short of completely releasing the content into the public domain. The CC licensing process is carried out by choosing from

[24] https://www.copyright.gov/title17/

[25] https://www.copyright.gov/title17/92chap1.html

[26] https://fairuse.stanford.edu/overview/fair-use/

[27] http://www.copyright.com/

[28] https://creativecommons.org/

Table 6.2 What is and is not protected copyright (Adapted from the Copyright Clearance Center)

Protected by copyright
• Literary works—all works expressed in writing both in print and digital form
• Computer software—considered to be literary works
• Pictorial, graphic, and sculptural works—paintings, drawings, carvings, photographs, clothing designs, textiles, etc.
• Architectural works—buildings blueprints, drawings, diagrams, models, etc.
• Sound recordings—songs, music, spoken word, sounds, and other recordings
• Audiovisual works—live action movies, animation, television programs, video games, etc.
• Pantomimes and choreographic works—art of imitating or acting out situations and the composition of dance movements and patterns, including those accompanied by music
• Dramatic works and accompanying music—plays and musicals
Not protected by copyright
• Works that have not been fixed in a tangible medium of expression—not written, recorded or captured electronically
• Titles, names, short phrases, and slogans; familiar symbols or designs; mere variations of typographic ornamentation, lettering, or coloring; mere listings of ingredients or contents
• Ideas, procedures, methods, systems, processes, concepts, principles, discoveries, or devices, as distinguished from a description, explanation, or illustration
• Works consisting entirely of information that are natural or self-evident facts, containing no original authorship, such as the white pages of telephone books, standard calendars, height and weight charts, and tape measures and rulers
• Works created by the US government
• Works for which copyright has expired, works in the public domain

https://www.copyright.com/learn/what-isnt-protected-copyright/

four conditions that apply to the work, giving rise to six CC licenses.[29] (A seventh license, CC 0, indicates a work is in the public domain.) The CC Web site provides a license deed as well as legal code for each of the license types. The four conditions for specifying a CC license are shown in Table 6.3, while the six CC license types are shown in Table 6.4.

CC supports a number of other initiatives. For example, it provides a search interface for images that have a CC license specified.[30] It also has collaborated with a number of well-known Web sites to facilitate the use of CC licenses, such as YouTube[31] and Wikipedia.[32] CC also supports initiatives for:

- Open educational resources[33]
- Open data[34]
- Open science[35]

[29] https://creativecommons.org/use-remix/cc-licenses/

[30] https://search.creativecommons.org/

[31] https://www.youtube.com/

[32] https://www.wikipedia.org/

[33] https://creativecommons.org/about/program-areas/education-oer/

[34] https://creativecommons.org/about/program-areas/open-data/

[35] https://creativecommons.org/about/program-areas/open-science/

Table 6.3 Conditions for specifying a Creative Commons license

Option	Condition
Attribution	Others may copy, distribute, and display the copyrighted work—and derivatives of it—but must give credit
Noncommercial	Others may copy, distribute, and display the copyrighted work but only for noncommercial purposes
No derivative works	Others may copy, distribute, and display only unmodified versions of the copyrighted work
Share alike	Others can distribute derivative works only under a license identical to the one governing the original work

https://creativecommons.org/use-remix/cc-licenses/

Table 6.4 Creative Commons license types

License type	Description
Attribution (CC BY)	Others may distribute, remix, tweak, and build upon a work, even commercially, as long as they credit the original creation
Attribution-ShareAlike (CC BY-SA)	Others may remix, tweak, and build upon a work even for commercial purposes, as long as they credit and license their new creations under the identical terms
Attribution-NoDerivs (CC BY-ND)	Others may reuse the work for any purpose, including commercially; however, it cannot be shared with others in adapted form, and credit must be provided
Attribution-NonCommercial (CC BY-NC)	Others may remix, tweak, and build upon a work noncommercially, and although their new works must also acknowledge original work and be noncommercial, they do not have to license their derivative works on the same terms
Attribution-NonCommercial-ShareAlike (CC BY-NC-SA)	Others may remix, tweak, and build upon a work noncommercially, as long as they credit original work and license their new creations under identical terms
Attribution-NonCommercial-NoDerivs (CC BY-NC-ND)	Most restrictive, others may download a work and share it with others as long as they credit the originator, but they cannot change the work in any way or use it commercially

https://creativecommons.org/use-remix/cc-licenses/

6.3.2 Digital Rights Management

The area of protecting online intellectual property (IP) is commonly called *digital rights management* (DRM). There are a number of ongoing open and proprietary efforts in this field, which are mired in political and economic struggles among commercial content producers (e.g., the Recording Industry Association of America, Microsoft Corp., etc.). The DRM issue remains a thorny one, not only for protecting IP but also for allowing fair use and respecting the privacy rights of users [42]. It is certainly understandable that publishers wish to protect their IP. The question is how to provide them the tools to protect that property while expanding the market for their content, which may in turn allow them to lower the unit price of access.

A particular challenge is how to serve the single users or those in small groups. While those at academic and other large medical centers often have direct access to resources based on their Internet Protocol (IP) addresses, practitioners who do not reside at such centers usually do not. Even clinicians at large centers want to access resources that their institutions do not provide and are inconvenienced by the usual authentication schemes.

A framework for an inventory of digital rights was developed by Rosenblatt, who defined categories of rights and user actions within them [43]:

- Render rights—print, view, play
- Transport rights—copy, move, loan
- Derivative work rights—extract, edit, embed
- Utility rights—backup, cache, insure data integrity

6.4 Open Access and Open Science

The electronic publishing of scientific journals has resulted in some reduction of costs needed for printing and mailing of journals. There is also a growing awareness that scientific research is mostly funded by government agencies, such as the National Institutes of Health (NIH) and the National Science Foundation (NSF) in the United States, yet the results are not readily accessible by the taxpayers who funded it due to its sequestering in copyrighted publications.[36] This all led to the rise in advocacy for unimpeded access to scientific information, giving rise to the notion of *open-access* (OA) publishing. Such publishing is guided by the philosophy that access to scientific archives should be free and unimpeded, with other means used to finance its cost, such as the grant funding that pays for most research. By easing dissemination, OA publishing may reduce waste of duplicated research and positively impact policy [44].

Some have extended this notion to that of *open science*. This notion was originally proposed by Pontika et al. [45], leading to the FOSTER project[37] funded by the European Union and including, in addition to OA:

- Open data—all data collected in research
- Open source—all software code developed and used
- Open reproducible research—clear and detailed description, all surveys and other tools
- Open science evaluation, including open peer review—all comments of peer reviewers
- Open science policies
- Open science tools

---

[36] https://www.taxpayeraccess.org/

[37] https://www.fosteropenscience.eu/

Pakenham-Walsh and Godlee argue there is a moral imperative to timely accurate healthcare information for people around the world [46]. One example of open science implementation has been described in the neuroscience community by Wiener [47]. The US National Academies of Sciences, Engineering, and Medicine also issued a report endorsing movement toward open science [48]. A major requirement for open science is interoperability of all resources [49].

Biomedical and health science increasingly relies on publicly available data resources, especially in the -omics sciences. Many of these resources have been built with public grant funding and used by many researchers, although their maintenance competes with funding for new research [50]. While many advocate for an Open Science "Commons," some are concerned a lack of coordination will lead to a so-called anti-commons, with resources so distributed, each with different rules for access and use, such that their collective integration and value becomes impossible [51, 52].

6.4.1 Open-Access Publishing

Although in existence for nearly two decades, there is still debate over the merits of OA publishing, including discussion of its financial feasibility as well as the issue of who controls scientific literature. The typical solution for OA publishing is "author pays," based on the notion that most research is funded by grants, and a small additional charge for publishing should not adversely affect their budgets. (In fact, most researchers with grants consider the time they spend writing papers about the research to be part of their salary time that is funded.) Most OA journals usually have provisions for those who cannot afford the page charges, especially scientists from developing countries.

The original open-access publishing effort in biomedicine was developed by BioMed Central (BMC).[38] Since its inception, BMC has expanded to over 250 journals. Most BMC journals are indexed in MEDLINE and archived in PMC. The main source of revenue for BMC is article processing charges, which authors pay after their article is accepted for publication. BMC was acquired by the commercial publisher Springer in 2008, but no changes have been made to its OA model. Another prominent OA journal family is the Public Library of Science (PLoS).[39] Starting with *PLOS Biology*, which began publication in 2003, PLoS has subsequently launched *PLOS Medicine*, *PLOS Computational Biology*, *PLOS Genetics*, *PLOS Pathogens*, *PLOS Neglected Tropical Diseases*, and the broad multidisciplinary *PLOS One*.

Most other biomedical journals have maintained the copyright and subscription-based approach, although a number of them offer an OA option for authors willing to pay, usually in the range of \$2000–\$3000. Some journals have created OA

[38] https://www.biomedcentral.com/

[39] https://www.plos.org/

counterparts to their tradition journals, such as *JAMIA* (*JAMIA Open*), *JAMA* (*JAMA Network Open*), *Applied Clinical Informatics* (*ACI Open*), and *Lancet* (*EBioMedicine*).

In the early days of OA, some publishers argued against its use. Lancet noted that the up-front page charges may limit venues of publishing for resource-poor scientists (although BMC and PLoS waive fees for such scientists) and that OA threatened the survival of nonprofit presses, such as university presses [53]. The leadership of JAMA expressed concern that the article processing charges of BMC and PLoS may not cover the costs of the publishing process, meaning that their business models are not sustainable, especially for journals with low acceptance rates like *JAMA* at 8% [54]. They also expressed concern that this model may provide incentive for journals to publish more and, as a result, lower their quality. The publisher of BMC, on the other hand, retorted that journals still need to maintain their quality if they want to provide incentive for scientists to publish there (J Velterop, founder of BMC, personal communication).

Despite those early arguments, OA has maintained a foothold in electronic published, with about 20% of all biomedical articles published under this model [55, 56]. There are two models of OA publishing that have emerged:

- Gold—"author pays" model, i.e., research funding cover costs
- Green—author required to deposit manuscript in public repository, e.g., PubMed Central

One alternative that emerged to OA, mainly from nonprofit publishers (typically professional societies), was the *Washington DC Principles for Free Access to Science*. Although no longer active, these publishers reaffirmed their view that they maintain the copyright on their publications but advocated a number of principles:

- Selected important articles available free online when published
- Complete contents freely available within months of publication
- Complete contents available for free to scientists in low-income countries
- Content available through online reference linking and major search engines

As such, articles older than 6–12 months continue to be made freely available on most of the Web sites of these journals, which include *JAMA*, *NEJM*, and *Annals of Internal Medicine*.

6.4.2 NIH Public Access Policy

In 2004, the NIH Director released an analysis of the cost of publishing of NIH research results [57]. Based on an estimate that 0.32% of grant funding was devoted to publication costs, he noted that the NIH already provided about $30 million in direct costs for publications through its funded research grants. Zerhouni asserted that adopting a plan to archive all publications in PubMed Central (PMC) would add only another $2–4 million per year, since it would be built on top of the existing

NIH information technology infrastructure. The RFC drew over 6000 responses. Many were in favor, but both commercial and nonprofit publishers raised concerns about the plan. Among the latter were public documents from the American College of Physicians [58] and *The New England Journal of Medicine* [59].

A number of public and private funding agencies started requiring their funded researchers to submit their papers to public repositories. In 2008, the NIH launched its Public Access Policy, requiring all manuscripts emanating from funded research to be submitted to PMC within 12 months of publication, with instructions on the NIH Public Access Web site.[40] This brought the NIH into line with other public (the UK Medical Research Council) and private funding agencies (Wellcome Trust[41] and Howard Hughes Medical Institute[42]) [60].

According to the NIH Public Access Policy,[43] authors must comply via four steps:

1. Determine Applicability—applies to any manuscript that
   (a) Is peer-reviewed
   (b) Is accepted for publication in a journal on or after April 7, 2008
   (c) Arises from:
      - Any direct funding from an NIH grant or cooperative agreement active in Fiscal Year 2008 or beyond
      - Any direct funding from an NIH contract signed on or after April 7, 2008
      - Any direct funding from the NIH Intramural Program.
      - An NIH employee
2. Address Copyright—ensure that the journal's publishing agreement allows the paper to be posted to PubMed Central in accordance with the NIH Public Access Policy
3. Submit Papers—submit final submitted manuscript or published paper to PubMed Central
4. Cite Papers—include the PMCID at the end of the full citation of the article whenever it is cited

Now that the OA movement has been around for several years, overviews and research about it have begun to emerge [61]. It is known that a large number of authors post (or "self-archive") their manuscripts, which have been found to have higher rates of citation that is attributed to their quality and not bias of being more available [62]. Some publishers post guidelines for authors for sharing publications, such as Elsevier[44] and Springer Nature.[45]

[40] https://publicaccess.nih.gov/

[41] https://www.wellcome.ac.uk/

[42] https://www.hhmi.org/

[43] https://publicaccess.nih.gov/policy.htm

[44] https://www.elsevier.com/about/policies/sharing

[45] https://www.springernature.com/gp/authors/research-data-policy

6.4.3 Predatory Journals

One of the unintended consequences of the OA movement has been the emergence of the so-called predatory journals, which offer inexpensive publishing but mainly exist to make money [63, 64]. Such journals often have names that sound similar to well-known journals but are characterized by minimal if any peer review, rapid turnaround, poor-looking Web sites with grammatical errors and generic (e.g., Gmail) email address domains [65]. Their use varies around the world, with the highest update in Asian and African countries [66]. Related predatory activities include invitations for researchers to serve on editorial boards, which give predatory journals some appearance of legitimacy [67], and the parallel growth of "fake conferences," which also serve as vehicles to make money for those who organize them [68].

Some researchers have spoofed predatory journals by publishing "fake papers" to demonstrate their fraudulence by using the autocomplete function of the Apple iPhone [69] or based on themes from the television series *Seinfeld* [70] and the movie *Star Wars* [71]. The consequences of predatory journals are real, however, as some researchers, intending to adhere to policies such as the NIH Public Access Policy, unknowingly publish in such journals and then submit manuscripts from them to repositories such as PMC [72]. This has led the NIH to post a notice strongly discouraging publishing in these kinds of journals and providing recommendations on publishing in "credible" journals [73]. (One tip-off of these journals this author has noted is lack of link to unsubscribe from the repetitive emails they send.)

Another concern is articles in predatory journals being cited and having impact in scientific fields. One analysis of 250 papers published in 2014 found a rate of 2.6 citations per article and 60% having no citations at all, which was much less than a representative sample of articles in the Scopus database of 18.1 citations with only 9% receiving no citations [74]. Thus, while the citation rate of articles in predatory journals is small, it is not zero.

There have been many approaches to alert those who perform and/or read scientific research about predatory journals. There have been calls in prominent journals for researchers and readers to avoid predatory journals [75, 76]. A Web site focused on predatory journals maintains a list of such journals.[46] This site superseded an earlier site that maintained a similar inventory, called *Beall's List* [77]. Another site, the Directory of Open Access Journals (DOAJ),[47] maintains a list of known high-quality OA journals.

[46] https://predatoryjournals.com/journals/

[47] https://doaj.org/

6.5 Preservation

As noted earlier in this chapter, libraries had always been the major organizations tasked with preservation of scholarly materials. In the twenty-first century, however, libraries tend to function more as intermediaries and facilitators in providing access to materials that reside on the servers of publishers and others. Even more concerning is that in the digital era, there are fewer "copies" of important scholarly works, as most scholars do not typically maintain their own archives. A leader in digital preservation efforts is the US Library of Congress.[48]

There are a number of issues specific to the preservation of digital materials [78]. One concerns the size of such materials. Although hard disk space is, in modern times, considered "cheap," the computer size of objects becomes important in determining how to store massive collections as well as transmit them across networks. Lesk compared the longevity of digital materials, noting that the longevity for magnetic materials was the least, with the expected lifetime of magnetic tape being 5 to 10 years [2]. Optical storage has somewhat better longevity, with an expected lifetime of 30 to 100 years depending on the specific type.

Others have noted that more traditional, non-digital sources of information have much more longevity. Lesk also pointed out that paper has a life expectancy well beyond the above digital media [2]. A more recent technology, microfilm, has at least a half century of life expectancy [79]. There is also the Rosetta Stone, which provided help in interpreting ancient Egyptian hieroglyphics and has survived over 20 centuries [80]. The latter author noted another problem familiar to most longtime users of computers, namely, that data can become obsolete not only owing to the medium but also as a result of data format. He pointed out that storage devices as well as computer applications, such as word processors, have seen their formats change significantly over the last couple of decades. Indeed, it may be harder in the future to decipher a document stored in an early version of Microsoft Word than an ancient stone or paper document.

One initiative aiming to preserve content is the Lots of Copies Keep Stuff Safe (LOCKSS)[49] project. As the name implies, numerous digital copies of important documents can be maintained. But the project further concerns itself with the ability to detect and repair damaged copies as well as to prevent subversion of the data. This is done via hashing schemes that assess the integrity of the data in the multiples caches of content and "fix" altered copies. An extension of LOCKSS project is Controlled Lots of Copies Keep Stuff Safe (CLOCKSS),[50] a global

---

[48] https://www.loc.gov/preservation/digital/

[49] https://www.lockss.org/

[50] https://clockss.org/

archive governed by scholarly publishers and top research libraries [81]. Another effort to preserve scholarly electronic journals, books, and digital collections is Portico.[51]

Of course, some content such as that on the Web is highly dynamic and undergoes constant change. An early analysis of the Web found that the lifetime of an average Web page was 44 days and the "half-life" of the survival of Web pages may actually be somewhat longer, at roughly 2 years [82]. This interest in the changing nature of Web pages led Kahle to undertake a project to archive the Internet[52] on a periodic basis. A popular feature of this Web site is the Internet Wayback Machine, which allows entry of a URL and its display at different points in time. Another site that provides access to distinct archived collections is Archive-It.[53]

A number of initiatives have been undertaken to insure preservation of scientific information. An effort of the LOC, replaced by current efforts, was the National Digital Information Infrastructure Preservation Program (NDIIPP)[54] of the US Library of Congress [83]. Another effort, still active, is the Digital Preservation Coalition in the United Kingdom[55] [84]. A related initiative is an effort to preserve computer software code, especially that which is used for scholarly purposes [85].

6.6 Librarians, Informationists, and Other Professionals

One concern about libraries is access to the professionals who have always aided their patrons. For example, reference librarians are still key to assisting researchers, especially when exhaustive searching is required, such as in systematic reviews. One challenge to the role of library professionals is an economic one: as the amount of online content increases in availability to users and it is used directly with increasing frequency, the amount of time that can be devoted to any user and/or resource shrinks. However, the value of professional assistance to users cannot be denied. A systematic review of studies of librarian-provided services in healthcare setting found documented benefit for participants in training programs (e.g., students and residents) in improving skills in searching the literature to use research evidence for clinical decision-making [14]. It also found studies showing that services provided to clinicians were effective in time-saving for healthcare professionals and providing relevant information for decision-making. A couple studies showed that such

[51] https://www.portico.org/

[52] https://archive.org/

[53] https://archive-it.org/

[54] http://www.digitalpreservation.gov/

[55] https://www.dpconline.org/

services led to decreased patient length of stay when literature searches related to a patient's case were performed for clinicians. There were no studies that assessed the value of these services for researchers or patients.

One proposal that caused a stir when it was promoted in an *Annals of Internal Medicine* editorial is the notion of a new information professional for the clinical setting, the *informationist* [86]. The medical library community responded to this call by touting the virtue of clinical librarianship and affirming the value of library science training [87]. This term was actually introduced by Garfield [88] in the context of having information professionals who understood the laws of information science and advocated in the early 1990s by Quint [89]. A recent book describes the knowledge and skills required for the informationist beyond search, such as data management and visualization, current awareness, and roles in evidence-based practice [90].

Although there has been little research assessing the efficacy of the informationist approach (e.g., in terms of improved clinical care or reduced information-seeking time by clinicians), several models have been developed. The most mature of these is the clinical informationist, with the informationist helping to optimize the use of not only evidence-based information but also informatics tools at the point of care [91]. Another approach has been to adapt the model to the biomedical research environment, leading to the clinical bioinformationist model, focusing on molecular biology, genetic analysis, biotechnology, research literature, and databases [92]. Florance et al. described the challenges of integrating information specialists into various biomedical settings [93]. Rosenbloom et al. found that informationists have skill levels comparable to physicians trained in research methodology and better than general physicians for selecting pertinent articles for clinical questions [94]. A further evolution of the informationist concept has been an entire service devoted to not only answering the complex clinical questions of care teams but also helping to develop clinical order sets as well as a patient portal [95]. An evaluation study based on focus groups and interviews found clinical teams valued their expertise and increased the use of information resources [96].

6.7 Future Directions

This chapter brings to an end our exploration of the state of the art for IR. Although access to knowledge-based information is common and even ubiquitous across the globe, the chapters in this section have demonstrated that there are still challenges to improve these systems. In the remainder of the book, we will explore major threads of research in IR, from evaluating the use of systems to developing new approaches for systems and their users.

References

1. Hildreth C. The online catalogue: developments and directions. The Library Association: London, England; 1989.
2. Lesk M. Understanding Digital Libraries. 2nd ed. San Francisco, CA: Morgan Kaufmann; 2005.
3. Price D. Little science, big science. New York: Columbia University Press; 1963.
4. Anonymous. The deterioration and preservation of paper: some essential facts. Washington, DC: Library of Congress; 2019.
5. Borgman C. What are digital libraries? Competing visions. Inf Process Manag. 1999;35:227–44.
6. Weise F. Being there: library as place. J Med Libr Assoc. 2004;92:6–13.
7. Monastersky R. Publishing frontiers: the library reboot. Nature. 2013;495:430–2.
8. Arms W. Digital Libraries. Cambridge, MA: MIT Press; 2001.
9. Witten I, Bainbridge D, Nichols D. How to build a digital library. 2nd ed. San Francisco: Morgan Kaufmann; 2010.
10. Purcell A. Digital library programs for libraries and archives: developing, managing, and sustaining unique digital collections. American Library Association: Chicago, IL; 2016.
11. Banerjee K, Reese T. Building digital libraries 2nd edition. Amazon Digital Services; 2018.
12. Anonymous. Mass digitization: implications for information policy. Washington, DC: U.S. National Commission on Libraries and Information Science 2006 May 9, 2006.
13. Fox E, Goncalves M, Shen R. Theoretical foundations for digital libraries: the 5S (societies, scenarios, spaces, structures, streams) approach. Morgan & Claypool: San Rafael, CA; 2012.
14. Perrier L, Farrell A, Ayala A, Lightfoot D, Kenny T, Aaronson E, et al. Effects of librarian-provided services in healthcare settings: a systematic review. J Am Med Inform Assoc. 2014;21:1118–24.
15. Wilkinson M, Dumontier M, Aalbersberg I, Appleton G, Axton M, vander Lei J, et al. The FAIR guiding principles for scientific data management and stewardship. Scientific Data. 2016;3:160018.
16. Haendel M, Su A, McMurry J. FAIR-TLC: metrics to assess value of biomedical digital repositories: response to RFI NOT-OD-16-133. Zenodo. 2016 December;15:2016.
17. Sollins K, Masinter L. Functional requirements for uniform resource names: internet engineering task force 1994 July 1, 2002.
18. Hersh W, Müller H, Jensen J, Yang J, Gorman P, Ruch P. Advancing biomedical image retrieval: development and analysis of a test collection. J Am Med Inform Assoc. 2006;13:488–96.
19. Miller P. Z39.50 for all. Ariadne. 1999;21.
20. Masys D. An evaluation of the source selection elements of the prototype UMLS information sources map. Proceedings of the 16th Annual Symposium on Computer Applications in Medical Care; 1992; Baltimore, MD: McGraw-Hill.
21. Miller P, Frawley S, Wright L, Roderer N, Powsner S. Lessons learned from a pilot implementation of the UMLS information sources map. J Am Med Inform Assoc. 1995;2:102–15.
22. Mendonça E, Cimino J. Evaluation of the information sources map. Proceedings of the AMIA 1999 annual symposium. Washington, DC: Hanley & Belfus; 1999.
23. Arms W, Hillmann D, Lagoze C, Krafft D, Marisa R, Saylor J et al. A spectrum of interoperability: the site for science prototype for the NSDL. D-Lib Magazine 2002;8.
24. Lagoze C, Vande Sompel H. The Open Archives Initiative: building a low-barrier interoperability framework. Proceedings of the First ACM/IEEE-CS Joint Conference on Digital Libraries; 2001; Roanoke, VA: ACM Press.
25. Vande Sompel H, Nelson M, Lagoze C, Warner S. Resource harvesting within the OAI-PMH framework. D-Lib Magazine. 2004;10(12)
26. Vasilevsky N, Johnson T, Corday K, Torniai C, Brush M, Segerdell E, et al. Research resources: curating the new eagle-i discovery system. Database. 2012;2012:bar067.
27. Vasilevsky N, Brush M, Paddock H, Ponting L, Tripathy S, Larocca G, et al. On the reproducibility of science: unique identification of research resources in the biomedical literature. PeerJ. 2013;5(1):e148.

28. Hersh W. Meeting My Doppelgänger (Googlegänger). Infromatics Professor 2015.
29. Cimino J. Linking patient information systems to bibliographic resources. Methods Inf Med. 1996;35:122–6.
30. Powsner S, Miller P. Linking bibliographic retrieval to clinical reports: Psychtopix. Proceedings of the 13th Annual Symposium on Computer Applications in Medical Care; 1989; Washington, DC: IEEE.
31. Miller R, Gieszczykiewicz F, Vries J, Cooper G. CHARTLINE: providing bibliographic references relevant to patient charts using the UMLS Metathesaurus knowledge sources. Proceedings of the 16th Annual Symposium on Computer Applications in Medical Care; 1992; Baltimore, MD: McGraw-Hill.
32. Cimino J, Aguirre A, Johnson S, Peng P. Generic queries for meeting clinical information needs. Bull Med Libr Assoc. 1993;81:195–206.
33. Cimino J, Johnson S, Aguirre A, Roderer N, Clayton P. The MEDLINE button. Proceedings of the 16th Annual Symposium on Computer Applications in Medical Care; 1992; Baltimore, MD: McGraw-Hill.
34. Cimino J, Socratorus S, Clayton P. Internet as clinical information system: application development using the world wide web. J Am Med Inform Assoc. 1995;2:273–84.
35. Cimino J, Li J, Bakken S, Patel V. Theoretical, empirical and practical approaches to resolving the unmet information needs of clinical information system users. Proceedings of the 2002 AMIA Annual Symposium; 2002; San Antonio, TX: Hanley & Belfus.
36. Heale B, Overby C, DelFiol G, Rubinstein W, Maglott D, Nelson T, et al. Integrating genomic resources with electronic health records using the HL7 infobutton standard. Appl Clin Inform. 2016;7:817–31.
37. Strasberg H, DelFiol G, Cimino J. Terminology challenges implementing the HL7 context-aware knowledge retrieval ('Infobutton') standard. J Am Med Inform Assoc. 2013;20:218–23.
38. Cook D, Teixeira M, Heale B, Cimino J, DelFiol G. Context-sensitive decision support (infobuttons) in electronic health records: a systematic review. J Am Med Inform Assoc. 2017;24:460–8.
39. Teixeira M, Cook D, Heale B, DelFiol G. Optimization of infobutton design and implementation: a systematic review. J Biomed Inform. 2017;74:10–9.
40. Adler P, Aufderheide P, Butler B, Jaszi P. Code of best practices in fair use for academic and research libraries, vol. 2012. Washington, DC: Association of Research Libraries; 2012 January.
41. Anonymous. So, what is (and Isn't) protected by copyright? Where copyright protection begins and ends. Danvers, MA: Copyright Clearance Center; 2017.
42. Tyrväinen P. Concepts and a design for fair use and privacy in DRM. D-Lib Magazine. 2005;11(2).
43. Rosenblatt B, Trippe B, Mooney S. Digital rights management–business and technology. New York: M&T Books; 2002.
44. Spedding S. Open access publishing of health research: does open access publishing facilitate the translation of research into health policy and practice? Publications. 2016;4(1):2.
45. Pontika N, Knoth P, Cancellieri M, Pearce S. Fostering Open Science to research using a taxonomy and an eLearning portal. Milton Keynes, UK: Open University; 2015.
46. Pakenham-Walsh N, Godlee F. Healthcare information for all. Br Med J. 2020;368:m759.
47. Wiener M, Sommer F, Ives Z, Poldrack R, Litt B. Enabling an open data ecosystem for the neurosciences. Neuron. 2016;92:617–21.
48. Anonymous. Open Science by design–realizing a vision for 21st century research. Washington, DC: National Academies Press; 2018.
49. Sansone S, Rocca-Serra P. Interoperability standards–digital objects in their own right. London, England Wellcome Trust 2016 October, 2016.
50. Kaiser J. Funding for key data resources in jeopardy. Science. 2016;351:14.
51. Heller M. The tragedy of the anticommons: a concise introduction and lexicon. The Modern Law Review. 2013;76(1):6–25.

52. Contreras J. The anticommons at 20: concerns for research continue. Science. 2018;361:335–7.
53. Horton R. 21st-century biomedical journals: failures and futures. Lancet. 2003;362:1510–2.
54. DeAngelis C, Musacchio R. Access to JAMA. J Am Med Assoc. 2004;291:370–1.
55. Laakso M, Welling P, Bukvova H, Nyman L, Björk B, Hedlund T. The development of open access journal publishing from 1993 to 2009. PLoS One. 2011;6(6):e20961.
56. Frank M. Open but not free--publishing in the 21st century. N Engl J Med. 2013;368:787–9.
57. Zerhouni E. Access to biomedical research information. National Institutes of Health: Bethesda, MD; 2004.
58. Tooker J. ACP comments on proposed NIH public access policy. Philadelphia, PA: American College of Physicians 2004 November 18, 2004.
59. Drazen J, Curfman G. Public access to biomedical research. N Engl J Med. 2004;351:1343.
60. Kaiser J. Scientific publishing. Uncle Sam's biomedical archive wants your papers. Science. 2008;319:266.
61. Miguel S, Tannuridede Oliveira E, CabriniGrácio M. Scientific production on open access: a worldwide bibliometric analysis in the academic and scientific context. Publications. 2016;4(1):1.
62. Gargouri Y, Hajjem C, Larivière V, Gingras Y, Carr L, Brody T, et al. Self-selected or mandated, open access increases citation impact for higher quality research. PLoS One. 2010;5(10):e13636.
63. Haug C. The downside of open-access publishing. N Engl J Med. 2013;368:791–3.
64. Beall J. Predatory journals exploit structural weaknesses in scholarly publishing. 4Open. 2018;1.
65. Shamseer L, Moher D, Maduekwe O, Turner L, Barbour V, Burch R, et al. Potential predatory and legitimate biomedical journals: can you tell the difference? A cross-sectional comparison. BMC Med. 2017;15:28.
66. Shen C, Björk B. 'Predatory' open access: a longitudinal study of article volumes and market characteristics. BMC Med. 2015;13:230.
67. Sorokowski P, Sorokowska A, Pisanski K. Predatory journals recruit fake editor. Nature. 2017;543:481–3.
68. Grant A. The proliferation of questionable conferences. Phys Today. 2018.
69. Bartneck C. iOS just got a paper on Nuclear Physics accepted at a scientific conference. Christoph Bartneck. 2016.
70. McCool J. Opinion: why I published in a predatory journal. The Scientist. 2017 April;6:2017.
71. Anonymous. Predatory Journals Hit by 'Star Wars' Sting. Neuroskeptic 2017.
72. Manca A, Moher D, Cugusi L, Dvir Z, Deriu F. How predatory journals leak into PubMed. Can Med Assoc J. 2018;190:E1042–E5.
73. Anonymous. Statement on article publication resulting from NIH Funded Research. Bethesda, MD: National Institutes of Health 2017 November 3, 2017 Contract No.: NOT-OD-18-011.
74. Björk B, Kanto-Karvonen S, Harviainen JT. How frequently are articles in predatory open access journals cited. arXivorg. 2019:arXiv:1912.10228.
75. Moher D, Moher E. Stop predatory publishers now: act collaboratively. Ann Intern Med. 2016;164:616–7.
76. Moher D, Shamseer L, Cobey K. Stop this waste of people, animals and money. Nature. 2017;549:23–5.
77. Straumsheim C. No more 'Beall's list. Inside Higher Ed. 2017 January;18:2017.
78. Kirchhoff A, Morrissey S, Wittenberg K. Networked Information's risky future: the promises and challenges of digital preservation. Educ Rev. 2015 March;2:2015.
79. Saper G. Microfilm lasts half a millennium. The Atlantic. 2018 July;22:2018.
80. Rothenberg J. Ensuring the longevity of digital information. RAND Corporation. 1999;. http://www.clir.org/pubs/archives/ensuring.pdf
81. Rosenthal DSH, Vargas DL. LOCKSS Boxes in the Cloud. LOCKSS Program, Stanford University Libraries: Palo Alto, CA, 2012. http://www.lockss.org/locksswp/wpcontent/uploads/2012/09/LC-final-2012.pdf.
82. Kahle B. Preserving the internet. Sci Am. 1997;276(3):82–3.
83. Friedlander A. The National Digital Information Infrastructure Preservation Program: expectations, realities, choices, and progress to date. D-Lib Magazine. 2002;8.

84. Beagrie N. An update on the digital preservation coalition. D-Lib Magazine. 2002;8.
85. Aufderheide P, Butler B, Cox K, Jaszi P. Code of best practices in fair use for software preservation, vol. 2019. Washington, DC: Association of Research Libraries; 2019 February.
86. Davidoff F, Florance V. The informationist: a new health profession? Ann Intern Med. 2000;132:996–8.
87. Schacher L. Clinical librarianship: its value in medical care. Ann Intern Med. 2001;134:717–20.
88. Garfield E. Bradford's law and related statistical patterns. In: Garfield E, editor. Essays of an information scientist: 1979–1980. Philadelphia: Institute for Scientific Information; 1979. p. 476–83.
89. Quint B. The last librarians: end of a millennium. Canadian Journal of Information Science. 1992;17:33–40.
90. DeRosa A, editor. A practical guide for Informationists: supporting research and clinical practice: Elsevier; 2018.
91. Giuse N, Koonce T, Jerome R, Cahall M, Sathe N, Williams A. Evolution of a mature clinical informationist model. J Am Med Inform Assoc. 2005;12:249–55.
92. Lyon J, Giuse N, Williams A, Koonce T, Walden R. A model for training the new bioinformationist. J Med Libr Assoc. 2004;92:188–95.
93. Florance V, Giuse N, Ketchell D. Information in context: integrating information specialists into practice settings. J Med Libr Assoc. 2002;90:49–58.
94. Rosenbloom S, Giuse N, Jerome R, Blackford J. Providing evidence-based answers to complex clinical questions: evaluating the consistency of article selection. Acad Med. 2005;80:109–14.
95. Giuse N, Williams A, Giuse D. Integrating best evidence into patient care: a process facilitated by a seamless integration with informatics tools. J Med Libr Assoc. 2010;98:220–2.
96. Grefsheim S, Whitmore S, Rapp B, Rankin J, Robison R, Canto C. The informationist: building evidence for an emerging health profession. J Med Libr Assoc. 2010;98:147–56.

Chapter 7
Evaluation

A recurring theme throughout the book thus far is that the information retrieval (IR) world changed substantially through the various editions of this book, particularly with the ubiquity of the World Wide Web and the growth of available information. From this, one might have expected a substantial increase in the amount and quality of evaluation research. However, this is not the case. While a modest number of new evaluation studies have appeared since the last edition, growth of evaluation research has not paralleled the explosion of new content and systems. This may well be due to the overall maturity and ubiquity of IR systems in the Web era, i.e., such systems are so ingrained in the lives of users that few believe that the need to evaluate them still exists. This is of course not the case, for much can be learned from looking at how IR systems are used and where they can be improved.

In this chapter, we will mainly focus on the evaluation of operational IR systems. (Research system evaluation will be discussed in the context of the research presented in the next chapter.) One challenge with operational systems is that some systems are discontinued, while others change in substantial ways. As such, the evaluation of a given system at a given time may not reflect the performance or value of that system at present or future times. The chapter closes with some discussion of research on relevance and then summarizes lessons learned and directions for future research.

For the evaluation of operational systems, our discussion will be organized around six questions developed for a systematic review of physician use of IR systems, although they can really apply to all IR systems and users [1]:

1. Was the system used?
2. For what was the system used?
3. Were the users satisfied?
4. How well did they use the system?
5. What factors were associated with successful or unsuccessful use of the system?
6. Did the system have an impact?

W. Hersh, *Information Retrieval: A Biomedical and Health Perspective*,
Health Informatics, https://doi.org/10.1007/978-3-030-47686-1_7

7.1 Usage Frequency

One of the best measurements of the value of any computer system is whether it is actually used by its intended audience. One can hypothesize about the pros and cons of different IR systems, but the discussion is moot if the system does not sustain the interest of users in the real world. This is certainly an important issue for developers of commercial systems, since unused systems are unlikely to last long in the marketplace. Clearly IR systems are used by many people. As noted in Chap. 1, nearly all physicians were using the Internet by 2012 [2], while by 2013 about 72% of US adult Internet users (59% of all US adults) reported looking for health information in the previous year [3]. Another indicator of massive uptake comes from the National Library of Medicine (NLM), which reported 3.3 billion searches of PubMed in fiscal year 2019.[1]

A number of usage studies were done in the 1980s and 1990s when IR systems were first becoming available in medical settings. Somewhat ironically, such studies were easier to do at that time, since most IR systems required logging in and there were fewer locations where they could be accessed, all of which allowed easier tracking of users and usage. Now, of course, IR systems are available almost everywhere, from desktop computers to wireless laptops and mobile devices. As such, measuring how often an IR system is used, let alone for health or biomedical information needs, can be challenging in modern times.

There were lessons to be learned from the early studies, which were summarized in the systematic review by Hersh and Hickam [1]. A review of about a dozen studies, in a variety of settings and with a variety of users, found usage to be only on the order of 0.3–6.0 times per user per month. This was noted to be in stark contrast with the known two-questions-per-three-patients information needs of clinicians noted around the same time [4]. In addition, a novelty effect was noted, in that usage was lower with a longer duration of observation. Another usage-related finding was a propensity for use of bibliographic resources, in particular MEDLINE, as opposed to full-text resources (such as CD-ROM textbooks).

These usage amounts have probably increased substantial in present times, with the proliferation of computer terminals in clinical and personal settings and the near-universal adoption of mobile devices by the population. Some newer studies provide an inkling of this. One study of internal medicine residents at three sites found that nearly all responding to the survey searched daily, with the most common resource searched being the comprehensive clinical reference, UpToDate [5]. The next most frequent source of information was consultation with attending faculty, followed by the Google search engine, the Epocrates drug reference, and various other "pocket" references. Another study of a family medicine practice

[1] https://www.nlm.nih.gov/bsd/medline_pubmed_production_stats.html

found that all physicians in the practice used a smartphone and/or tablet PC during daily practice and reported the reason of use was commonly for communication and Internet search purposes. Usage during working hours was limited, but medical apps were perceived mainly positively for receiving medical information via the Internet.

A pair of studies assessed a system of care process models (CPMs) that integrated current guidelines, recent evidence, and local expertise to represent cross-disciplinary best practices for managing clinical problems that were integrated with the EHR at Mayo Clinic. The first study found the resource to be used at least once by 71% of staff physicians, 66% of midlevel providers, and 75% of residents and fellows [6]. In any given month, about 10% of providers used the system two or more times. General internal medicine physicians were found to use the system most, with about five uses over a 1-year period. A more comprehensive follow-up study of over 4000 clinicians (2014 physicians in practice, 1117 resident physicians, and 878 nurse practitioners/physician assistants [NPs/PAs]) found that 140 CPMs were viewed a total of 81,764 times [7]. Usage varied from 1 to 809 views per person and from 9 to 4615 views per CPM. Residents and NPs/PAs viewed CPMs more often than practicing physicians. Generalist clinicians were found to use the CPMs more often than specialists, with topics accessed by specialists mostly aligned with topics within their specialties. The top 20% of available CPMs (28/140) accounted for 61% of uses. Generalists revisited topics more often than specialists (mean of 8.8 vs. 5.1 views per topic).

Patient and consumer searching of the Web for health information also continues to be reported high. In the most recent update of her ongoing survey of health-related searching, Fox found that 72% of US adult Internet users (59% of all US adults) had looked for health information in the last year [3].

Another usage analysis focused on a query log of PubMed rather than a population of individual users [8]. A single day's log from around October 2005 was made available to these researchers. They were able to determine "individuals" by Internet Protocol (IP) address. They eliminated from their analysis all users with over 50 queries during the time period, figuring that these were "bot" queries. For the remainder of the data, they determined that there were about 2.7 million queries posed by 624,514 users. The mean number of queries per user was 4.21, while the median number of queries was 2. The three most commonly used words were the PubMed tags [author], [au], and [pmid]. These were followed in frequency by the words, `cancer`, `cell`, `review`, and `2005`. A more focused analysis was carried out on 2272 randomly selected queries. These queries were classified as *informational* (74.4%) versus *navigational* (22.1%), with the latter appearing to be seeking specific articles. The number of articles in the result set of these queries varied widely (1 to 4.8 million), with an average of 14,050 and median of 68.

7.2 Types of Usage

In addition to knowing the frequency of system usage, it is also valuable to know what types of information need users' address. Many of the early studies assessed in the Hersh and Hickam systematic review also investigated this issue [1]. Since information resources, users, and settings were heterogeneous, direct comparison is difficult. But taken as a whole, the studies found a relatively consistent picture that questions of therapy are most frequent, followed by overview (or review) and diagnosis.

A more recent study analyzed 695 structured queries from users of McMaster Premium LiteratUre Service Federated Search (MacPLUS FS), an online search system offering access to summary, pre-appraised, and original literature [9]. Overall, queries were found to be based on background questions 56.5% of the time and foreground questions 43.5% of the time, distributed among therapy (30.6%), diagnosis (6.9%), etiology (3.5%), and prognosis (2.5%) questions. There was little difference of distribution among types of queries between residents and faculty physicians.

There have also been some more recent studies that have looked at consumer searching coming from Mayo Clinic. One convened three focus groups and asked consumers about their online searching use and needs [10]. Subjects reported searching, filtering, and comparing information retrieved, with the process stopping due to saturation and fatigue. Another study analyzed search queries submitted through general search engines but leading users into a consumer health information portal from computers and mobile devices [11]. The most common types of searches were on symptoms (32–39%), causes of disease (19–20%), and treatments and drugs (14–16%). Health queries tended to be longer and more specific than general (non-health) queries. Health queries were somewhat more likely to come from mobile devices. Most searches used keywords, although some were also phrased as questions (wh- or yes/no).

Some older Pew reports on consumer searchers of the Web assessed the most common types of searches done by such users [12]. Ranking first was searching for a specific disease or medical condition followed by a certain medical treatment or procedure. A more recent analysis found a wide divergence between what consumers die from, what they search Google for, and what is published in the news media (see Fig. 7.1) [13].

One study of usage logs focused on how medical professionals and laypeople use a variety of search systems [14]. Their analysis found it was possible to distinguish between medical experts and laypeople based on search behavior characteristics, with experts issuing more queries and modifying their queries more often, which the researchers concluded to show they were either more persistent than laypeople or that their information needs were more complex and more difficult to reach. They also found, contrary to some other studies, that diseases were the focus of the largest number of search sessions as opposed to symptoms.

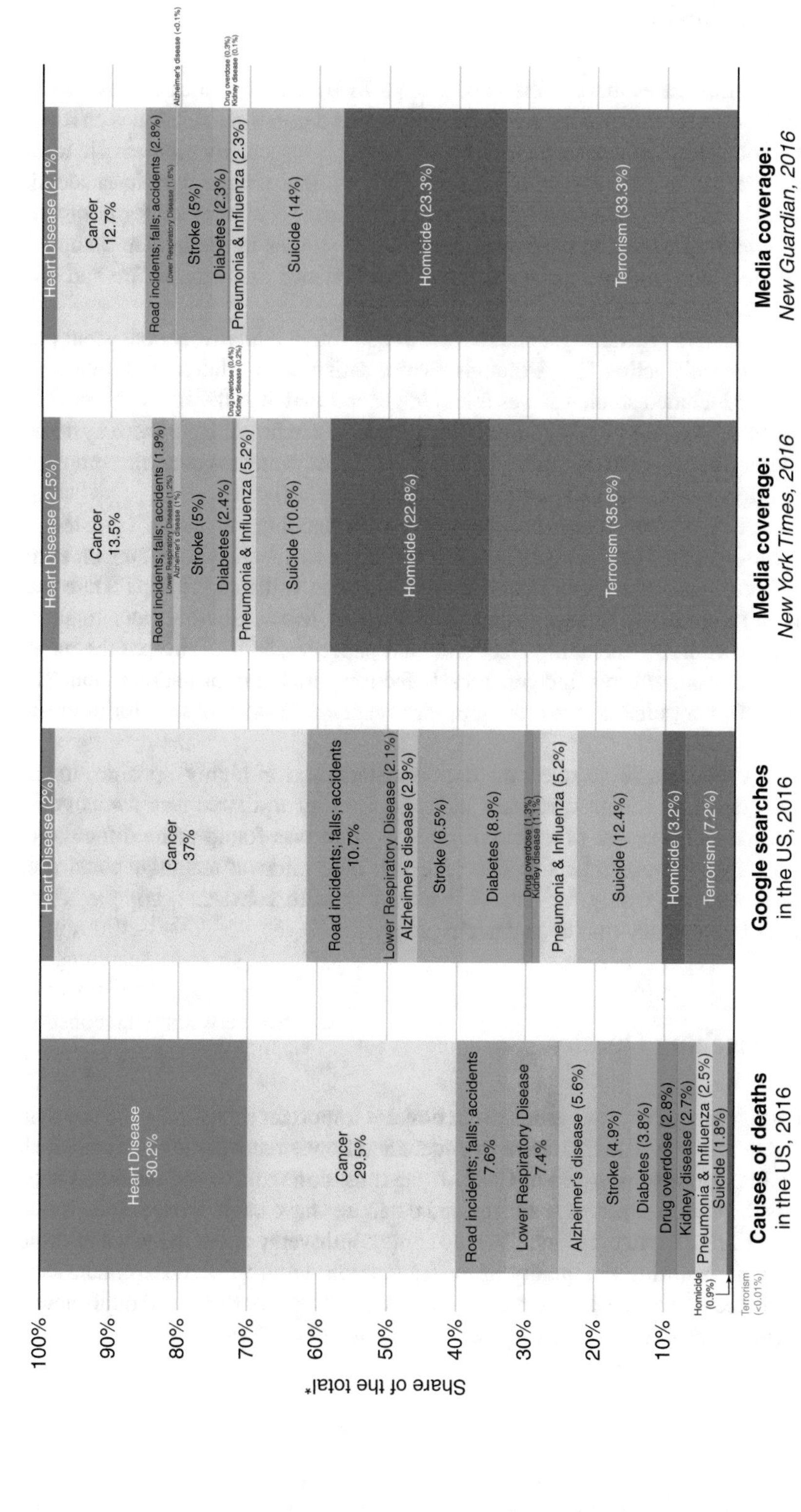

Fig. 7.1 What people die from, search for, and is reported in the news, CC-BY [13]

7.3 User Satisfaction

Another method of evaluating the impact of an IR system is to measure user satisfaction. Of course, researchers are never certain that a user's satisfaction with a system is associated with successful use of it. This may be especially problematic when systems are made available with great fanfare, without charge, and in academic settings where peer pressure might motivate their use. Nonetheless, for computer applications in general, an early meta-analysis of studies in the human-computer interface literature showed a general correlation between user satisfaction and successful use of systems [15].

The Hersh and Hickam systematic review also found a relatively consistent picture for user satisfaction [1]. Although diverse satisfaction-related questions were asked in the included studies, it was found in general that 50–90% of users were satisfied with the system provided them. When users were not satisfied with systems, the general reasons were the time required to use them, concerns over the completeness of information, and difficulties in navigating the software.

There are few new studies of satisfaction with searching or use of knowledge-based resources. In their study of internal medicine residents, Duran-Nelson et al. assessed attributes of search systems that users found valuable [5]. UpToDate was valued for its speed and linkage to the medical record. Most resources were noted for their trustworthiness, including electronic and paper textbooks. Most of the major surveys of consumer users find general satisfaction with the information found. The survey by Taylor noted that searching is very successful (44%) or successful (46%) for all users [16].

Some studies have focused on user satisfaction for highly specific search resources, such as a data discovery index to identify available sets for possible research use [17]. Usage of a data discovery index was found to be difficult for users, leading the researchers to conclude that new retrieval techniques and user interfaces were necessary for dataset exploration, with consistent, complete, and high-quality metadata vital to enable the process.

7.4 Searching Quality

While usage frequency and user satisfaction are important components in any system evaluation, it is also important to understand how effectively users search with IR systems. As was discussed in Chap. 1, the most commonly used measures used to assess the effectiveness of searchers and databases have been the relevance-based measures of recall and precision. Despite some controversy about the value of these measures in capturing the quality of the interaction with the IR system, considerable knowledge about IR systems has been gained by their use, although newer approaches to evaluation have provided additional perspective.

This section of the chapter is divided into two parts: evaluations that focus on performance of the system and those that focus on the user. As with many classifications in this book, the line between the two is occasionally fuzzy. Within each category, the studies are divided into those that focus on different types of usage and categories of resources. While the discussion focuses on health-related studies, a few important non-health evaluation studies are described as well.

7.4.1 System-Oriented Performance Evaluations

System-oriented studies are those that focus on some aspect of the system. That is, even though the searches may have been originated by real users, the research question was oriented toward some aspect of system performance. Many system-oriented retrieval studies were undertaken in the late 1950s and 1960s, but two stand out as setting the historical groundwork for such evaluations. The first of these was actually a series of experiments, commonly called the Cranfield studies, conducted by Cleverdon and associates at the Cranfield College of Aeronautics in England [18]. While these studies were criticized for some of the methods and assumptions used [19], they provided a focus for retrieval performance research and the limitations of such studies. The second study, performed by Lancaster, was the first IR evaluation to provide insight into the success and failure of IR systems [20]. Commissioned by the NLM, this study assessed MEDLINE as it was available at the time: with searches composed by librarians on forms that were mailed to the NLM, which ran the actual searches and returned the results by mail. Preceding the advent of interactive searching, this access to MEDLINE was markedly different than from what is available today.

Lancaster's study assessed a total of 299 searches from 21 different academic, research, and commercial sites in 1966–1967. In his protocol, users first completed a searching form and mailed it to the NLM, where librarians undertook a second, manual search on the topic, using *Index Medicus*. The results of both searches were combined and returned to the searcher by mail. The user then judged the combined set of results for relevance. The results showed that the recall and precision for the computer-based searches were 57.7 and 54.4%, respectively, indicating that the manual searches identified many articles that the computer searches did not (and vice versa). For "value" articles (i.e., only those denoted "highly relevant"), recall and precision for the computer-based searches were 65.2 and 25.7%. Lancaster also performed a failure analysis, which is described below.

System-oriented evaluations of bibliographic databases have focused on issues such as comparability across different databases, comparability of different approaches with the same database, and optimal strategies for finding articles of specific types. A number of early studies were important for that time, but their results probably have little pertinence to modern databases and retrieval systems. Some of these studies measured recall for searches in one or more databases [21,

22]. Other early studies assessed the value of resources (many vastly different now or no longer available) or systems (very different from modern Web-based systems) to answer clinical questions [23–25]. Additional research focused on comparing different systems accessing the same database, such as a study comparing the performance and time required of around a dozen different access routes to MEDLINE available in 1986 and in 1994 [26, 27]. It was found that most systems yielded the same quantity of articles both directly and generally relevant, though there were substantial differences in cost, online time required, and ease of use.

A well-known early study of full-text retrieval was carried out by Blair and Maron [28]. These investigators used the IBM STAIRS system, a full-text, word-based, Boolean system, to evaluate a legal document database of 40,000 documents. Fifty-one searches were posed by two attorneys and carried out by paralegal assistants. Searching was repeated until a satisfactory document collection was obtained for a query. After this, additional searching was done by logical (changing ANDs to ORs) and semantic (adding synonyms) expansion. The attorneys who originated the searches made relevance judgments using a four-point scale: vital, satisfactory, marginally relevant, or not relevant. The results (see Table 7.1) showed that recall was low, far below the 75% level that the attorneys felt was required for optimal searching results.

Full-text searching in early systems was also assessed in the biomedical domain. McKinin et al. compared searching in two full-text medical databases and MEDLINE [29]. They took 89 search requests from a university medical library and performed each one on all three systems. Only documents present in all three were used for recall and precision calculations. The articles were judged for relevance by the original requester on a four-point scale: relevant, probably relevant, probably not relevant, not relevant. Their results found that full-text searching by word-based Boolean methods led to higher recall at the expense of lower precision in comparison to abstract (i.e., MEDLINE) searching (see Table 7.1).

Another line of system-oriented research with bibliographic databases has focused on the ability to retrieve articles of a specific type. This approach to searching is most commonly done in the context of evidence-based medicine (EBM), where the searcher is seeking to identify the "best evidence" for a given question.

Table 7.1 Results of full-text versus abstract searching in some early studies

Database and condition	% Recall	% Precision
Legal document database [28]		
All articles	20	79
Vital and satisfactory articles	25	57
Vital articles only	48	18
Medical databases [29]		
MEDLINE—indexing terms	42	55
MEDLINE—text words	41	62
MEDIS—full text	78	37
CCML—full text	76	37

As noted in Chap. 2, what constitutes the best evidence varies according to the question being asked. In the case of articles about interventions, the most common type of question asked of retrieval systems (see Sect. 7.2), the best evidence comes from a randomized controlled trial (RCT). Early work in this era leveraged the decision to add the publication type field to the MEDLINE database and the development of filters for the Clinical Queries feature of the PubMed system.[2]

More recent work in this area has focused on assessing the value of evidence-based search filters. Lokker et al. assessed the search results of 40 physicians who searched PubMed on the topic of their choice, with their results sent to the standard PubMed interface or to the Clinical Queries filter [30]. For searches on treatment topics, the number of relevant articles retrieved was not significantly different between the two types of search processing, although a higher proportion of articles from the Clinical Queries searches met methodologic criteria and were published in core internal medicine journals. For diagnosis topics, the Clinical Queries results returned more relevant articles and fewer nonrelevant articles. Participants were noted to vary greatly in their search performance.

Another study of search filters focused on Canadian nephrologists searching on aspects of renal therapy [31]. The searchers entered topics into PubMed. Further analysis of the search output was done with filters for best evidence (PubMed Clinical Queries) and pertinence to nephrology, each in a "broad" and "narrow" configuration. Recall and precision were measured for the first 40 articles in the retrieval output as well as all articles retrieved. Consistent with other studies, the total search output had relatively high recall (45.9%) and very low precision (6.0%). The narrow Clinical Queries filter was most effective in raising precision (22.9%), with no additional benefit provided by the narrow subject filter. The nephrology subject filter did, however, raise recall to as high as 54.5%. Also consistent with other research, the search limited to the first 40 articles retrieved had lower baseline recall (12.7%) with little change in precision (5.5%). Similar to the full retrieval, the narrow Clinical Queries filter was most effective in raising precision (to 23.1%) and also in raising recall (to 26.1%).

Some recent studies have found the process of developing search filters more difficult for other types of information needs. Wilczynski et al. reported difficulty creating filters for nursing, which they attributed to the overlapping and expanding scope of practice for nurses compared to other health professionals, and for rehabilitation, due to its broad scope and its practitioners varying definitions of "health and ability" [32]. Likewise, Neilson reported on an unsuccessful attempt to develop a search filter for systematic review methodology articles in the EMBASE bibliographic database [33].

Another comparison of different strategies for retrieval of evidence was carried in a study that looked at retrieval of articles included in systematic reviews [34]. For 30 clinical questions derived from systematic reviews on the topic, searches were composed using a variety of approaches, from publication type limits to the PICO

[2] https://www.ncbi.nlm. nih.gov/books/NBK3827/#pubmedhelp.Clinical_Queries_Filters

framework to the PubMed clinical queries. Output was assessed based on the results from the first 2 pages (40 articles) of the standard PubMed output. Searches using the Clinical Queries narrow filter and the PICO framework had the best overall results, although there was substantial variation across topics.

Additional studies have focused on whether two different systems, PubMed and an EBM-oriented search system, Epistemonikos,[3] could reliably retrieve "gold standard" clinical recommendations [35]. Both systems were able to answer 100 questions with both methods. Of 200 recommendations obtained, 6.5% were classified as potentially misleading and 93.5% as reasonable. Six of the 13 potentially misleading recommendations could have been avoided by the appropriate usage of the Epistemonikos matrix tool or by constructing summary of findings tables.

Some additional system-oriented research has focused on coverage of different databases and other resources. One analysis of different resources for searching concluded that optimal searches for systematic reviews should search at least EMBASE, MEDLINE, Web of Science, and Google Scholar to guarantee adequate and efficient coverage [36]. A study assessing clinical questions posed for the United Kingdom's National Institute for Health and Clinical Excellence (NICE) clinical guidelines found that searching CINAHL did not add value [37]. Another study comparing size estimates of academic search systems found that Google Scholar, with 389 million records, was the most comprehensive academic search engine, well beyond all other commercial systems [38].

Another aspect assessed in system-oriented evaluation focused on timeliness of results, searching for 200 clinical topics in 4 online textbooks [39]. The number of topics for which there was one or more recently published articles found in a continuous online evidence rating system (McMaster PLUS) that had evidence that differed from the textbooks' treatment recommendations varied from 23–60% depending on the product used. They also found that the time of last update for each textbook varied from 170 to 488 days for different products, indicating that even in the era of instant information, timeliness of information is still a challenge.

Some studies have looked at the impact of different approaches to indexing and retrieval. One newer study in this area compared retrieval results searching over the full text of articles versus only titles and abstracts for articles in the Text REtrieval Conference (TREC) 2007 Genomics Track collection [40]. (Most coverage of the TREC Genomics Track is provided in Chap. 8, but this study is presented here because it compares retrieval based on titles and abstracts versus full text.) Two retrieval algorithms (standard Lucene and BM25) and three retrieval measures (mean average precision, precision at 20 retrieved, and IP@R50) were assessed, with results showing that searching the full text outperformed searching titles and abstracts, especially when the former used spans within the text as retrieval units as opposed to the entire document.

Finally, an additional study looked at the volatility of the output of Web search engines, which change constantly due to such factors as their discovery of new

[3] https://www.epistemonikos.org/

content, changes to output ranking, and even differences between content retrieved through the search interface versus use of application programming interface (API) options [41]. Analyzing the Microsoft Bing search engine, this study found that on average over 64 days, search engine results changed by about 10% every 2 days. For any given set of results, normalized discounted cumulative gain (NDCG) over the top ten results varied by about 20%.

7.4.2 User-Oriented Performance Evaluations

Studies assessing the ability of users with IR systems have looked at a variety of measures to define performance. A great many have focused on the retrieval of relevant documents, usually as measured by recall and precision, although these measures have been criticized for being less pertinent to user success (see Chap. 1). Other studies have attempted to measure how well users were able to complete a prescribed task, such as answering clinical questions.

This section of the chapter groups studies into early studies, those with a focus on question-answering, studies assessing other clinician searching, and those with a focus on consumer searching.

7.4.2.1 Early User-Oriented Studies

In summarizing the research from 1960 to 1980 on user-oriented evaluation, Fenichel noted several consistent findings across studies that may still be pertinent today [42]:

1. There was a correlation between search success, measured in terms of recall, and "search effort," which included number of commands used and time taken.
2. There was considerable variation across users, even with the same system and database. Even experienced users made mistakes that affected searching performance.
3. New users could learn to perform good searches after minimal training.
4. The major problems were related more to the search strategy than to the mechanics of using the system. Users made few errors related to use of the command language.

The main approach to user-oriented evaluation has been through the use of relevance-based measures. One of the original studies measuring searching performance in clinical settings was performed by Haynes et al. [43]. This study also compared the capabilities of librarian and clinician searchers. In this study, 78 searches were randomly chosen for replication by both a clinician experienced in searching and a medical librarian. During this study, each original ("novice") user had been required to enter a brief statement of information need before entering the search program. This statement was given to the experienced clinician and librarian for searching on MEDLINE. All the retrievals for each search were given to a subject domain expert, blinded with respect to which searcher retrieved which reference. Recall and precision were calculated for each query and averaged. The results (Table 7.2) showed that the experienced clinicians and librarians achieved comparable recall, although the librarians had statistically significantly better precision. The novice clinician searchers had lower recall and precision than either of the other groups. This study also assessed user satisfaction of the novice searchers, who despite their recall and precision results said that they were satisfied with their search outcomes. The investigators did not assess whether the novices obtained enough relevant articles to answer their questions or whether they would have found additional value with the ones that were missed.

A follow-up study yielded some additional insights about the searchers [44]. Different searchers tended to use different strategies on a given topic. The different approaches replicated a finding known from other searching studies in the past, namely, the lack of overlap across searchers of overall retrieved citations as well as relevant ones. Figure 7.2 shows overlap diagrams, pointing out that the majority of both retrieved documents and relevant documents were retrieved by one searcher only. Thus, even though the novice searchers had lower recall, they did obtain a great many relevant citations not retrieved by the two expert searchers. Furthermore, fewer than 4% of all the relevant citations were retrieved by all three searchers. Despite the widely divergent search strategies and retrieval sets,

Table 7.2 Results from an early study comparing Grateful Med users, adapted from [43]

	Results (%)	
Users	Recall	Precision
Novice clinicians	27	38
Experienced clinicians	48	49
Medical librarians	49	58

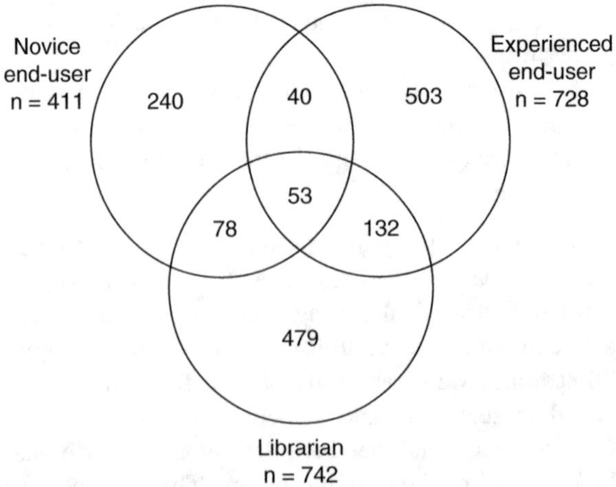

Fig. 7.2 Overlap of relevant articles retrieved by three MEDLINE searchers, adapted from [44]

overall recall and precision were quite similar among the three classes of users. A later study by this group found that relatively simple training of novice searchers could make them as effective as experts [45].

Another large-scale attempt to assess recall and precision in clinician searchers was carried out by Hersh and Hickam [46]. They not only assessed the capability of expert versus novice searchers but also compared the latter with access to MEDLINE via a Boolean versus natural language system. The latter system was Knowledge Finder (KF; Aires Systems), which represented one of the first commercial implementations of that approach for medical content. Hersh and Hickam also compared the performance of the experienced searchers using the full MEDLINE feature set and just text words from the title, abstract, and MeSH heading fields. The KF system used in this study was a CD-ROM version containing MEDLINE references from 270 core primary care journals covering a period of 5 years. As with Haynes et al., relevance was assessed by clinicians blinded to the searcher.

One challenge with the results of this study (and in fact any study comparing Boolean and natural language searching) was the large retrieval set obtained by using KF. While advocates of this approach argue that a large output of relevance-ranked documents allows the searcher to choose their own recall and precision (i.e., there are usually more relevant documents near the top of the list, so the further one looks down the retrieval list, the more likely it is that recall will increase and precision will decrease), direct comparison of recall and precision with sets generated from Boolean retrieval is difficult. As seen in Table 7.3, the clinicians who were novices were able to retrieve much higher recall than any of the expert searchers, although they paid a price in precision (and most likely would not look at all 100 references on the retrieval list anyway). To give a comparison of the novice searchers with retrieval at a level more comparable to that of the experienced searchers, a second set of recall and precision values was calculated with KF's default retrieval lowered to 15, the average size of Boolean retrieval sets. The levels of recall and precision were still comparable among all groups of expert searchers, with no statistically significant differences. Thus, the approach used by KF clearly showed the potential to be of value to searchers, certainly novices.

Overlap among retrieval of relevant articles was also assessed, with results similar to those of Haynes et al. As shown in Table 7.4, over half of all relevant references were retrieved by only one of the five searchers, while another quarter were retrieved by two searchers. Well under 10% of relevant references were retrieved by four or five searchers.

This study also compared the searching performance of experienced clinician and librarian searchers. It showed that the difference between both these groups and inexperienced clinician searchers was small and not statistically significant. Related to this finding, there appeared to be no benefit associated with the use of advanced MEDLINE searching features, since both experienced clinicians and librarians achieved comparable recall and precision using text-word searching only. In fact, experienced physicians showed a trend toward better recall when they used text words. There was a statistically significant difference for librarians using

Table 7.3 Comparison of Knowledge Finder and ELHILL users, adapted from [46]

		Results definitely relevant only (%)		Results definitely/ possibly relevant (%)	
Group	Retrieved	Recall	Precision	Recall	Precision
Novice physicians, using KF	88.8	68.2	14.7	72.5	30.8
Novice physicians, KF top 15	14.6	31.2	24.8	25.5	43.8
Librarians, full MEDLINE	18.0	37.1	36.1	30.8	59.4
Librarians, text words only	17.0	31.5	31.9	27.0	50.3
Experienced physicians, full MEDLINE	10.9	26.6	34.9	19.8	55.2
Experienced physicians, text words only	14.8	30.6	31.4	24.1	48.4

Table 7.4 Overlap among relevant references retrieval by up to five users, adapted from [46]

Number of searchers	Relevant references retrieved
1	957 (53.2%)
2	474 (26.4%)
3	190 (10.6%)
4	99 (5.5%)
5	42 (2.3%)

MEDLINE features over clinicians using MEDLINE features, indicating that these features are of most benefit to librarians.

Another limitation of these studies was the unrealistic situation in which the librarian searcher was assessed. As most librarians will note, their work involves more than just the search itself. An equally important aspect is the interview with the user, during which the information needs are explicitly gleaned. Indeed, the study by Saracevic and Kantor, discussed shortly, notes that performing this interview or having access to it doubles the intermediary searcher's recall [47]. However, most of these studies (and their searches) took place in clinical settings, where detailed interviews by librarians are impractical. Thus it was valid to compare the end user and the librarian in these settings, if only to use the latter as a point of reference for searching quality.

A number of other studies have focused on recall and precision obtained by clinicians using different IR systems or approaches. Hersh and Hickam evaluated medical students searching an online version of the textbook, *Scientific American Medicine*, with a Boolean or natural language interface (as well as an experimental system whose results are discussed in Chap. 8) [48]. Twenty-one students searched on 10 queries, which were randomly allocated for each from the 106 queries of the same researchers' study described earlier [46]. The users obtained comparable recall (75.3 vs. 70.6%, not statistically significant) and precision (14.8 vs. 18.9%, not statistically significant) for the natural language interface. This study also analyzed the relationship between the number of relevant documents and recall, finding that a larger number of relevant documents led, on the average, to users obtaining a lower level of recall.

7.4.2.2 User Studies Focused on Answering Questions

One approach to system-oriented evaluation has been to focus on the use of "task-oriented measures," in particular how well users can find the answers to questions, which is of course a common use of IR systems. As mentioned at the end of Chap. 1, a number of investigators looked for alternatives to relevance-based measures for measuring the quality of IR system performance. One approach has been to give users tasks, such as answering a question. Egan et al. piloted this approach with a statistics textbook, finding significant performance differences with changes in the user interface [49]. Mynatt et al. used a similar approach to assess the ability of college students to find answers to questions in an online encyclopedia [50].

Hersh and colleagues carried out a number of studies assessing the ability of IR systems to help students and clinicians answer clinical questions. The rationale for these studies was that the usual goal of using an IR system is to find an answer to a question. While the user must obviously find relevant documents to answer that question, the quantity of such documents is less important than whether the question is successfully answered. In fact, recall and precision can be placed among the many factors that may be associated with ability to complete the task successfully. Other researchers have adopted variations of this methodology.

The first study by Hersh et al. using the task-oriented approach compared Boolean versus natural language searching in the textbook, *Scientific American Medicine* [51]. Thirteen medical students were asked to answer 10 short-answer questions and rate their confidence in their answers. The students were then randomized to one or the other interface and asked to search on the five questions for which they had rated confidence the lowest. The study showed that both groups had low correct rates before searching (average 1.7 correct out of 10) but were mostly able to answer the questions with searching (average 4.0 out of 5). There was no difference in ability to answer questions with one interface or the other. Most answers were found on the first search to the textbook. For the questions that were incorrectly answered, the document with the correct answer was actually retrieved by the user two-thirds of the time and viewed more than half the time.

Another study compared Boolean and natural language searching of MEDLINE with two commercial products, CD Plus (now Ovid) and KF [52]. These systems represented the ends of the spectrum in terms of using Boolean searching on human-indexed thesaurus terms (CDP) versus natural language searching on words in the title, abstract, and indexing terms (KF). Sixteen medical students were recruited and randomized to 1 of the 2 systems and given 3 yes/no clinical questions to answer. The students were able to use each system successfully, answering 37.5% correct before searching and 85.4% correct after searching. There were no significant differences between the systems in time taken, relevant articles retrieved, or user satisfaction. This study demonstrated that both types of system can be used equally well with minimal training.

Further research by this group expanded the analysis to include nurse practitioner (NP) students and a myriad of factors that could influence successful use of the IR system. Most of the results concerning the latter are presented in Sect. 7.5.

However, the searching success rates are noted here. Each of these studies used only one IR system, the Ovid system used to search MEDLINE that also had links to about 80 full-text journals. The first study focused solely on NP students and used multiple-choice questions from the *Medical Knowledge Self-Assessment Program* (MKSAP, American College of Physicians, Philadelphia) [53]. Each of the 24 subjects answered 3 out of the 8 questions used. Before searching, 25 of the 72 questions (34.7%) were answered correctly, and after searching the total of correct responses increased to 42 out of 72 (58.3%). The second study assessed both medical and NP students, with 29 subjects answering 3 questions each out of a group of 30 [54]. The questions, which were phrased in a short-answer format, were obtained from three sources: MKSAP, the Cochrane Database of Systematic Reviews, and a set expressed in actual clinical practice [55]. The main success-related results showed that medical students scored higher before and after searching but that both groups improved their scores by the same amount.

In the final study, which was probably the largest study of medical searchers to date at the time, 66 medical and NP students searched 5 questions each [56]. This study used a multiple-choice format for answering questions that also included a judgment about the evidence for the answer. Subjects were asked to choose from one of three answers:

- Yes, with adequate evidence
- Insufficient evidence to answer question
- No, with adequate evidence

Table 7.5 shows the results from this study and several studies we will subsequently discuss that applied this methodology. As can be seen in the results in the table from this study, both groups achieved a pre-searching correctness on questions about equal to chance (32.3% for medical students and 31.7% for NP students). However, medical students improved their correctness with searching (to 51.6%), whereas NP students hardly did at all (to 34.7%). Table 7.5 shows that NP students changed with searching from incorrect to correct answers as often as they did from correct to incorrect. These results were further assessed to determine whether NP students had trouble answering questions or judging evidence (unpublished data). To assess this, a two-by-two contingency table was constructed that compared designating the evidence correctly (i.e., selecting yes or no when the answer was yes or no and selecting indeterminate when the answer was indeterminate) and incorrectly (i.e., selecting yes or no when the answer was indeterminate and selecting indeterminate when the answer was yes or no). As seen in Table 7.6, NP students had a higher rate of incorrectly judging the evidence. Thus, since medical and NP students had virtually identical rates of judging the evidence correct when answering the question incorrectly, the major difference with respect to questions answered incorrectly between the groups was incorrect judgment of evidence.

Other researchers adapted variants of this study methodology. Westbrook et al. used clinical scenarios with 44 physicians and 31 clinical nurse consultants (CNCs)

Table 7.5 Cross-tabulation of number and percentage of answers correct vs. incorrect before and after searching for various subjects in different studies using methodology developed by [56]

	Pre-searching		Post-searching	
			Incorrect	Correct
Hersh et al. [56]	Incorrect	All	133 (41%)	87 (27%)
		Medical	81 (36%)	70 (31%)
		NP	52 (52%)	17 (17%)
	Correct	All	41 (13%)	63 (19%)
		Medical	27 (12%)	45 (20%)
		NP	14 (14%)	18 (18%)
McKibbon and Fridsma [57]	Incorrect	All	22 (48%)	5 (11%)
	Correct	All	6 (13%)	13 (28%)
Westbrook et al. [58]	Incorrect	All	220 (39%)	184 (33%)
		Hospital	66 (35%)	61 (33%)
		FP	47 (35%)	34 (25%)
		CNC	107 (45%)	89 (38%)
	Correct	All	39 (7%)	114 (20%)
		Hospital	17 (9%)	43 (23%)
		FP	8 (6%)	45 (34%)
		CNC	14 (6%)	26 (11%)
Van Der Vegt et al. [59]	Incorrect	All	578 (35%)	513 (31%)
		High time pressure	260 (45%)	142 (25%)
		Med time pressure	157 (33%)	150 (32%)
		Low time pressure	161 (27%)	221 (37%)
	Correct	All	189 (11%)	373 (23%)
		High time pressure	82 (14%)	96 (17%)
		Med time pressure	57 (12%)	111 (23%)
		Low time pressure	50 (8%)	166 (28%)

Table 7.6 Cross-tabulation of number and percentage of evidence judgments correct vs. incorrect before and after searching for all (A), medical (M), and NP (N) students. Percentages represent percent correct within each group of students, adapted from [56]

Answer		
Evidence	Incorrect	Correct
Incorrect	138 (42.6%)	0%
A	84 (37.7%)	0%
M	54 (53.5%)	0%
N		
Correct	36 (11.1%)	150 (46.3%)
A	24 (10.8%)	115 (51.6%)
M	12 (11.9%)	35 (34.7%)
N		

to assess an online evidence retrieval system [60]. They assessed practicing physicians and consulting nurses using a suite on full-text evidence-based resources in addition to MEDLINE. As seen in Table 7.5, Westbrook et al. found that physicians started with a higher pre-searching rate of correctness on the clinical tasks (37% vs. 18%) but that the retrieval system brought both groups up to the same level (50%). They also found that confidence in answers was likely to be higher for correct vs. incorrect answers, although over half of those who had persistently incorrect answers (before and after searching) were likely to have confidence in their answers. In addition, those who answered the scenario incorrectly initially had the same confidence in their answer after searching whether it was correct or incorrect. Both the Hersh et al. and the Westbrook et al. studies demonstrate that retrieval systems, and the confidence they engender, are far from perfect.

McKibbon and Fridsma used the same questions as Hersh et al. and obtained somewhat similar results [57]. As shown in Table 7.5, practicing clinicians were given the questions and allowed to search all of their "usual" resources. The results found that the addition of the search system did not improve their answers, as 39.1% of questions were answered correctly before searching and 42.1% were answered correctly after searching. Users went from incorrect to correct answers with searching at the same frequency of going from correct to incorrect answers. The researchers found great variation in the ability of different resources to answer questions, with Google/Web and the Cochrane Database more likely to lead to correct answers and PubMed, UpToDate, and InfoPOEMS more likely to lead to incorrect answers.

More recently, Van der Vegt et al. performed a study using a similar methodology and a search system containing the TREC 2014–2015 Clinical Decision Support (CDS) Track open-access subset of PubMed Central [59, 61]. An additional goal of the study aimed to understand the impact of realistic time pressures on clinicians by varying the search time available to find clinical answers and randomizing subjects to carrying out their searching under low (9 min), medium (6 min), and high (3 min) time pressure. They also assessed the impact of improvements in search system effectiveness on the same clinical decisions. A total of 85 final-year medical students, 16 physicians, and 8 nurses searched on 16 questions based on clinical scenarios. Six of the questions were adapted from the Westbrook et al. [60], four from Hersh et al. [56], three from the TREC 2015 CDS Track [62], and three developed by a physician de novo. Identical to the previous studies, users gave answers of yes, no, or conflicting evidence.

Similar to the previous studies and seen in Table 7.5, Van der Vegt et al. found a near-random rate of correctness before searching. Also comparable to the earlier studies, searching led to a 54% rate of correct answering, with 11% of searches going from the answer correct to incorrect after searching. Searching done under higher time pressure had higher rates of going from correct to incorrect answering: 14% for high time pressure, 12% for medium time pressure, and 8% for low time pressure. Higher time pressure was also associated with decreased confidence by the searcher in the answer, increased perceived difficulty of the question, and higher overall stress.

The systems had also been further randomized to use different output of the ranking [63]. They compared an adaptation of the best-performing approach of the TREC 2015 CDS Track and showed a 33–84% improvement in batch searching over standard BM25 ranking [62]. In the hands by real searchers, the differences in ranking output were much smaller, on the order of 9%. Furthermore, this difference in systems had no impact on correctness of answers by users. Further analysis found that users providing incorrect answers were more likely to look at fewer "turning point" documents and to interpret such documents incorrectly.

7.4.2.3 Other User-Oriented Studies of Clinicians

Several studies have looked at attributes of point-of-care (POC) information resources such as quality, timeliness, and comprehensiveness. Ahmadi et al. compared four resources touted as evidence-based for rate of answer retrieval and mean time taken to obtain it with 112 residents in training, each of whom answered 3 of 24 questions [64]. The resources that were most successful in answering questions also tended to have shortest time to answer (some no longer produced), i.e., UpToDate (86% answered, 14.6 min to answer), First Consult (69%, 15.9 min), ACP PIER (49%, 17.3 min), and Essential Evidence (45%, 16.3 min). The differences were statistically significant. Prorok et al. performed a similar study, also noting differences in timeliness, breadth, and quality, with Dynamed and UpToDate ranking highest overall [65].

A survey of European physicians found that all were frequent users of Internet medical resources [66]. The most common resources for which they reported use were general search engines (e.g., Google), research databases (e.g., PubMed), Wikipedia, and specialty society resources. Academic physicians and those in training made higher use of research databases and Wikipedia, while practicing physicians made more use of specialty society sites and those targeted to their practice specialty. The use of resources requiring subscription fees (e.g., UpToDate) was relatively low.

Kim et al. looked at the ability of internal medicine interns to answer questions starting from Google vs. an evidence-based summary resource developed by a local medical library [67]. Ten questions were given to each subject, with each participant randomized to start in either Google or the summary resource for half of the questions. Answers were found for 82% of the questions administered, with no difference between groups in correct answers (58–62% correct) and time taken (136–139 sec). While those starting in the summary resource mostly found answers in resources that were part of the summary system 93% of the time, those starting with Google found answers in commercial medical portals (25.7%), hospital Web sites (12.6%), Wikipedia (12.0%), US government Web sites (9.4%), PubMed (9.4%), evidence-based summary resources (9.4%), and others (18%).

A similar study compared Google, Ovid, PubMed, and UpToDate for answering clinical questions among trainees and attending physicians in anesthesiology and critical care medicine [68]. Users were allowed to select which tool to use for a first set of four questions to answer, while 1–3 weeks later they were randomized to only a single tool to answer another set of eight questions. For the first set of questions, users most commonly selected Google (45%), followed by UpToDate (26%), PubMed (25%), and Ovid (4.4%). The rate of answering questions correctly in the first set was highest for UpToDate (70%), followed by Google (60%), Ovid (50%), and PubMed (38%). The time taken to answer these questions was lowest for UpToDate (3.3 min), followed by Google (3.8 min), PubMed (4.4 min), and Ovid (4.6 min). In the second set of questions, the correct answer was most likely to be obtained by UpToDate (69%), followed by PubMed (62%), Google (57%), and Ovid (38%). Subjects randomized a new tool generally fared comparably, with the exception of those randomized from another tool to Ovid.

Another study compared searching UpToDate and PubMed Clinical Queries at the conclusion of a course for 44 medical residents in an information mastery course [69]. Subjects were randomized to one system for two questions and then the other system for another two questions. The correct answer was retrieved 76% of the time with UpToDate versus only 45% of the time with PubMed Clinical Queries. Median time to answer the question was less for UpToDate (17 min) than PubMed Clinical Queries (29 min). User satisfaction was higher with UpToDate.

The study described above of users of MacPLUS FS also assessed query structure and information accessed [9]. Foreground queries tended to have more terms than background queries, with a median of four vs. two terms, respectively. Queries were assessed for how often they included the population, intervention, comparator, and outcome (PICO) elements for EBM questions. Of background queries, 71.2% included a population term, 24.7% an intervention term, 1.0% an etiology term, 6.1% a diagnostic term, and 2.5% an outcome term. Foreground queries contained 74.2% with a population term, 73.5% with an intervention term, 21.5% an outcome term, 16.2% a diagnostic term, and 7.6% an etiology term. Overall, about 51.5% of information accessed was from summary sources, with 24.4% pre-appraised literature and 24.1% original research. Summary information was more likely to be accessed by faculty and less by residents, with original research accessed more by the latter.

Some user evaluation studies have focused on specific resources. Markonis et al. performed a user-oriented evaluation of a text- and content-based medical image retrieval system [70]. They assessed the performance of 16 radiologists searching for individual images and for patient cases containing images relevant to the search topic. The success rates in finding relevant information were on average 87% and 78% for image and case retrieval tasks, respectively. The average time for a successful search was less than 3 min in both cases. Users felt quickly comfortable with the novel techniques and tools (after 5 to 15 min), such as content-based image retrieval and relevance feedback. User satisfaction measures showed a very positive attitude toward the system's functionalities.

Another system-specific study focused on use of Wikipedia by medical students [71]. Students assigned to search different resources had comparable pre-search knowledge (43.9–45.5% correct on a multiple-choice test). Wikipedia users had slightly higher post-search knowledge (61.0%) than those using UpToDate (55.3%, not statistically significant) or an online textbook (49.2%, statistically significant from Wikipedia). Access to hyperlinks, search functions, and open-source editing were rated significantly higher for Wikipedia than the other resources.

Other studies have focused on search system features that are used (or not used). Lau et al. compared the search behaviors of resource-based vs. task-based systems, with the former allowing the user to select one of six information resources (e.g., PubMed, a pharmaceutical database, evidence-based guidelines, etc.) and the latter allowing the user to select one of six tasks (e.g., diagnosis, therapy, drug information, etc.) [72]. A total of 44 physicians and 31 senior nurse consultants were randomized to 1 approach or the other. Clinicians randomized to the resource-based system tended to use a "breadth-first" strategy of entering the same query into different databases, whereas those randomized to the task-based system tended to use a "depth-first" strategy of entering and refining queries into single resources.

7.4.2.4 User-Oriented Studies of Consumers

A number of user-oriented evaluation studies have focused on consumers. One study applied a variant of the task-oriented approach to healthcare consumers searching the Web [73]. This study of 17 users given health questions to search on and found an answer was successfully obtained in 4 to 5 min. Although participants were aware of quality criteria for health-related Web sites (e.g., source, professional design, scientific language), they did not appear to apply these criteria when actually visiting sites.

Lau et al. found that use of a consumer-oriented medical search system that included PubMed, MedlinePlus, and other resources by college undergraduates led to answers being correct at a higher rate after searching (82.0%) than before searching (61.2%) [74, 75]. Providing a feedback summary from prior searches boosted the success rate of using the system even higher, to 85.3%. Confidence of user answers was not found to be highly associated with correctness of the answer, although confidence was likely to increase for those provided with feedback from other searchers on the same topic.

Van Deursen assessed a variety of computer-related and content-related skills from randomly selected subjects in the Netherlands [76]. Older age and lower educational level were associated with reduced skills, including use of search engines. While younger subjects were more likely to have better computer and searching skills than older subjects, they were more likely to use nonrelevant search results and unreliable sources in answering health-related questions. This latter phenomenon has also been seen outside the health domain among the "millennial" generation, sometimes referred to as "digital natives" [77].

Another line of consumer-oriented health searching research has focused on retrieval of "health cards," which are provided when the Google search engine detects a search on a health topic. An initial study assessed 48 searchers performing 8 tasks each, with half randomized to an interface with the health cards and half without [78]. For users shown health cards, they selected to look at them in their results about half the time, and for the four searches done with them in the results, 72% of searchers clicked on the cards for at least one of their searches. Correctness of the evidence retrieved was not associated with the health cards being retrieved, nor was the time taken to complete the search task different when they were retrieved. However, searchers were more satisfied with their results when a health card was retrieved.

An additional study added the retrieval of up to 4 health cards per query and assessed 64 users in their ability to discern a self-diagnosis and rate its urgency for seeking medical care for 8 tasks each [79]. Participants were more likely to get the diagnosis correct when a health card was retrieved and most likely to get it correct when a single correct card was retrieved. They misestimated the rate of urgency of seeking care about half the time, which was unchanged whether or not one or more health cards were retrieved.

7.5 Factors Associated with Success or Failure

Although determining how well users can perform with IR systems is important, additional analysis focusing on why they succeed or fail is important, not only in figuring out how to best deploy such systems but also for the sake of determining how to improve them. This section focuses on two related groups of analyses. In the first group are studies attempting to determine the factors associated with successful use of systems, while the second group consists of analyses of why users fail to obtain optimal results.

7.5.1 Predictors of Success

One of the earliest and most comprehensive analyses of predictors of success was from outside the healthcare domain, but its results set the stage for further work. Saracevic et al. recruited 40 information seekers, each of whom submitted a question to a search intermediary, underwent a taped interview with a reference librarian to describe his or her problem and intended use of the information, and evaluated the retrieved items for relevance as well as the search in general [47, 80, 81]. Each question was searched by nine intermediaries. Up to 150 retrieved items were returned to the users, who rated them as relevant, partially relevant, or not relevant to their information need.

All results were framed in the context of the odds that retrieved items would be judged relevant by the users. Some of the factors that led to statistically significantly higher odds of documents being judged relevant were a well-defined problem posed by a user who was very certain the answer would be found, searches limited to answers in English and requiring less time to complete, questions that were initially not clear or specific but were complex and had many presupposed concepts, and answers that had high utility for the user, as measured by benefits in time, money, or problem resolution. Another finding of interest in this study was a low overlap in search terms used (27%) and items retrieved (17%) for a given question, a finding similar to that of McKibbon et al. for healthcare searchers [44]. However, Saracevic and Kantor did determine that the more searchers a document was retrieved by, the more likely that document was to be judged relevant.

The most comprehensive analysis of factors relating to searching success in biomedicine was carried out by Hersh and colleagues [56]. They developed a comprehensive model of factors that might influence the success of searching. Successful use of the IR system, defined in the study to be the task of successfully answering the clinical question, was the dependent (outcome) variable. The elements of the model made up the independent (predictor) variables and were grouped in several different categories. The first consisted of identifiers for the user and question searched, as well as the order of the question. The next category covered demographic variables, some of which were generic (e.g., age and sex), while others were specific to the study population (e.g., school enrolled and years worked as a nurse). There were also categories for computer experience, computer attitudes, and searching experience. The searching experience factors included not only general amounts of literature and Web searching but also specific knowledge of and experience with advanced features of MEDLINE.

The model also included assessment of cognitive factors, since these had been shown to be associated with searching performance not only in the studies of Saracevic et al. cited earlier but in others as well. Three factors were included because they had been found to be associated with successful use of computer systems in general or retrieval systems specifically. The cognitive traits were assessed by validated instruments from the Educational Testing Service (ETS) Kit of Cognitive Factors [82]. The three factors were:

- Spatial visualization—ability to visualize spatial relationships among objects, measured by the *Paper Folding Test*
- Logical reasoning—ability to reason from premise to conclusion, measured by the *Nonsense Syllogisms Test*
- Verbal reasoning—ability to understand vocabulary, measured by the *Advanced Vocabulary Test I* to assess verbal reasoning

Other categories in the model included intermediate search results (i.e., results of searching performance that ultimately influence the user's ability to successfully answer the question). One of these was search mechanics, such as the time taken, the number of Boolean sets used in the searching process, the number of articles retrieved in the "terminal" set, and the number of MEDLINE references and full-text articles viewed by the user. Another intermediate category was user satisfaction, which was measured with the Questionnaire for User Interface Satisfaction (QUIS) 5.0 instrument that measured user satisfaction with a computer system, providing a score from zero (poor) to nine (excellent) on a variety of user preferences [83]. The overall user satisfaction is determined by averaging the scores of all the preferences.

The next group of factors addressed the relevance of the retrieval set. These measures, including recall and precision, were considered to be intermediate outcome measures relative to the ultimate outcome measure of successfully answering the question. This is in distinction to the many retrieval studies that assess recall and precision as the final outcome measures. The final category of factors contains variables associated with the answer, such as the answer itself, the EBM type, whether the user gave the correct answer before or after searching, and the user's certainty of the answer.

As noted in Sect. 7.4, 66 searchers, 45 medical students, and 21 NP students, performed 5 searches each. There were 324 searches analyzed. Several differences between medical and NP students were seen. The use of computers and use of productivity software were higher for NP students, but searching experience was higher for medical students. Medical students also had higher self-rating of knowledge and experience with advanced MEDLINE features. The NP students tended to be older, and all were female (whereas only half the medical students were female). Medical students also had higher scores on the three cognitive tests. In searching, medical students tended to have higher numbers of sets but lower numbers of references viewed. They also had a higher level of satisfaction with the IR system, as measured by QUIS.

Further analysis determined the factors associated with successful searching, as defined by the outcome variable of correct answer after searching. The final model showed that knowing the correct answer before searching, score on the *Paper Folding Test*, past usage of advanced MEDLINE features, and EBM question type were statistically significantly different. For the EBM question type, questions of prognosis had the highest likelihood of being answered correctly, followed by questions of therapy, diagnosis, and harm. The analysis also found that the *Paper Folding Test* and searcher type (medical vs. NP student) demonstrated multicollinearity; that is, they were very highly correlated, and once one was in the model, the other did not provide any additional statistical significance. Next, a similar analysis was done to find the best model using the 220 searches when the subject did not have the right answer before the MEDLINE search. The final best model was very similar to the model for all questions, with pre-searching correctness obviously excluded. Again, the *Paper Folding Test* and searcher type demonstrated high multicollinearity.

One surprising finding was that there was virtually no difference in recall and precision between medical and NP students. Likewise, there was no difference in recall and precision between questions that were answered correctly and incorrectly. Other variables having no association with successful searching included time taken to complete the question and certainty that the searcher had in their answer.

A number of conclusions were drawn from this study. First, users spent an average of more than 30 min conducting literature searches and were successful at correctly answering questions less than half the time. Whereas medical students were able to use the IR system to improve question-answering, NP students were led astray by the system as often as they were helped by it. The study also found that experience in searching MEDLINE and spatial visualization ability were associated with being successful in answering questions. A final finding was that the often-studied measures of recall and precision were virtually identical between medical and NP students and had no association with correct answering of questions. Possible reasons for the limited success of question-answering include everything from inadequate training to an inappropriate database (i.e., a large bibliographic database instead of more concise, synthesized references) to problems with the retrieval system to difficulties in judging evidence.

Magrabi et al. looked at the factors that make IR systems likely to be used by clinicians [84]. In a survey of 227 Australian general practitioners with access to the Quick Clinical system described earlier, they found that few factors were associated with usage, including age, level of clinical training, experience, or hours worked. They did find, however, that female clinicians were slightly more likely to search than male physicians. Not surprisingly, those who believed the system improved care were more likely to use it.

Another study using the collection from the TREC Genomics Track assessed the value of MeSH terms for different types of searchers [85]. The researchers recruited four types of searchers:

- Search Novice (SN)—undergraduates with no formal search training or advanced knowledge in biomedicine
- Domain Expert (DE)—biomedical graduate students
- Search Expert (SE)—library and information science graduate students
- Medical Librarian (ML)

The searchers used a digital library system to search on 20 of the 50 topics from the original test collection (see Table 7.7). Searchers assigned to search with MeSH were provided access to a MeSH browser. As with other studies, recall and precision were relatively close across different groups. MeSH terms had little impact upon recall in the four groups, but they were found to substantially increase precision in search novices (SN and DE) and decrease it in search experts (SE and ML) (recall and precision with MeSH; without MeSH). User characteristics that improved precision were number of undergraduate and graduate biology courses for SN and DE, respectively. User characteristics associated with improved recall included having had online search courses and MeSH use experience. Other factors having no association with search results included gender, native language, age, or experience or frequency with database searching.

Table 7.7 Recall and precision results for various academic-environment searchers, adapted from [85]

	Overall		With MeSH		Without MeSH	
Group	Recall	Precision	Recall	Precision	Recall	Precision
Search novice (SN)	0.21	0.29	0.21	0.36	0.20	0.23
Domain expert (DE)	0.15	0.40	0.15	0.29	0.15	0.51
Search expert (SE)	0.15	0.30	0.13	0.38	0.16	0.21
Medical librarian (ML)	0.23	0.35	0.24	0.42	0.22	0.28

Another study carried out a detailed analysis of search by four clinicians, who were provided queries and performed relevance assessments [86]. Among the study findings were that query formulation had more impact on retrieval effectiveness than particular retrieval systems used. The most effective queries were short, ad hoc keyword queries. Different clinicians were observed to consistently adopt specific query formulation strategies. The most effective searchers were found to be those who inferred novel keywords most likely to appear in relevant documents.

A study of consumers assessed the extent to which users can be influenced by search engine results [87]. In a controlled laboratory study, the researchers biased search results toward correct or incorrect information for ten different medical treatments. They found that search engine results can significantly influence people both positively and negatively. Study participants made more incorrect decisions when they interacted with search results biased toward incorrect information than when they had no interaction with search results at all. Some nonrelevant information is incorrect and potentially harmful when people use it to make decisions that may negatively impact their lives.

7.5.2 *Analysis of Failure*

The attempt to determine why users do not obtain optimal results with IR systems is called *failure analysis*. A number of such analyses have been carried out over the years. In his original MEDLINE study, Lancaster performed a detailed failure analysis, which he divided into recall (failure to retrieve a relevant article) and precision (retrieval of nonrelevant article) failures [20]. For both types of failure, Lancaster cataloged problems related to indexing (i.e., problems with the indexing language or assignment of its terms) and retrieval (i.e., problems with search strategy). The particular problems, along with their frequencies, are shown in Table 7.8.

Table 7.8 Recall and precision failures in MEDLINE, adapted from [20]

Recall failures
Indexing language—lack of appropriate terms (10.2%)
Indexing—indexing not sufficiently exhaustive (20.3%), indexer omitted important concept (9.8%), indexing insufficiently specific (5.8%)
Retrieval—searcher did not cover all reasonable approaches to searching (21.5%), search too exhaustive (8.4%), search too specific (2.5%), selective printout (1.6%)
Precision failures
Indexing language—lack of appropriate specific terms (17.6%), false coordinations (11.3%), incorrect term relationships (6.8%)
Indexing—too exhaustive (11.5%)
Retrieval—search not specific (15.2%), search not exhaustive (11.7%), inappropriate terms or combinations (4.3%)
Inadequate user-system interaction (15.3%)

A number of early failure analyses focused on the NLM's Grateful Med, which was one of the first systems designed for end users. A large study at the NLM focused on searches retrieving no articles ("no postings") [88]. This was found to occur with 37% of Grateful Med searches performed in April 1987 and 27% of searches from September 1992. The 1987 searches were analyzed in more detail, with the finding that 51% of searches used excessive ANDs, in that no documents contained the intersection of all search terms ANDed together by the searcher. Other reasons for empty sets include inappropriate entering of author names (15%), term misspellings (13%), punctuation or truncation errors (11%), and failed title searches (6%). The investigators did not assess how many "no postings" were due to an absence of material on the topic. Other errors made included the following:

1. Inappropriate use of specialty headings (e.g., using the term `Pediatrics`, which is intended to represent the medical specialty, to search for children's diseases)
2. Incorrect use of subheadings (e.g., using `Management` instead of `Therapy` when searching for articles about treatment of a disease).
3. Not using related terms, either in the form of text words (e.g., adding a term like `cerebr:` or `encephal:` to the MeSH heading `Brain`) or MeSH cross-references (e.g., adding terms like `Bites and Stings` or `Dust` to `Allergens`).

Walker et al. assessed 172 "unproductive" Grateful Med searches at McMaster University in 1987–1988, dividing problems into the categories of search formulation (48%), the Grateful Med software itself (41%), and system failure (11%) [89]. While half the search formulation problems were due to an absence of material on the topic, the most common errors were found to be use of low posting terms, use of general terms instead of subheadings, and excessive use of AND. Problems specific to Grateful Med included inappropriate use of the title line (i.e., unwittingly typing a term on the title line, thus limiting retrieval to all articles with that term in the title) and the software's automatic combining of words on the subject line(s) with OR, so that the phrase `inflammatory bowel disease` was searched as `inflammatory` OR `bowel` OR `disease`.

Not all failure analyses have looked at bibliographic databases. In their study of full-text retrieval performance described earlier, McKinin et al. also assessed the reasons for full-text retrieval failures [29]. About two-thirds of the problems were due to search strategy, in that the concepts from the search were not explicitly present in the document or an excessively restrictive search operator was used. The remaining third were due to natural language problems, such as use in the documents of word variants, more general terms, synonyms, or acronyms.

A more recent study assessed search system features desired by the most meticulous searchers, namely, medical librarians and other healthcare information professionals [90]. Over 100 respondents to an email survey indicated that their search process relied on the use of complex, repeatable, and transparent search strategies. On average, searching was reported to require 60 min to formulate a search strategy, with the entire search task taking 4 h and consisting of 15 strategy lines.

Respondents reviewed a median of 175 results per search task, far more than they would ideally like (100). The most desired features of a search system were merging search queries and combining search results. Respondents provided examples of search functionality they believed to require advanced query formulation support, including:

- Syntax checking—"automate checking of parentheses, operators, and field codes"
- Truncation—"wildcards at beginning of words; wildcard within a word to replace single or multiple letters"
- Misspellings—"account for misspellings" and "UK/American spelling"
- Proximity—"interpreting proximity within sentence rather than crossing punctuation limits"
- Term frequency and location—"terms in the first and/or last sentence of the abstract only"
- Negation—"a negation that doesn't exclude articles where the negated concept is preceded"

Little research has been done of users outside academic medical centers. One exception is a study by McCray and Tse, who assessed search failures (i.e., queries yielding no retrievals) in the NLM's consumer-oriented resources, MedlinePlus and ClinicalTrials.gov [91]. About 77% of the MedlinePlus queries and 88% of the ClinicalTrials.gov queries were "in scope." Over two-thirds of these in-scope queries were error-free but just retrieved no matches. The most common errors were the same with both databases: misspelled words (16% in MedlinePlus and 27% in ClinicalTrials.gov), use of non-alphanumeric characters (14% and 21%, respectively), and inappropriate search operators (14% and 15%, respectively). Another interesting finding of these queries was the minimal use of "consumer" terms, e.g., `nose bleed` and `tube tied`, which were used less than 0.4%.

7.6 Assessment of Impact

It was first noted in Chap. 1 that the true measure of an IR system's success should be how much impact it has on the searcher's information problem, be it improving clinical care or the ability to perform research. As we have seen, there have been far more studies of the details of the user-system interaction than of how well that interaction assists in solving a problem, making a correct decision, and so forth. This state of affairs is understandable, given that studies of impact are not only costly and time-consuming but also are potentially contaminated by confounding variables unrelated to the system. Many variables play a role in the outcome of a medical diagnosis and intervention, and even if the use of IR systems is controlled (i.e., physicians are randomized to one system or another), there may be other differences in patients and/or healthcare providers that explain differences in outcome independent of IR system use.

The main approach to assessing impact has been the use of questionnaires asking providers questions such as whether the system led to a change in a decision, action, or outcome. The limitations of this approach, of course, are related to selective recall of those who reply to such surveys and/or potential differences among those who do and do not reply.

Several studies have involved administering questionnaires to clinician users of hospital library services, validating the value of such libraries and the services they provide [92–95]. The latter conducted a Web-based survey of physicians, residents, and nurses at 56 library sites serving 118 hospitals, along with 24 follow-up telephone interviews. Those who were surveyed were asked to respond based on a recent episode of seeking information for patient care. Over 16,000 individuals responded, with about three quarters indicating that the library resources led them to handle the patient care episode in a different manner. The reported changes included advice given to the patient (48%), diagnosis (25%), choice of drugs (33%), other treatment (31%), and tests (23%). Nearly all respondents (95%) said the information resulted in a better-informed clinical decision. Respondents also reported that the information allowed them to avoid different types of adverse events, including patient misunderstanding of their disease (23%), additional tests (19%), misdiagnosis (13%), adverse drug reactions (13%), medication errors (12%), and patient mortality (6%). An additional pair of studies found that provision of a rapid evidence-based question-answering service by librarians led to clinician satisfaction [96] and potential cost savings due to time efficiency [97].

Another approach to assessing impact is the "critical incident technique," in which users are prompted to recall a recent search that was effective or not. Lindberg et al. analyzed 86% of searches deemed effective by a sample of 552 end-user physicians, scientists, and others [98]. The most common impact of the information obtained was to develop an appropriate treatment plan (45%), followed by recognizing or diagnosing a medical problem or condition (22%), implementing a treatment plan (14%), and maintaining an effective patient-physician relationship (10%).

A more recent application of this technique was used by Westbrook et al., who performed semi-structured interviews which were done with 29 clinicians that generated 85 episodes where the system provided tangible benefit [99]. One quarter of these led to better provision of clinical care. They also identified a process of "journey mapping" that showed the "journey" clinicians could take from their first initial experiences with systems to their use as key knowledge tools. In another study, these same researchers also surveyed 55,000 users of their system, finding that 41% reported direct experience of a benefit.

Pluye and colleagues performed research looking at the impact of IR and other informatics applications on physicians. They began by developing a taxonomy of system impact based on an organizational case study and grouped six types of impact into broader categories of whether the impact was positive or negative [100]:

- High-positive impact
  - Practice improvement
  - Learning
  - Recall

- Moderate-positive impact
  - Reassurance
  - Confirmation
- No impact
- Negative impact
  - Frustration

Next they performed a systematic review that gathered studies assessing the impact of IR systems on physicians and classified them as to whether they had the above impacts [101]. A number of 26 studies that met their inclusion criteria showed impact in each of the positive categories, with an estimated one-third of searches having a positive impact. Many searches, however, showed no impact and a few showed negative impact. Further work compared the impact of IR systems versus decision support systems, noting that the former were more likely to cause learning and recall, while the latter were associated with practice improvement [102].

Some recent studies have assessed the impact of IR systems for a variety of outcomes. Although the cause and effect were unknown, hospitals having UpToDate available were found to have better patient outcomes in the form of shorter length of stay, reduced risk-adjusted mortality rates, and improved performance on quality indicators [103]. Bringing UpToDate on beside rounds showed it being used 157 times over a 3-month period [104]. Searches took a median time of 3 min, providing a useful answer 75% of the time, a partial answer 17% of the time, and no answer 9% of the time. The search results led to a change of diagnosis or management plans 37% of the time, confirmed original plans 38% of the time, and had no effect 25% of the time. In the Reed et al. study of nearly 4000 internal medicine physicians who took the IM–MOCE exam between 2006 and 2008 and who held individual licenses to ACP PIER and/or UpToDate, more frequent usage of electronic information resources was associated with modestly higher exam scores [105].

Another line of work has focused on analysis of user search logs to understand aspects of health-related searching. Early work focused on processing search logs, mostly from Microsoft Bing to understand users' characteristics and intentions [106, 107]. This approach has uncovered "cyberchondria," defined as unnecessary escalation of health-related concern when searching [108], and "Web-scale pharmacovigilance," the uncovering of drug interactions from search logs [109, 110]. This approach has also been used to identify patients who have a higher likelihood to develop pancreatic carcinoma [111] and lung carcinoma [112]. Some limitations of these approaches are the retrospective nature of the data and the inferring of user actions and intent solely from the search logs, although Yom Tov has documented the various ways that consumer searching can benefit their health [113].

7.7 Research on Relevance

To this point, relevance has merely been defined as a document meeting an information need that prompted a query. This fixed view of relevance makes recall and precision very straightforward to calculate. But as it turns out, relevance is not quite so objective. For example, relevance as judged by physicians has a moderately high degree of variation, as shown in experiments measuring the overlap between judges in assigning relevance of MEDLINE references to queries generated in a clinical setting [114]. This level of disagreement has been verified in similar assessments [43, 48, 115, 116]. In each of these studies, the kappa statistic was used to measure interrater reliability. This statistic, described in Sect. 7.3, is commonly used to assess agreement in diagnostic evaluations, such as X-ray or pathology specimen reading [117].

Interest in relevance has waxed and waned over the years. There was a great deal of theoretical thinking and research into relevance in the 1960s, culminating in Saracevic's seminal review paper [118]. That paper summarized all the classifications and research data to that time. Two basic problems, Saracevic noted, were the lack of agreement on the definition of relevance (he identified seven different views of it) and the paucity of experimental data supporting either those definitions or how relevance was being applied in evaluation studies.

There was a rekindling of interest in relevance in the 1990s, most likely owing to the increasing prevalence of IR systems, with a resultant increase in claims and counterclaims about their performance. Schamber et al. attempted to resurrect debate over the theoretical notions of relevance in the 1990s [119]. Their approach pared Saracevic's categories of relevance down to two: a system-oriented topical view and a user-oriented situational view. These two views are not at odds with Saracevic's classification, since the situational category encompasses several of Saracevic's views that were conceptually similar. The categories of Schamber et al. will be used for the following discussion. Saracevic recently published a monograph updating research on relevance [120].

7.7.1 *Topical Relevance*

The original view of relevance is that of topical relevance, which Saracevic called the system's view of relevance. In this view, a document is relevant because part or all of its topical coverage overlaps with the topic of the user's information need. There is a central but questionable assumption that underlies this view of relevance, noticed by Meadow [121], which is that the relevance relationship between query and document is fixed. But just because a document is "about" an information need does not mean that it is relevant. A clinician with a patient care problem incorporating the treatment of hypertension with a certain drug most likely will not want to retrieve an article dealing with the use of that drug to treat hypertension in rats. Likewise, a research pharmacologist studying the molecular mechanisms of blood pressure reductions with that drug probably will not want articles about clinical trials with the drug. Furthermore, a medical student or a patient, who knows far less than the clinician or researcher, may not want to retrieve this article at all because its language is too technical.

The topical view of relevance persists, however, for several reasons. First, it is associated with a perception of objectivity, hence reproducibility. Another reason is that quantitative methods to assess IR systems with situational relevance are difficult to perform and interpret. But perhaps the main reason for the survival of topical relevance is that this view has led to relatively easy measures for quantifying performance in IR systems. The notion of a fixed relevance between query and document greatly simplifies the task of IR evaluation, since if the relevance of a document with respect to a document is fixed, then evaluation can be simulated (without human users) quite easily once relevance judgments have been made.

This approach to evaluation has been the modus operandi of a large segment of the IR research world, particularly among those who advocate automated approaches to IR. This approach makes the task of evaluation quite easy in that system users are unnecessary. All that is needed is a test collection consisting of queries, documents, and relevance judgments. When a new system is implemented or an existing one is modified, evaluation is a simple matter of running the existing queries into the new system and measuring recall and precision. There is reason, however, to question the external validity of the results obtained with this sort of evaluation, which will be explored in greater detail later in this chapter and in Chap. 7.

7.7.2 Situational Relevance

The second category of relevance attempts to incorporate the user's situation into the judgment. Saracevic called this view the destination's view, while others have termed variations of it "situational" [119], "logical" [122], or "psychological" [123] relevance. The major underlying assumption in this view is that the user's situation and needs cannot be separated from the relevance judgment. Rees [124] said, "There is no such thing as *the* relevance of a document to an information requirement, but rather the relevance judgment of an individual in a specific judging situation …. at a certain point in time." Cooper defined the difference between (topical) relevance and utility, arguing that the latter could be measured to assess what value information was actually provided to the user [122].

Situational relevance can be challenged from two perspectives. The first is in fact very pertinent to IR in the healthcare domain, which is that the user may be distinctly *unqualified* to judge relevance. It was noted in the last chapter, for example, that many physicians lack the skills to critically appraise the medical literature

[125]. Thus, a user may deem an article relevant to a given issue yet be unable to recognize that it is flawed or that the results described do not justify the conclusions published.

The second challenge is whether the variance of the situational picture has an impact on retrieval performance measurements. Lesk and Salton carried out a study in which users originated a query and judged their retrieved documents for relevance [126]. Relevance judgments were also made by another subject expert. Additional sets of relevance judgments were created by taking the intersection and union of both judges' relevance assessments. Recall and precision were then measured based on the original retrieval results, showing that the different judgment sets had little effect on overall results. In other words, algorithms that performed well under one set of relevance judgments performed well under all of them, with the poorly performing algorithms faring poorly under all sets as well.

Voorhees noted this constancy with data from TREC [127], although Bailey et al. found the relationship broke down with the use of "bronze standard" judges, who were those who did not define topics and were not experts in the task [128]. Overall results were more consistent when so-called "gold standard" judges, who were topic originators and experts in a particular information-seeking task, and "silver standard" judges, who were task experts but did not create topics, were used.

7.7.3 Research About Relevance Judgments

Despite all the disagreement about the nature of relevance, few studies have actually attempted to investigate the factors that influence relevance judgment. Early insights on relevance judgments came from two large studies done in the 1960s [129, 130]. Cuadra and Katter developed a five-category classification scheme of the factors that could affect relevance judgments [130], which Saracevic later used in a review paper to summarize the results of research from these studies and others [118].

The first category was type of document, such as its subject matter and the quantity of it available to the relevance judge. It was found that subject content was the most important factor influencing relevance judgments, indicating that topical relevance does have importance. It was also discovered that specific subject content in a document led to higher agreement among judges. Regarding the amount of document representation available to the relevance judge, it was clear that the title alone led to poor agreement; there were conflicting results with respect to whether abstract text or increasing amount of full text was better.

The second category was the query or information needs statement. In general, the more judges knew about a user's information need, the more agreement they had. However, the less they knew about the query, the more likely they were to classify documents as relevant. It was also found that statements in documents that resembled the query statement increased the likelihood of a positive relevance judgment.

The third category was the relevance judge. Increased subject knowledge of the judge and his or her familiarity with subject terminology correlated with consistency of agreement but varied inversely with number of documents judged relevant. Professional or occupational involvement with users' information problem also led to higher rates of agreement, regardless of specific subject knowledge. Differences in intended use of documents (i.e., use for background, updating, etc.) also produced differences in relevance judgments. Level of agreement of the relevance judgment was found to be greater for nonrelevant than for relevant documents.

The fourth category was judgment conditions, such as different definitions of relevance or varied pressures on the judges. Changing the definition of relevance did not appear to lead to different relevance judgments. However, greater time or stringency pressures did have an effect, causing more positive relevance judgments.

In the last category, judgment mode, it was found that judges tend to prefer (i.e., to feel more "comfortable" or "at ease" with) more categories in a rating scale. It was also noted that the end points of scales (i.e., very relevant or very nonrelevant) tended to be used most heavily, although ratings were not normally distributed but rather skewed in one direction. Another finding was that relative scores for a group of document judgments were more consistent than absolute scores. That is, users tended to rank documents for relevance in the same order, even if they chose different categories or scores of relevance.

Research in relevance judgments did not pick up again until the mid-1980s, when Eisenberg began to investigate methods for estimating relevance [131]. Concerned that fixed, named categories of relevance were problematic, he adapted the technique of *magnitude estimation*, where subjects made their judgments on analog scales without named points. In particular, he used a 100 mm line, with the categories of relevant and nonrelevant as the end points. This approach was found to lessen the problem of relevance judges spreading out their judgments across the fixed, labeled categories of a traditional relevance scale.

This technique has also been used to assess how the order of presentation of documents influences relevance judgments. Eisenberg and Barry gave subjects a set of 15 documents and an information needs statement [132]. Based on earlier work, the relative relevance of each document was known. The documents were presented in either random, high to low, or low to high order. A "hedging phenomenon" was observed, wherein judges tended to overestimate the relevance of initial documents in the set ordered "low to high" and to underestimate relevance for the initial documents in the other set. Parker and Johnson, using 47 queries into a database of computer science journal references, found that no difference in relevance judgments occurred with retrieval sets less than or equal to 15 documents (which was the size of Eisenberg's set) [133]. But for larger sets, relevant articles ranked beyond the fifteenth document were slightly less likely to be judged relevant than if they had occurred in the first 15.

Florance and Marchionini provided additional insight into relevance by assessing how three physicians processed the information in a group of retrieved articles on six clinical topics [134]. The order of the presentation not only had a dramatic effect on relevance but also showed that the information in the articles was complementary and interrelated. The authors identified two strategies these physicians used to process the information. In the *additive* strategy, information from each successive paper reinforced what was present in preceding ones. In the *recursive* strategy, on the other hand, new information led to reinterpretation of previously seen information and reconsideration of the data in the light of new evidence. This work demonstrated that simple topical relevance oversimplifies the value of retrieved documents to users.

Another line of research of relevance judgments looks at the consistency of judges in assigning them. Many studies measuring recall and precision have looked at this phenomenon, obtaining results comparable to those shown in Table 7.9 from a study of Hersh and Hickam [114]. We will discuss these results further in the context of measuring consistency via the kappa statistic in Sect. 7.7.6.

Some more recent research into relevance judgments found that topical relevance is a part of but not a complete predictor of situational relevance [135]. This study also found that a measurement of usefulness correlated more with user satisfaction than topical relevance. Another study compared judgments of actual users in a user study versus judgments done by others "out of context" [136]. While topical relevance was found to be relatively consistent across the two types of judgements, there were other aspects of the retrieval experience—novelty, understandability, reliability, and effort—that were not captured well by external judges. Likewise, click dwell time was found to predict some of these factors (topical relevance, novelty, and effort) better than others (reliability and effort). Finally, Zuccon developed a model that found understandability of documents by the user was complementary to topical relevance [137].

7.7.4 Limitations of Relevance-Based Measures

If relevance judgments are situational and inherently variable across judges, then what does this say about the use of recall and precision? One of the harshest critics of these measures has been Swanson, who argued that, "An information need cannot be fully expressed as a search request that is independent of innumerable presuppositions of context—context that itself is impossible to describe fully, for it includes

Table 7.9 Overlap of judges on assigning relevance to documents retrieved by clinical questions using MEDLINE, adapted from [114]. Judgments were rated on a three-point scale: definitely relevant, possibly relevant, and not relevant

	Judge 2			
Judge 1		Definitely relevant	Probably relevant	Not relevant
	Definitely relevant	127	112	96
	Probably relevant		97	224
	Not relevant			779

among other things the requester's own background of knowledge" [138]. Harter likewise argued that fixed relevance judgments cannot capture the dynamic nature of the user's interaction with an IR system [123].

Even if relevance were a relative concept that existed between certain bounds so that measures based on it, such as recall or precision, could be made, there are still a number of limitations associated with the use of these measures to assess user-system interaction. Hersh noted that the magnitude of a significant difference (such as between systems) is not known [139]. Just because statistical significance exists for a research result does not mean that a difference is meaningful. Using a medical example, consider a new drug being used to treat diabetes, and suppose it lowers blood sugar by an average of 5 mg/dL. Readers with a medical background will note that this value is insignificant in terms of treatment of diabetes or its long-term outcome. Yet one could design a study with a very large sample size that could show statistical significance for the results obtained with this clinically meaningless difference. Yet, clinical significance between different levels of recall and precision has never really been defined for IR. In other words, it is unknown whether the difference between, say, 50 and 60% recall has any significance to a real user whatsoever.

Related to this issue is the assumption that more relevant and fewer nonrelevant articles are better. For example, in some instances, complete precision is not totally desired. Belkin and Vickery noted that users often discover new knowledge by "serendipity" [140]. A famous newspaper columnist, the late Sydney Harris, used to periodically devote columns to "things I learned while looking up something else." Sometimes there is value in learning something new that is peripheral to what one is seeking at the moment. Similarly, at times complete recall is not desired and may even be a distraction, for example, the busy clinician who seeks a quick answer to a question.

A final problem with recall and precision is that they are often applied in a context different from that of the original experiments, or more problematically, in no context at all. The latter case may be akin to testing a medical therapy without a disease. While simulation can be used to achieve meaningful results in IR evaluation, it must go beyond simple batching of queries into a retrieval system. There must be some interaction with the user, even if that user is acting within a simulated setting.

Relevance-based retrieval evaluation has clearly had many benefits, allowing assessment, at least superficially, the value of different approaches to indexing and retrieval. It is clearly useful in the early stages of system development when trying to assess from which indexing and retrieval approaches to choose. Hersh stated that conventional recall-precision studies with topical relevance should be done in the early evaluation of a system [139]. The problem comes when investigators attempt to draw conclusions about indexing and retrieval approaches based solely on recall and precision results.

7.7.5 Automating Relevance Judgments

Another limitation of relevance judgments is the time and cost it takes to obtain them. A number of researchers have explored whether they, or surrogates for them, can be collected in an automated manner. Soboroff et al. proposed the measurement of recall and precision without human relevance judgments [141]. Noting past work by Voorhees demonstrating that differences in judgments did not affect the relative performance of systems [127], they selected random documents from the retrieval pool of multiple searches on each topic. Their results were most effective when they did not eliminate duplicates from selection (in essence giving more frequently retrieved documents a more likely chance to be selected as relevant). They found that their results were most effective in separating high-performing and low-performing systems from those in the middle but that they were less successful at identifying the truly best (or worst) systems from among the top (or bottom) performing systems. Aslam et al. developed methods for sampling very small numbers of documents (4% of usual pool size) that led to estimates of relevance for the remaining retrieved documents comparable to if they were judged by relevance judges [142].

Another concern about recall and precision is the completeness of relevance judgments. When using relative recall, we cannot be certain that enough relevant documents have been identified to give a close approximation to absolute recall. Buckley and Voorhees introduced a new measure, binary preference (bpref), which was based on the number of times judged nonrelevant documents are retrieved before known relevant ones (that, of course, have been judged) [143]. Experiments showed that the measure was highly correlated with existing measures, such as mean average precision (MAP), when judgments were complete and more robust to incomplete judgments. Stated simplistically, bpref essentially is a measure that uses only the retrieved documents that have been judged for relevance.

Joachims introduced a new approach to evaluation for the Web based on *click-through data* [144, 145]. It was based on the premise that the links a user clicks on in the results listing from a Web search engine are a measure of relevance. A search engine or system is therefore "better" if more links are clicked from the output of one over the other. He proposed two types of experiments:

1. Regular click-through data—the user's query is sent to two search engines, with the complete rankings from one system or the other randomly presented to the user.
2. Unbiased click-through data—the user's query is sent to two search engines, but in this approach the results are mixed (although order within each set is maintained) together.

In both types of experiments, one system was deemed superior to the other when more Web pages from its output are clicked through by users.

In follow-up work, Joachims et al. looked at eye movements and click-through behavior of real users, comparing them with the relevance judgments of other real users [146]. They found that the user click-through was relatively highly associated with relevance but was subject to two modest biases:

1. Trust bias—users are influenced by the ranking order of the search engine, i.e., how much they trust its output.
2. Quality bias—users are influenced by the overall quality of the search engine, i.e., better actual ranking actually influences users' clicking.

They concluded that while clicks cannot be thought of as absolute relevance judgments, they were a highly effective relative approximation.

7.7.6 Measures of Agreement

Much IR evaluation involves human judgments. Such judgments may consist of determining whether documents are relevant or indexing terms are appropriately assigned by a person or computer. There are a variety of measures for assessing how well humans agree on these judgments. Probably the best-known and most widely used among these is the *kappa statistic* [147, 148]. There are other measures of agreement and reliability for judgments, which have been described in the textbook by Friedman and Wyatt [149].

The kappa statistic measures the difference between observed concordance (OC) and expected concordance (EC). Although the kappa statistic can be calculated for more than dichotomous variables, the example here will use a variable that can only have two values (such as relevant or nonrelevant). Table 7.10 defines the variables used in the following formulas:

$$\mathrm{OC} = \frac{a+d}{a+b+c+d} \tag{7.1}$$

$$\mathrm{EC} = \frac{\dfrac{(a+b)(a+c)}{a+b+c+d} + \dfrac{(b+d)(c+d)}{a+b+c+d}}{a+b+c+d} \tag{7.2}$$

Table 7.10 Table to calculate kappa statistic for two observers judging whether an event is X or Y

	Observer 2			
Observer 1		*X*	*Y*	Total
	X	*a*	*b*	*a* + *b*
	Y	*c*	*d*	*c* + *d*
	Total	*a* + *c*	*b* + *d*	*a* + *b* + *c* + *d*

Table 7.11 Sample data to calculate kappa

	Observer 2			
Observer 1		Relevant	Nonrelevant	Total
	Relevant	75	3	78
	Nonrelevant	2	20	22
	Total	77	23	100

$$\text{Kappa} = \frac{\text{OC} - \text{EC}}{1 - \text{EC}} \tag{7.3}$$

In general, the following kappa values indicate the stated amount of agreement [147]:

- Poor <0.4
- Fair 0.4–0.6
- Good 0.6–0.8
- Excellent >0.8

Table 7.11 presents sample data to calculate kappa for relevance judgments. The OC is 95/100 = 0.95. The EC is [(77*78/100) + (23*22/100)]/100 = 0.65. The kappa is therefore (0.95–0.65)/(1–0.65) = 0.86. The kappa value for the relevance judgments presented in Table 7.11 above was 0.41 [114], with comparable results obtained in other studies [43, 48, 115, 150].

Hripcsak and Rothschild investigated the relationship of kappa to the F measure [151]. They showed that when the number of negative cases is large and the probability of chance agreement on positive cases is very small, then the two measures will approach each other mathematically. This is therefore useful in situations (more common in assessment of natural language understanding systems) where the true number of negative cases is unknown but large. In addition, there are actually variants of the kappa measure whose assumptions lead to different results in some cases [152].

7.8 What Has Been Learned About IR Systems?

Although the scope of IR evaluation research does not tell us everything we might wish to know about system use, efficacy, and outcomes, the sum of what has been done provides many insights into how systems are used, how often they are successful, and where they can be improved. We can end this chapter with a review of the research findings in the context of the six questions around which the main sections of the chapter are organized.

We certainly now know that IR systems are ubiquitous in their use for biomedical and health information needs, both by professionals and consumers. The quantity of their use is difficult to measure in modern times with so many avenues for their availability, from linkage out of EHRs to mobile devices that most people carry. User satisfaction with IR systems tends to be high.

System-oriented studies of searching quality have shown that databases vary in coverage by topic. They also show that searching the same database with a different system can give divergent results, an outcome perhaps exacerbated by the new features modern systems have added to make searching simpler for end users. In addition, achieving maximum recall, as needed for identifying studies such as RCTs for systematic reviews, continues to be challenging. The capabilities of Web search engines are not known for all tasks, but their ubiquitous use indicates they are likely important for those seeking information.

User-oriented studies have shown that searchers are generally able to learn to search effectively, although they make significant numbers of errors and missed opportunities. Studies of recall and precision show that most user searches do not come anywhere close to retrieving all the relevant articles on a given topic. Of course, most searchers do not need to obtain all the relevant articles to answer a clinical question (unless they are doing a systematic review). These studies also find lack of overlap in the relevant articles retrieved when different users search on the same topic. This can be important, especially since the quality of the evidence in studies can vary widely, as described in Chap. 2. These studies also show that the type of indexing or retrieval interface may not have as large an impact on user performance as attributes of the user himself or herself.

Task-oriented studies show that users improve their ability to answer clinical questions with IR systems, but sometimes those systems lead them to overturn the correct answer. However the quality of searching by users is assessed, and systems take a long time to use. Large bibliographic databases such as MEDLINE may be inappropriate for most questions generated in the clinical setting, and the move to "synthesized," evidence-based resources has been helpful in this regard.

Searching ability is influenced by a variety of factors. Although further research is needed to make more definitive statements, the abilities of healthcare personnel vary, with one or more specific cognitive traits (e.g., spatial visualization) possibly explaining the difference. Factors that may not play a significant role at all in search success are recall and precision. Although a searcher obviously needs to retrieve reasonable amounts of relevant documents and not be inundated by nonrelevant ones, the small differences across IR systems and users may not be significant. It is also clear that searchers make frequent mistakes and have missed opportunities that might have led to better results.

Finally, although healthcare IR systems are widely distributed and commercially successful, their true impact on healthcare providers and patient care is unknown. Demonstrating their benefit in the complex healthcare environment is difficult at best, with RCTs showing benefits in patient outcomes unlikely to be performed. On the other hand, as noted in the keynote address at the 1991 *Symposium on Computer Applications in Medical Care* by David Eddy, no one has ever assessed the impact of elevators on patient care, though they are obviously important. Analogously, no one can deny that biomedical and health IR systems are important and valuable, so further research should focus on how they can be used most effectively by clinicians, patients, and researchers.

References

1. Hersh W, Hickam D. How well do physicians use electronic information retrieval systems? A framework for investigation and review of the literature. J Am Med Assoc. 1998;280:1347–52.
2. Anonymous. From screen to script: the Doctor's digital path to treatment. New York, NY: Manhattan Research; 2012.
3. Fox S, Duggan M. Health online 2013. Washington, DC: Pew Internet & American Life Project; 2013 January 15.
4. Gorman P. Information needs of physicians. J Am Soc Inf Sci. 1995;46:729–36.
5. Duran-Nelson A, Gladding S, Beattie J, Nixon L. Should we Google it? Resource use by internal medicine residents for point-of-care clinical decision making. Acad Med. 2013;88:788–94.
6. Cook D, Sorensen K, Nishimura R, Ommen S, Lloyd F. A comprehensive information technology system to support physician learning at the point of care. Acad Med. 2014;90:33–9.
7. Cook D, Sorensen K, Linderbaum J, Pencille LJ, Rhodes D. Information needs of generalists and specialists using online best-practice algorithms to answer clinical questions. J Am Med Inform Assoc. 2017;24:754–61.
8. Herskovic J, Tanaka L, Hersh W, Bernstam E. A day in the life of PubMed: analysis of a typical day's query log. J Am Med Inform Assoc. 2007;14:212–20.
9. Seguin A, Haynes R, Carballo S, Iorio A, Perrier A, Agoritsas T. Physicians' translation of clinical questions into searchable queries: an analytical survey. JMIR Medical Education. 2020:Epub ahead of print.
10. Fiksdal A, Kumbamu A, Jadhav A, Cocos C, Nelsen L, Pathak J, et al. Evaluating the process of online health information searching: a qualitative approach to exploring consumer perspectives. J Med Internet Res. 2014;16(10):e224.
11. Jadhav A, Andrews D, Fiksdal A, Kumbamu A, McCormick J, Misitano A, et al. Comparative analysis of online health queries originating from personal computers and smart devices on a consumer health information portal. J Med Internet Res. 2014;16(7):e160.
12. Fox S. Health topics. Washington, DC: Pew Internet & American Life Project; 2011 February 1.
13. Ritchie H. Does the news reflect what we die from? Our world in data 2019.
14. Palotti J, Hanbury A, Muller H, Kahn C. How users search and what they search for in the medical domain - understanding laypeople and experts through query logs. Information Retrieval Journal. 2016;19:189–224.
15. Nielsen J, Levy J. Measuring usability: preference vs. performance. Commun ACM. 1994;37:66–75.
16. Taylor H. The growing influence and use of health care information obtained online. New York, NY: Harris Interactive 2011 September 15. Contract No.: Harris Poll #98.
17. Dixit R, Rogith D, Narayana V, Salimi M, Gururaj A, Ohno-Machado L, et al. User needs analysis and usability assessment of data med–a biomedical data discovery index. J Am Med Inform Assoc. 2018;25:337–44.
18. Cleverdon C, Keen E. Factors determining the performance of indexing systems (Vol. 1: design, Vol. 2: results). Aslib Cranfield Research Project: Cranfield, England; 1966.
19. Swanson D. Information retrieval as a trial-and-error process. Libr Q. 1977;47:128–48.
20. Lancaster F. Evaluation of the MEDLARS demand search service. Bethesda, MD: National Library of Medicine; 1968.
21. McCain K, White H, Griffith B. Comparing retrieval performance in online databases. Inf Process Manag. 1987;23:539–53.
22. Gehanno J, Paris C, Thirion B, Caillard J. Assessment of bibliographic databases performance in information retrieval for occupational and environmental toxicology. Occup Environ Med. 1998;55:562–6.
23. Alper B, Stevermer J, White D, Ewigman B. Answering family physicians' clinical questions using electronic medical databases. J Fam Pract. 2001;50:960–5.
24. Koonce T, Giuse N, Todd P. Evidence-based databases versus primary medical literature: an in-house investigation on their optimal use. J Med Libr Assoc. 2004;92:407–11.

25. Trumble J, Anderson M, Caldwell M, Chuang F, Fulton S, Howard A, et al. A systematic evaluation of evidence based medicine tools for point-of-care Houston. TX: Texas Health Science Libraries Consortium; 2007.
26. Haynes R, McKibbon K, Walker C, Mousseau J, Baker L, Fitzgerald D, et al. Computer searching of the medical literature: an evaluation of MEDLINE searching systems. Ann Intern Med. 1985;103:812–6.
27. Haynes R, Walker C, McKibbon K, Johnston M, Willan A. Performance of 27 MEDLINE systems tested by searches with clinical questions. J Am Med Inform Assoc. 1994;1:285–95.
28. Blair D, Maron M. An evaluation of retrieval effectiveness for a full-text document-retrieval system. Commun ACM. 1985;28:289–99.
29. McKinin E, Sievert M, Johnson E, Mitchell J. The MEDLINE/full-text research project. J Am Soc Inf Sci. 1991;42:297–307.
30. Lokker C, Haynes R, Chu R, McKibbon K, Wilczynski N, Walter S. How well are journal and clinical article characteristics associated with the journal impact factor? A retrospective cohort study. J Med Libr Assoc. 2012;100:28–33.
31. Shariff S, Sontrop J, Haynes R, Iansavichus A, McKibbon K, Wilczynski N, et al. Impact of PubMed search filters on the retrieval of evidence by physicians. Can Med Assoc J. 2012;184:E184–E90.
32. Wilczynski N, Lokker C, McKibbon K, Hobson N, Haynes R. Limits of search filter development. J Med Libr Assoc. 2016;104:42–6.
33. Neilson C. A failed attempt at developing a search filter for systematic review methodology articles in Ovid Embase. J Med Libr Assoc. 2019;107:203–9.
34. Agoritsas T, Merglen A, Courvoisier D, Combescure C, Garin N, Perrier A, et al. Sensitivity and predictive value of 15 PubMed search strategies to answer clinical questions rated against full systematic reviews. J Med Internet Res. 2012;14(3):e85.
35. Izcovich A, Criniti J, Popoff F, Ragusa M, Gigler C, Malla C, et al. Answering medical questions at the point of care: a cross-sectional study comparing rapid decisions based on PubMed and Epistemonikos searches with evidence-based recommendations developed with the GRADE approach. BMJ Open. 2017;7:e016113.
36. Bramer W, Rethlefsen M, Kleijnen J, Franco O. Optimal database combinations for literature searches in systematic reviews: a prospective exploratory study. Syst Rev. 2016;6:245.
37. Beckles Z, Glover S, Ashe J, Stockton S, Boynton J, Lai R, et al. Searching CINAHL did not add value to clinical questions posed in NICE guidelines. J Clin Epidemiol. 2013;66:1051–7.
38. Gusenbauer M. Google scholar to overshadow them all? Comparing the sizes of 12 academic search engines and bibliographic databases. Scientometrics. 2019;118:177–214.
39. Jeffery R, Navarro T, Lokker C, Haynes R, Wilczynski N, Farjou G. How current are leading evidence-based medical textbooks? An analytic survey of four online textbooks. J Med Internet Res. 2012;14(6):e175.
40. Lin J. Is searching full text more effective than searching abstracts? BMC Bioinformatics. 2009;10:46.
41. Jimmy, Zuccon G, Demartini G. On the volatility of commercial search engines and its impact on information retrieval research. Proceedings of the 41st International ACM SIGIR Conference on Research & Development in Information Retrieval; 2019; Ann Arbor, MI.
42. Fenichel C. The process of searching online bibliographic databases: a review of research. Library Res. 1980;2:107–27.
43. Haynes R, McKibbon K, Walker C, Ryan N, Fitzgerald D, Ramsden M. Online access to MEDLINE in clinical settings. Ann Intern Med. 1990;112:78–84.
44. McKibbon K, Haynes R, Dilks CW, Ramsden M, Ryan N, Baker L, et al. How good are clinical MEDLINE searches? A comparative study of clinical end-user and librarian searches. Comput Biomed Res. 1990;23(6):583–93.
45. Haynes R, Johnston M, McKibbon K, Walker C, Willan A. A randomized controlled trial of a program to enhance clinical use of MEDLINE. Online J Curr Clin Trials. 1992;Doc No 56.
46. Hersh W, Hickam D. The use of a multi-application computer workstation in a clinical setting. Bull Med Libr Assoc. 1994;82:382–9.

47. Saracevic T, Kantor P. A study of information seeking and retrieving. III. Searchers, searches, and overlap. J Am Soc Inf Sci. 1988;39:197–216.
48. Hersh W, Hickam D. An evaluation of interactive Boolean and natural language searching with an on-line medical textbook. J Am Soc Inf Sci. 1995;46:478–89.
49. Egan D, Remde J, Gomez L, Landauer T, Eberhardt J, Lochbaum C. Formative design-evaluation of Superbook. ACM Trans Inf Syst. 1989;7:30–57.
50. Mynatt B, Leventhal L, Instone K, Farhat J, Rohlman D. Hypertext or book: which is better for answering questions? Proceedings of Computer-Human Interface 92; 1992.
51. Hersh W, Elliot D, Hickam D, Wolf S, Molnar A, Leichtenstein C, Towards new measures of information retrieval evaluation. Proceedings of the 18th Annual Symposium on Computer Applications in Medical Care; 1994; Washington, DC: Hanley & Belfus.
52. Hersh W, Pentecost J, Hickam D. A task-oriented approach to information retrieval evaluation. J Am Soc Inf Sci. 1996;47:50–6.
53. Rose L. Factors influencing successful use of information retrieval systems by nurse practitioner students [M.S.]. Portland, OR: Oregon Health Sciences University; 1998.
54. Hersh W, Crabtree M, Hickam D, Sacherek L, Rose L, Friedman C. Factors associated with successful answering of clinical questions using an information retrieval system. Bull Med Libr Assoc. 2000;88:323–31.
55. Gorman P, Helfand M. Information seeking in primary care: how physicians choose which clinical questions to pursue and which to leave unanswered. Med Decis Mak. 1995;15:113–9.
56. Hersh W, Crabtree M, Hickam D, Sacherek L, Friedman C, Tidmarsh P, et al. Factors associated with success for searching MEDLINE and applying evidence to answer clinical questions. J Am Med Inform Assoc. 2002;9:283–93.
57. McKibbon K, Fridsma D. Effectiveness of clinician-selected electronic information resources for answering primary care physicians' information needs. J Am Med Inform Assoc. 2006;13:653–9.
58. Westbrook J, Coiera E, Gosling A. Do online information retrieval systems help experienced clinicians answer clinical questions? J Am Med Inform Assoc. 2005;12:315–21.
59. van der Vegt A, Zuccon G, Koopman B. Do better search engines really equate to better clinical decisions? If not, why not? J Am Soc Inf Sci. 2020; in press.
60. Westbrook J, Gosling A, Coiera E. The impact of an online evidence system on confidence in decision making in a controlled setting. Med Decis Mak. 2005;25:178–85.
61. vander Vegt A, Zuccon G, Koopman B, Deacon A. Impact of a search engine on clinical decisions under time and system effectiveness constraints: research protocol. JMIR Research Protocols. 2019;8(5):e12803.
62. Roberts K, Simpson M, Voorhees E, Hersh W. Overview of the TREC 2015 clinical decision support track. The Twenty-Fourth Text REtrieval Conference (TREC 2015) Proceedings; 2015; Gaithersbug, MD.
63. vander Vegt A, Zuccon G, Koopman B. Do better search engines really equate to better clinical decisions? If not, why not? J Am Soc Inf Sci. 2020:In review.
64. Ahmadi S, Faghankhani M, Javanbakht A, Akbarshahi M, Mirghorbani M, Safarnejad B, et al. A comparison of answer retrieval through four evidence-based textbooks (ACP PIER, essential evidence Plus, first consult, and UpToDate): a randomized controlled trial. Med Teach. 2011;33:724–30.
65. Prorok J, Iserman E, Wilczynski N, Haynes R. The quality, breadth, and timeliness of content updating vary substantially for 10 online medical texts: an analytic survey. J Clin Epidemiol. 2012;65:1289–95.
66. Kritz M, Gschwandtner M, Stefanov V, Hanbury A, Samwald M. Utilization and perceived problems of online medical resources and search tools among different groups of European physicians. J Med Internet Res. 2013;15(6):e122.
67. Kim S, Noveck H, Galt J, Hogshire L, Willett L, O'Rourke K. Searching for answers to clinical questions using Google versus evidence-based summary resources: a randomized controlled crossover study. Acad Med. 2014;89:940–3.

68. Thiele R, Poiro N, Scalzo D, Nemergut E. Speed, accuracy, and confidence in Google, Ovid, PubMed, and UpToDate: results of a randomised trial. Postgrad Med J. 2010;86:459–65.
69. Ensan L, Faghankhani M, Javanbakht A, Ahmadi S, Baradaran H. To compare PubMed clinical queries and UpToDate in teaching information mastery to clinical residents: a crossover randomized controlled trial. PLoS One. 2011;6:e23487.
70. Markonis D, Holzer M, Baroz F, DeCastaneda R, Boyer C, Langs G, et al. User-oriented evaluation of a medical image retrieval system for radiologists. Int J Med Inform. 2015;84:774–83.
71. Scaffidi M, Khan R, Wang C, Keren D, Tsui C, Garg A, et al. Comparison of the impact of Wikipedia, UpToDate, and a digital textbook on short-term knowledge acquisition among medical students: randomized controlled trial of three web-based resources. JMIR Med Educ. 2017;3(2):e20.
72. Lau A, Coiera E, Zrimec T, Compton P. Clinician search behaviors may be influenced by search engine design. J Med Internet Res. 2010;12(2):e25.
73. Eysenbach G, Kohler C. How do consumers search for and appraise health information on the world wide web? Qualitative study using focus groups, usability tests, and in-depth interviews. Br Med J. 2002;324:573–7.
74. Lau A, Coiera E. Impact of web searching and social feedback on consumer decision making: a prospective online experiment. J Med Internet Res. 2008;10(1):e2.
75. Lau A, Kwok T, Coiera E. How online crowds influence the way individual consumers answer health questions. Appl Clin Inform. 2011;2:177–89.
76. van Deursen A. Internet skill-related problems in accessing online health information. Int J Med Inform. 2012;81:61–72.
77. Taylor A. A study of the information search behaviour of the millennial generation. Inf Res. 2012;17:1.
78. Jimmy J, Zuccon G, Koopman B, Demartini G. Health cards for consumer health search. Proceedings of the 42nd International ACM SIGIR Conference on Research and Development in Information Retrieval; 2019; Paris, France.
79. Jimmy J, Zuccon G, Demartini G, Koopman B. Health cards to assist decision making in consumer health search. Proceedings of the AMIA 2019 Annual Symposium; 2019; Washington, DC.
80. Saracevic T, Kantor P, Chamis A, Trivison D. A study of information seeking and retrieving. I. Background and methodology. J Am Soc Inf Sci. 1988;39:161–76.
81. Saracevic T, Kantor P. A study in information seeking and retrieving. II. Users, questions, and effectiveness. J Am Soc Inf Sci. 1988;39:177–96.
82. Ekstrom R, French J, Harmon H. Manual for kit of factor-referenced cognitive tests. Princeton, NJ: Educational Testing Service; 1976.
83. Chin J, Diehl V, Norman K. Development of an instrument measuring user satisfaction of the human-computer interface. Proceedings of CHI '88 - Human Factors in Computing Systems; 1988; New York: ACM Press.
84. Magrabi F, Westbrook J, Coiera E. What factors are associated with the integration of evidence retrieval technology into routine general practice settings? Int J Med Inform. 2007;76:701–9.
85. Liu Y, Wacholder N. Evaluating the impact of MeSH (medical subject headings) terms on different types of searchers. Inf Process Manag. 2017;53:851–70.
86. Koopman B, Zuccon G, Bruza P. What makes an effective clinical query and querier? J Am Soc Inf Sci Tech. 2017;68:2557–71.
87. Pogacar F, Ghenai A, Smucker M, Clarke C. The positive and negative influence of search results on people's decisions about the efficacy of medical treatments. 2017 ACM SIGIR International Conference on the Theory of Information Retrieval; 2017; Amsterdam, Netherlands.
88. Kingsland L, Harbourt A, Syed E, Schuyler P. COACH: applying UMLS knowledge sources in an expert searcher environment. Bull Med Libr Assoc. 1993;81:178–83.
89. Walker C, McKibbon K, Haynes R, Ramsden M. Problems encountered by clinical end users of MEDLINE and grateful med. Bull Med Libr Assoc. 1991;79:67–9.
90. Russell-Rose T, Chamberlain J. Expert search strategies: the information retrieval practices of healthcare information professionals. JMIR Med Inform. 2017;5(4):e33.

91. McCray A, Tse T. Understanding search failures in consumer health information systems. Proceedings of the AMIA 2003 Annual Symposium; 2003; Washington, DC: Hanley & Belfus.
92. King D. The contribution of hospital library information services to clinical care: a study of eight hospitals. Bull Med Libr Assoc. 1987;75:291–301.
93. Marshall J. The impact of the hospital library on decision making: the Rochester study. Bull Med Libr Assoc. 1992;80:169–78.
94. Mathis Y, Huisman L, Swanson S, Griswold M, Salzwedel B, Watson M. Mediated literature searches. Bull Med Libr Assoc. 1994;69:360.
95. Marshall J, Sollenberger J, Easterby-Gannett S, Morgan L, Klem M, Cavanaugh S, et al. The value of library and information services in patient care: results of a multisite study. J Med Libr Assoc. 2013;101:38–46.
96. McGowan J, Hogg W, Rader T, Salzwedel D, Worster D, Cogo E, et al. A rapid evidence-based service by librarians provided information to answer primary care clinical questions. Health Inf Libr J. 2009;27:11–21.
97. McGowan J, Hogg W, Zhong J, Zhao X. A cost-consequences analysis of a primary care librarian question and answering service. PLoS One. 2012;7(3):e33837.
98. Lindberg D, Siegel E, Rapp B, Wallingford K, Wilson S. Use of MEDLINE by physicians for clinical problem solving. J Am Med Assoc. 1993;269:3124–9.
99. Westbrook J, Coiera E, Braithwaite J. Measuring the impact of online evidence retrieval systems using critical incidents and journey mapping. Stud Health Technol Inform. 2005;116:533–8.
100. Pluye P, Grad R. How information retrieval technology may impact on physician practice: an organizational case study in family medicine. J Eval Clin Pract. 2004;10:413–30.
101. Pluye P, Grad R, Dunikowski L, Stephenson R. Impact of clinical information-retrieval technology on physicians: a literature review of quantitative, qualitative and mixed methods studies. Int J Med Inform. 2005;74:745–68.
102. Grad R, Pluye P, Meng Y, Segal B, Tamblyn R. Assessing the impact of clinical information-retrieval technology in a family practice residency. J Eval Clin Pract. 2005;11:576–86.
103. Isaac T, Zheng J, Jha A. Use of UpToDate and outcomes in US hospitals. J Hosp Med. 2012;7:85–90.
104. Phua J, See K, Khalizah H, Low S, Lim T. Utility of the electronic information resource UpToDate for clinical decision-making at bedside rounds. Singap Med J. 2012;53:116–20.
105. Reed D, West C, Holmboe E, Halvorsen A, Lipner R, Jacobs C, et al. Relationship of electronic medical knowledge resource use and practice characteristics with internal medicine maintenance of certification examination scores. J Gen Intern Med. 2012;27:917–23.
106. Cartright M, White R, Horvitz E. Intentions and attention in exploratory health search. Proceedings of the 34th Annual International ACM SIGIR Conference on Research and Development in Information Retrieval (SIGIR 2011); 2011; Beijing, China.
107. White R, Horvitz E. Studies of the onset and persistence of medical concerns in search logs. Proceedings of the 35th Annual International ACM SIGIR Conference on Research and Development in Information Retrieval (SIGIR 2012); 2012; Portland, OR.
108. White R, Horvitz E. Cyberchondria: studies of the escalation of medical concerns in web search. ACM Trans Inf Syst. 2009;4:23–37.
109. White R, Tatonetti N, Shah N, Altman R, Horvitz E. Web-scale pharmacovigilance: listening to signals from the crowd. J Am Med Inform Assoc. 2013;20:404–8.
110. Nguyen T, Larsen M, O'Dea B, Phung D, Venkatesh S, Christensen H. Estimation of the prevalence of adverse drug reactions from social media. J Biomed Inform. 2017;102:130–7.
111. Paparrizos J, White R, Horvitz E. Screening for pancreatic adenocarcinoma using signals from web search logs: feasibility study and results. J Oncol Pract. 2016;12:737–44.
112. White R, Horvitz E. Evaluation of the feasibility of screening patients for early signs of lung carcinoma in web search logs. JAMA Oncol. 2017;3:398–401.
113. Yom-Tov E. Crowdsourced health: how what you do on the internet will improve medicine. Cambridge, MA: MIT Press; 2016.

114. Hersh W, Buckley C, Leone T, Hickam D. OHSUMED: an interactive retrieval evaluation and new large test collection for research. Proceedings of the 17th Annual International ACM SIGIR Conference on Research and Development in Information Retrieval; 1994; Dublin, Ireland: Springer-Verlag.
115. Hersh W, Hickam D. A comparison of two methods for indexing and retrieval from a full-text medical database. Med Decis Mak. 1993;13:220–6.
116. Hersh W, Hickam D, Haynes R, McKibbon K. A performance and failure analysis of SAPHIRE with a MEDLINE test collection. J Am Med Inform Assoc. 1994;1:51–60.
117. Kramer M, Feinstein A. Clinical biostatistics: LIV. The biostatistics of concordance. Clin Pharmacol Ther. 1981;29:111–23.
118. Saracevic T. Relevance: a review of and a framework for the thinking on the notion in information science. J Am Soc Inf Sci. 1975;26:321–43.
119. Schamber L, Eisenberg M, Nilan M. A re-examination of relevance: toward a dynamic, situational definition. Inf Process Manag. 1990;26:755–76.
120. Saracevic T. The notion of relevance in information science: everybody knows what relevance is. But, what is it really? San Rafael. CA: Morgan & Claypool; 2016.
121. Meadow C. Relevance? J Am Soc Inf Sci. 1985;36:354–5.
122. Cooper W. On selecting a measure of retrieval effectiveness. J Am Soc Inf Sci. 1973;24:87–100.
123. Harter S. Psychological relevance and information science. J Am Soc Inf Sci. 1992;43:602–15.
124. Rees A. The relevance of relevance to the testing and evaluation of document retrieval systems. ASLIB Proc. 1966;18:316–24.
125. Anonymous. Evidence-based medicine: a new approach to teaching the practice of medicine. Evidence-based medicine working group. J Am Med Assoc. 1992;268:2420–5.
126. Lesk M, Salton G. Relevance assessments and retrieval system evaluation. Information Storage and Retrieval. 1968;4:343–59.
127. Voorhees E. Variations in relevance judgments and the measurement of retrieval effectiveness. Proceedings of the 21st Annual International ACM SIGIR Conference on Research and Development in Information Retrieval; 1998; Melbourne, Australia: ACM Press.
128. Bailey P, Craswell N, Soboroff I. Relevance assessment: are judges exchangeable and does it matter? Proceedings of the 31st Annual International ACM SIGIR Conference on Research and Development in Information Retrieval; 2008; Singapore.
129. Rees A, Schultz D. A field experimental approach to the study of relevance assessments in relation to document searching. Cleveland, OH: Center for Documentation and Communication Research, Case Western Reserve University; 1967.
130. Cuadra C, Katter R. Experimental studies of relevance judgments. Santa Monica, CA: Systems Development Corp.1967. Report No.: TM-3520/001, 002, 003.
131. Eisenberg M. Measuring relevance judgments. Inf Process Manag. 1988;24:373–89.
132. Eisenberg M, Barry C. Order effects: a study of the possible influence of presentation order on user judgments of document relevance. J Am Soc Inf Sci. 1988;39:293–300.
133. Parker L, Johnson R. Does order of presentation affect users' judgment of documents? J Am Soc Inf Sci. 1990;41:493–4.
134. Florance V, Marchionini G. Information processing in the context of medical care. Proceedings of the 18th Annual International ACM SIGIR Conference on Research and Development in Information Retrieval; 1995; Seattle: ACM Press.
135. Mao J, Liu Y, Zhou K, Nie J, Song J, Zhang M et al. When does relevance mean usefulness and user satisfaction in web search? Proceedings of the 39th International ACM SIGIR conference on Research and Development in Information Retrieval; 2016; Pisa, Italy.
136. Jiang J, He D, Allan J. Comparing in situ and multidimensional relevance judgments. Proceedings of the 40th International ACM SIGIR Conference on Research and Development in Information Retrieval; 2017; Tokyo, Japan.
137. Zuccon G. Understandability biased evaluation for information retrieval. Advances in Information Retrieval: 38th European Conference on IR Research; 2016; Padua, Italy.

138. Swanson D. Historical note: information retrieval and the future of an illusion. J Am Soc Inf Sci. 1988;39:92–8.
139. Hersh W. Relevance and retrieval evaluation: perspectives from medicine. J Am Soc Inf Sci. 1994;45:201–6.
140. Belkin N, Vickery A. Interaction in the information system: a review of research from document retrieval to knowledge-based system. The British Library: London, England; 1985.
141. Soboroff I, Nicholas C, Cahan P. Ranking retrieval systems without relevance judgments. Proceedings of the 24th Annual International ACM SIGIR Conference on Research and Development in Information Retrieval; 2001; New Orleans, LA: ACM Press.
142. Aslam J, Pavlu V, Yilmaz E. A statistical method for system evaluation using incomplete judgments. Proceedings of the 29th Annual International ACM SIGIR Conference on Research and Development in Information Retrieval; 2006; Seattle, WA: ACM Press.
143. Buckley C, Voorhees E. Retrieval evaluation with incomplete information. Proceedings of the 27th Annual International ACM SIGIR Conference on Research and Development in Information Retrieval; 2004; Sheffield, England: ACM Press.
144. Joachims T. Optimizing search engines using clickthrough data. Proceedings of the ACM Conference on Knowledge Discovery and Data Mining; 2002; Edmonton, Alberta, Canada: ACM Press.
145. Joachims T. Evaluating retrieval performance using clickthrough data. Proceedings of the SIGIR Workshop on Mathematical/Formal Methods in Information Retrieval; 2002; Tampere, Finland: ACM Press.
146. Joachims T, Granka L, Pang B, Hembrooke H, Gay G. Accurately interpreting clickthrough data as implicit feedback. Proceedings of the 28th International ACM SIGIR Conference on Research and Development in Information Retrieval; 2005; Salvador, Brazil: ACM Press.
147. Cohen J. A coefficient of agreement for nominal scales. Educ Psychol Meas. 1960;20:37–46.
148. Fleiss J, Levin B, Paik M. The measurement of Interrater agreement. Statistical methods for rates and proportions. 3rd ed. Hoboken, NJ: Wiley; 2003. p. 598–626.
149. Friedman C, Wyatt J. Evaluation methods in biomedical informatics. New York, NY: Springer; 2006.
150. Hersh W, Hickam D. A comparison of retrieval effectiveness for three methods of indexing medical literature. Am J Med Sci. 1992;303:292–300.
151. Hripcsak G, Rothschild A. Agreement, the F-measure, and reliability in information retrieval. J Am Med Inform Assoc. 2005;12:296–8.
152. DiEugenio B, Glass M. The kappa statistic: a second look. Comput Linguist. 2004;30:95–101.

Chapter 8
Research

Just as operational information retrieval (IR) has changed profoundly over the editions of this book, so has IR research. Like many computational and informatics-related fields, research has pursued different paths and priorities. Some aspects of what used to be IR research are now in operational IR systems, often protected by trade secrets and desire to protect intellectual property. The growth of commercial IR systems has also led to a good deal of research being done by industry, where there has been criticism that not all results or datasets are published [1].

A number of books and overview articles have been published on IR research. Two volumes cover the major IR challenge evaluations, the Text REtrieval Conference (TREC)[1] [2] and the Conference and Labs of the Evaluation Forum[2] (CLEF, formerly Cross-Language Evaluation Forum) [3]. Harman has written monographs on evaluation [4] and an early history of the field, when it was research-oriented [5]. Other overview articles include one on a framework for evaluation [6] and another brief overview article [7]. More specific to biomedical and health informatics and going beyond IR is the Statement on the Reporting of Evaluation Studies in Health Informatics (STARE-HI), which provides recommendations on the report of evaluative research in informatics [8, 9].

8.1 Frameworks and Challenge Evaluations

One way to get a sense of the breadth of IR research is to look at various frameworks and challenge evaluations that categorize research. One framework comes from the annual ACM SIGIR conference,[3] with the most recent instance shown in Table 8.1.

[1] https://trec.nist.gov/.

[2] http://www.clef-initiative.eu/.

[3] https://sigir.org/sigir2019/calls/long/.

W. Hersh, *Information Retrieval: A Biomedical and Health Perspective*, Health Informatics, https://doi.org/10.1007/978-3-030-47686-1_8

Table 8.1 Areas of research focus in ACM SIGIR call for papers[a]

Search and ranking—Research on core IR algorithmic topics, including IR at scale, covering topics such as:

- Queries and query analysis
- Web search, including link analysis, sponsored search, search advertising, adversarial search and spam, and vertical search
- Retrieval models and ranking, including diversity and aggregated search
- Efficiency and scalability
- Theoretical models and foundations of information retrieval and access

Future directions—Research with theoretical or empirical contributions on new technical or social aspects of IR, especially in more speculative directions or with emerging technologies, covering topics such as:

- Novel approaches to IR
- Ethics, economics, and politics
- Applications of search to social good
- IR with new devices, including wearable computing, neuroinformatics, sensors, internet of things, vehicles

Domain-specific applications—Research focusing on domain-specific IR challenges, covering topics such as:

- Social search
- Search in structured data including email search and entity search
- Multimedia search
- Education
- Legal
- Health, including genomics and bioinformatics
- Other domains such as digital libraries, enterprise, news search, app search, archival search

Content analysis, recommendation, and classification—Research focusing on recommender systems, rich content representations, and content analysis, covering topics such as:

- Filtering and recommender systems
- Document representation
- Content analysis and information extraction, including summarization, text representation, readability, sentiment analysis, and opinion mining
- Cross- and multilingual search
- Clustering, classification, and topic models

Artificial intelligence, semantics, and dialog—Research bridging AI and IR, especially toward deep semantics and dialog with intelligent agents, covering topics such as:

- Question-answering
- Conversational systems and retrieval, including spoken language interfaces, dialog management systems, and intelligent chat systems
- Semantics and knowledge graphs
- Deep learning for IR, embeddings, and agents

Human factors and interfaces—Research into user-centric aspects of IR, including user interfaces, behavior modeling, privacy, and interactive systems, covering topics such as:

- Mining and modeling search activity, including user and task models, click models, log analysis, behavioral analysis, and attention modeling
- Interactive and personalized search
- Collaborative search, social tagging, and crowdsourcing
- Information privacy and security

Table 8.1 (continued)

Evaluation—Research that focuses on the measurement and evaluation of IR systems, covering topics such as:

- User-centered evaluation methods, including measures of user experience and performance, user engagement, and search task design
- Test collections and evaluation metrics, including the development of new test collections
- Eye-tracking and physiological approaches, such as fMRI
- Evaluation of novel information access tasks and systems such as multi-turn information access
- Statistical methods and reproducibility issues in information retrieval evaluation

[a]https://sigir.org/sigir2019/calls/long/

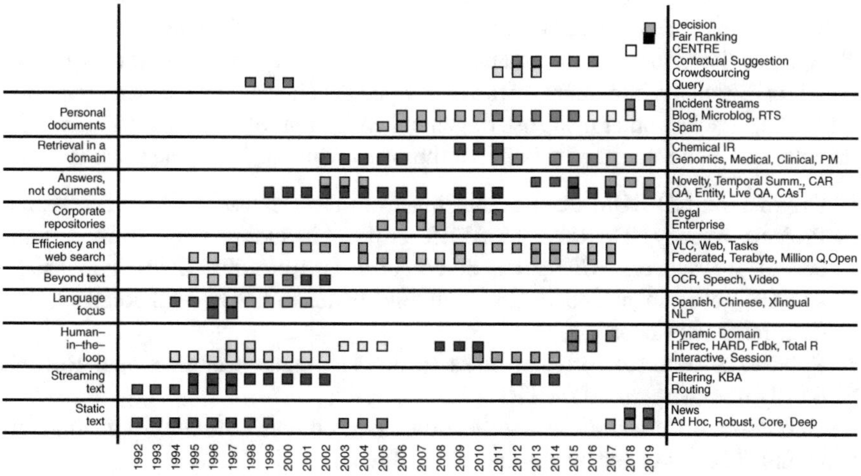

Fig. 8.1 TREC general areas and specific tracks over time (Courtesy, Ellen Voorhees, NIST)

Figure 8.1 shows a classification of TREC tracks with general areas and specific tracks classified within them, which will be explored in this section. Table 8.2 shows the priorities to emerge from the Strategic Workshop on Information Retrieval in Lorne (SWIRL) 2018 gathering of research leaders in the field [10].

The first TREC meeting was held in 1992 and featured two general IR tasks, retrieval of static text and of streaming text. The *ad hoc retrieval task* simulated an IR system, where a static set of documents was searched using new topics, similar to the way a user might search a database or Web search engine with an information need for the first time. The *routing task* simulated a standing query against an oncoming new stream of documents, similar to a topic expert's attempt to extract new information about his or her area of interest. The original tasks used queries created by US government information analysts, who also provided relevance judgments based on pooling of runs generated by TREC participants. By the fourth TREC conference (TREC-4), interest was developing in other IR areas besides ad

Table 8.2 Research priorities from Strategic Workshop on Information Retrieval in Lorne (SWIRL) 2018 [10]

• Conversational information seeking
• Fairness, accountability, confidentiality, and transparency in information retrieval
• IR for supporting knowledge goals and decision-making
• Evaluation
• Machine learning in information retrieval (learnable IR)
• Generated information objects
• Efficiency challenges
• Personal information access

hoc tasks and routing. At that time, the conference began to introduce *tracks* geared to specific interests, each of which developed one or more tasks in each annual cycle.

TREC aims to develop large, real-world test collections, the notion of which has changed as the amount of information and the ability to store and process it have grown over time. While many tracks developed specialized data sources (e.g., the biomedical tracks), other made use of general collections of news, government documents, and Web information. Some of the collections used over the years include:

- Original six CD-ROM disks emanating from the Defense Advanced Research Projects Agency (DARPA) TIPSTER project, including news from a number of newspapers; Computer Select articles from Ziff-Davis Publishing; and US government documents, including patients, the Federal Register, and Congressional Record.
- Robust04—subset of original disks (disks 4–5 minus Congressional Record, mostly newswire), used for TREC Robust Track.
- GOV2—first "terabyte"-level collection based on crawl of. GOV domain, containing 25 million documents and 426 GB in size.
- ClueWeb09—about 25 terabytes (five terabytes compressed) of one billion Web pages in ten languages collected in early 2009, with a subset of 50 million English-language pages (Category B) for smaller-scale experiments.
- ClueWeb12—a successor to ClueWeb09 with about 733 million Web pages and a smaller Category B collection that captured all textual pages (including XML, JavaScript, and CSS pages) and images, but omitted multimedia (e.g., Flash) and compressed (e.g., Zip) files.
- *The Washington Post* news corpus—608,180 news articles and blog posts from 2012 to 2017.
- Microsoft Machine Reading Comprehension (MS-MARCO)—8.8 million passages extracted from 3.6 million Web documents retrieved by Microsoft Bing, used for deep learning in passage and document retrieval.

The ad hoc retrieval task continued for the first eight TREC conferences. Tracks focused on static text searching that were later added included:

- Robust—focus on improving consistency in poorly performing topics [11, 12].
- Common Core—extension of Robust track to explore new methods to build depth and breadth of test collections through additional queries and relevance judgments.

- Deep Learning—using a well-labeled dataset to explore machine learning approaches to IR based on the MS-MARCO collection[4] [13, 14].
- News—supporting searching by both readers and writers of news, with tasks for background linking to a current story and identification of passages that should be linked to other articles.[5]

Additional tracks devoted to retrieval of streaming text were developed beyond the routing task [15]. The Filtering Track added time-stamped documents to add a temporal dimension to the task. A later Knowledge Base Acceleration Track focused on the use case of human knowledge base having the system suggest modifications and extensions to the knowledge base based on monitoring of data streams.

One early interest beyond ad hoc retrieval and filtering early in TREC was cross-language retrieval (CLIR), i.e., querying in one language to retrieve documents in another. This first began with development of parallel corpora and retrieval experiments in Spanish and Chinese, eventually expanding to multiple European languages in the Cross-Language Information Retrieval Track [16]. As noted earlier, this track spun off to become CLEF in 2000. Another language-oriented track in the early years of TREC was the Natural Language Processing (NLP) Track, which explored the use of NLP in retrieval on a subset of the original data. In addition, an Asian-language counterpart of TREC had been launched in 1997, the NII Test Collection for IR Systems (NCTIR),[6] which like CLEF is still running.

Another early interest in TREC was retrieval beyond text. This began with a focus on retrieval of text that had been scanned and processed with optical character recognition (OCR) in the Confusion Track [17, 18]. This was followed by tracks focusing on retrieval of speech and video, with the latter expanding into the still-active TREC Video Retrieval Evaluation (TRECVID).[7]

An additional early interest in TREC was the notion of systems returning answers to questions and just the documents that may contain them. This started with the Question-Answering Track [19]. A number of tracks subsequently adopted aspects of question-answering, including (but not limited to):

- Novelty—investigated systems' abilities to locate new (i.e., nonredundant) information.
- Temporal Summarization—monitor information associated with an event over time.
- Genomics Track in 2006 and 2007 [20].
- Entity—finding entities and properties of entities in Web search.
- Complex Answer Retrieval—collecting references, facts, and opinions into a single coherent summary.[8]

[4] https://microsoft.github.io/msmarco/.

[5] http://trec-news.org/.

[6] http://research.nii.ac.jp/ntcir/index-en.html.

[7] https://trecvid.nist.gov/.

[8] http://trec-car.cs.unh.edu/.

Even though TREC has mostly focused on system-oriented evaluation, there has been interest in interactive search evaluation since its early days. From the start of TREC, research groups had to characterize their runs as automatic or manual, with the latter involving some human modification of the topic text. The Interactive Track started with TREC-3 using a subset of the original TREC disks provided to users in experimental settings using interactive retrieval systems [21]. Starting with TREC-5, an instance recall task was adopted in TREC-5 that shifted the focus away from total numbers of relevant documents retrieval by users but rather instances of topics that more typically motivated real user searching [22].

A number of subsequent tracks have modeled aspects of interactive searching, including:

- High Precision—focusing on providing high precision results to a user.
- High Accuracy Retrieval from Documents (HARD)—aiming to leverage additional information about the searcher and/or search context [23].
- Feedback—evaluate relevance feedback with a single document.
- Session—develop methods for measuring multiple-query sessions where information needs change or get more or less specific over the user's session.
- Total Recall—evaluate methods for tasks that require high recall (e.g., production of systematic reviews), including methods that include a human assessor in the loop.
- Open Search—research groups providing interactive versions of their systems to real users.

Another early interest that has been maintained is search efficiency, especially among large Web collections. This began with the Very Large Collection (VLC) Track in TREC-5, which soon was renamed to the Web Track, reflecting the large quantity of information on the Web [24]. With such large collections, system efficiency became important. The Web Track ran in two different iterations, from 1999–2004 to 2009–2014. Additional tracks focused on large-scale data have included:

- Federated—selection and combination of search results from large number of real Web sites.
- Terabyte—effort to scale up sizes of collections with half-terabyte GOV2 collection [25].
- Million Queries—effort to scale up numbers of queries and determine efficacy of evaluation with small numbers of relevance judgments for each.
- Tasks—systems understanding the tasks that users might be trying to accomplish when they give a query.

An additional emphasis in TREC has been on various focused types of content, including corporate repositories, domain-specific retrieval, and personal documents. The Enterprise Track used a collection of a corporate organization and modeled user tasks typical to that organization.

Domain-specific retrieval in TREC has been focused over several tracks in biomedicine (discussed in the next section) along with those in chemical and legal IR. Personal document retrieval has focused on a number of tasks, such as:

- Spam—detection of unwanted email [26].
- Blog—tasks and search over blogs [27].
- Microblog—focus on real-time information needs and their satisfaction in context of microblogging environments such as Twitter.
- Real-Time Summarization (RTS)—evolution of the Microblog Track focused on real-time update summaries from Twitter streams.[9]
- Incident Streams—automatically process Twitter streams during emergency situations.[10]

A variety of other tracks have focused on other aspects of IR:

- Query—early track focused on impact of variability in queries for a given topic.
- Crowdsourcing—provide collaborative venue to explore crowdsourcing methods for evaluating search and performing search tasks.
- Contextual Suggestion—investigate search techniques for complex information needs highly dependent on context and user interests.[11]
- Health Misinformation—discerning authoritative from unreliable information and correct from incorrect information (originally called the Decision Track).[12]
- CENTRE—effort across TREC, CLEF, and NCTIR to investigate replicability and reproducibility of IR evaluation results.[13]
- Fair Ranking—focus on how well systems provide fair exposure to a variety of authors in an academic search engine,[14] based on a sampled version of the Semantic Scholar Open Research Corpus.[15]
- Conversational Assistance (CAsT)—with the growth of conversational IR, this track focuses on open-domain information-centric conversational search.

8.2 Biomedical and Health IR Research

Although a good deal of biomedical and health IR research was covered in Chap. 7, the focus there was mainly on the evaluation of operational systems and settings. Although the distinction is somewhat imprecise, this section focuses on research systems and how they are used. The section begins with a reporting on several early studies that, due to the functionality of the system or size of the collection, are mainly of historical interest. It then turns to an overview of the TREC biomedical tracks, which continue to influence current research. This is followed by a focus on

[9] http://trecrts.github.io/.

[10] http://dcs.gla.ac.uk/~richardm/TREC_IS/.

[11] https://sites.google.com/site/treccontext/.

[12] https://trec-health-misinfo.github.io/.

[13] https://www.centre-eval.org/.

[14] https://fair-trec.github.io/.

[15] http://api.semanticscholar.org/corpus/.

ad hoc retrieval, i.e., general use of search systems, mainly geared toward professionals. We then turn toward search aimed at specific audiences or tasks, namely, consumer, image, high recall, and electronic health record (EHR).

8.2.1 Early Studies

Biomedical and health uses of IR have been a focus of attention and research since the earliest systems. Some early work focused on improving hypertext capabilities [28], taking advantage of knowledge resources, such as the UMLS Metathesaurus [29, 30], and improving access to high-quality evidence [31]. A number of early test collections included MED [32], a collection from the NLM [33], and OHSUMED[16] [34], which was the largest of its kind at the time and is still used for research at present. The latter consists of about 350,000 MEDLINE with 106 topics judged for relevance.

Some early approaches attempted to map words and phrases in documents and queries into controlled vocabularies. One of the earliest efforts to do this in IR was the SAPHIRE system [35], which aimed to leverage the Unified Medical Language System (UMLS) Metathesaurus[17] and its rich synonym linkages across medical vocabularies (e.g., the MeSH term `Hypertension` was linked to the ICD-9 term `Elevated Blood Pressure`). Since many terms within these vocabularies contained synonyms, the grand sum of all synonymous terms was large, which enabled SAPHIRE to recognize a wide variety of string forms that mapped into concepts.

The original version of SAPHIRE employed a *concept-matching algorithm* in both indexing and retrieval [35]. The algorithm took as its input any string of text, such as a document sentence or a user query, and returned a list of all concepts found, mapped to their *canonical* or preferred form. This was done by detecting the presence of *word-level synonyms* between words in concepts (e.g., high and elevated) as well as *concept-level synonyms* between concepts (e.g., hypertension and high blood pressure). The concept-matching process was purely semantic, with no syntactic methods (e.g., parsing) used. In SAPHIRE's indexing process, the text to be indexed for each document was passed to the concept-matching algorithm. The indexing terms for each document were the concepts matched, which were weighted with IDF and TF redefined for concepts. For retrieval, the user entered a natural language query, and the text was passed to the concept-matching algorithm. Each document with concepts in the list then received a score based on the sum of the weights of terms common to the query and document, with the resulting list of matching documents was then sorted based on the score. SAPHIRE was comprehensively evaluated with databases of several different types and in both batch and

[16] https://dmice.ohsu.edu/hersh/ohsumed/.

[17] https://www.nlm.nih.gov/research/umls/knowledge_sources/metathesaurus/index.html.

interactive modes [36–40]. In all, SAPHIRE showed performance nearly comparable to, but not better than, word-based methods. While its use of synonyms was shown to be beneficial in some queries, the inability to map free text into vocabulary terms hindered it in others.

Another early approach used MEDLINE test collections to define measures of association between the words in the title and abstract of the MEDLINE record and its assigned MeSH terms [41, 42]. In this approach, each MEDLINE record is represented by two vectors, one for words and one for MeSH terms. Initial word-based queries against MEDLINE are expanded to include MeSH terms, which are then used for retrieval by means of the MeSH vectors. Experimental results showed modest performance gains (e.g., 8–9% in average precision), but even better results were obtained by query expansion using the MeSH terms from top-ranking relevant documents. Researchers at NLM also explored semantically assisted query expansion, with their approach processing queries using MetaMap to identify Metathesaurus terms, which were in turn used to expand queries by means of the INQUERY system [43].

Another line of work looked at methods for reordering search output to identify "important" articles in bibliographic databases such as MEDLINE. Bernstam et al. assessed a variety of citation-based algorithms that attempted to rank documents deemed important by inclusion in a bibliography about surgical oncology [44]. They compared eight different algorithms: simple PubMed queries, PubMed clinical queries (sensitive and specific versions), vector cosine, citation count, journal impact factor, PageRank, and a machine learning approach based on polynomial support vector machines. The citation-based algorithms were found to be more effective than noncitation-based algorithms at identifying important articles. The most effective strategies were simple citation count and PageRank, which on average identified over six important articles in the first 100 results compared to <1 for the best noncitation-based algorithm. Similar differences were observed between citation-based and noncitation-based algorithms at 10, 20, 50, 200, 500, and 1000 results. They also assessed citation lag, i.e., how it takes a period of time before citations to appear to an important article. This was found to affect performance of PageRank more than simple citation count. In spite of citation lag, however, the citation-based algorithms were still more effective than noncitation-based algorithms. They concluded that algorithms that were successful on the Web could be applied to biomedical information retrieval, helping to identify important articles within large sets of relevant results. Further work by Aphinyanaphongs et al. found even better performance with the addition of machine learning techniques [45].

Another system of historical interest that aimed to implement hypermedia capabilities was Frisse's Dynamic Medical Handbook project [28]. The system's retrieval approach began with a conventional word-based ranking approach but modified document weighting to account for terms in linked nodes. The system used two weighting components for ranking nodes. The *intrinsic* component of the weight consisted of the usual TF*IDF weighting for the words common to each node and the query. The *extrinsic* component, however, was the weights of all immediately linked nodes divided by the number of such nodes:

$$\text{WEIGHT}_i = \sum_j \text{WEIGHT}_{ij} + \frac{1}{y}\sum_d \text{WEIGHT}_d \quad (8.1)$$

where WEIGHT_i was the total weight of node i, j was the number of search terms, WEIGHT_{ij} was the weight of all the search terms j in node i, y was the number of immediately linked nodes, d was the index number of immediately linked nodes, and WEIGHT_d was the weight of each linked node.

8.2.2 Challenge Evaluations in Biomedicine and Health

The first biomedical track in any challenge evaluation was the TREC Genomics Track, which was introduced in 2003 and spawned an area of IR now generally called domain-specific IR. Three other biomedical and health-related tracks have followed. CLEF has also introduced biomedical and health tasks in imaging, consumer health search, and systematic review assistance.

8.2.2.1 TREC Genomics Track

The first biomedical track in TREC was the Genomics Track,[18] the results of which were summarized in an overview paper that was part of a special issue of the journal, *Information Retrieval* [20]. The tasks of the track for each year are shown in Table 8.3. In essence, the first 2 years focused on ad hoc retrieval of bibliographic references, while the next year focused on full-text ad hoc retrieval and the final year was devoted to passage retrieval and question-answering.

The first 2 years of the Genomics Track mainly focused on ad hoc retrieval in the genomics domain. The 2004 [52] and 2005 [49] tasks modeled the situation of a user with an information need using an IR system to access the biomedical scientific literature. The document collection was based on a 10-year subset of MEDLINE. Topics for the ad hoc retrieval task were based on information needs collected from real biologists.

In the 2004 track, the best results were obtained by a combination of Okapi weighting (BM25 for term frequency but with standard inverse document frequency), Porter stemming, expansion of gene names and symbols using a genome translation tool and MeSH, query expansion, and use of all three fields of the topic (title, need, and context) [53]. These achieved a MAP of 0.4075. Another group achieved high-ranking results with a combination of approaches that included Okapi weighting, query expansion, and various forms of domain-specific query expansion (including expansion of lexical variants as well as acronym, gene, and protein name synonyms) [54]. Approaches that attempted to map to controlled vocabulary terms did not fare as well [55–57].

[18] https://dmice.ohsu.edu/trec-gen/.

Table 8.3 Tasks of the TREC Genomics Track

Year	Task description	Document collection	Topics
2003 [46]	Ad hoc retrieval	A 1-year (4/2002–4/2003) subset of 525,938 MEDLINE records	Gene names, with the goal of finding all MEDLINE references that focus on the basic biology of the gene or its protein products from the designated organism
2003 [46]	GeneRIF [47] annotation from article titles and abstract	139 articles that had been assigned GeneRIFs, derived from all articles appearing in five journals during the latter half of 2002	Assigned GeneRIFs
2004 [48]	Ad hoc retrieval	A 10-year subset (1994–2003) of 4,591,008 MEDLINE records	50 information needs statements with title, information need, and context (background)
2004 [48]	Categorization of documents containing data about gene function suitable for "triage" to annotators assigning gene ontology (GO) codes for mouse genome informatics database	A 3-year set of 11,880 full-text articles for three journals obtained from HighWire press	N/A
2005 [49]	Ad hoc retrieval	A 10-year subset (1994–2003) of 4,591,008 MEDLINE records	50 information needs statements similar to 2004 but classified into one of five generic topic types (GTTs)
2005 [49]	Categorization of documents containing data about gene function suitable for "triage" to annotators assigning GO codes or identifying for inclusion into databases about tumor biology, embryologic gene expression, or alleles of mutant phenotypes for mouse genome informatics	A 3-year set of 11,880 full-text articles for three journals obtained from HighWire press	N/A
2006 [50]	Retrieval of passages (from part of sentence to paragraph in length) with linkage to 5 entities (e.g., genes, proteins) and the source article	Collection of 162,259 full-text HTML documents from 49 journals that publish electronically via HighWire press	28 question statements based on GTTs
2007 [51]	Entity-based question-answering based on retrieval of passages linked to 14 entities and the source article	Collection of 162,259 full-text HTML documents from 49 journals that publish electronically via HighWire press	36 question statements based on the 14 entities

Somewhat similar results were obtained in the 2005 track. As with 2004, the basic Okapi weighting gave good baseline performance, with manual synonym expansion of queries giving the highest MAP [58], although automated query expansion did not fare as well [59, 60]. Relevance feedback was found to be beneficial, but worked best without term expansion [61].

The first 2 years of the TREC Genomics Track also featured a text categorization task [49, 52]. The mail goal of the task was to "triage" articles for human annotators in the Mouse Genome Informatics (MGI) resource.[19] Systems were required to classify full-text documents from a 2-year span (2002–2003) of three journals, with the first year's (2002) documents comprising the training data and the second year's (2003) documents making up the test data.

In 2006 and 2007, the track shifted to a task of *entity-based question-answering* [50, 51]. The rationale for this was that many information seekers, especially users of the biomedical literature, desired a system that provided short, specific answers to questions and put them in context by providing supporting information and linking to original sources. As such, the track developed a task that focused on retrieval of short passages (from phrase to sentence to paragraph in length) that specifically addressed an information need, along with linkage to the location in the original source document.

8.2.2.2 TREC Medical Records Track

TREC launched its second biomedical track, the Medical Records Track, in 2011 [62]. The track ran again in 2012 although was not continued after that due to problems with the availability of the data [63]. The task of the TREC 2011–2012 Medical Records Tracks consisted of searching EHR documents in order to identify patients matching a set of clinical criteria, a use case that might be part of the identification of individuals eligible for a clinical study or trial [64]. The task's various topics each represented a different case definition, with the topics varying widely in terms of detail and linguistic complexity. This use case is one of a larger group that represent the reuse (or secondary use) of data in EHRs that facilitate clinical research, quality improvement, and the learning health system [65–67].

The corpus for the TREC Medical Records Track consisted of a set of 93,552 patient notes extracted from the EHR system of the University of Pittsburgh Medical Center (UPMC). Each note was part of an encounter that represented a visit to the hospital, either to the emergency department or an admission to the hospital, as depicted in Fig. 8.2. Hospital encounters contained multiple notes entered by clinicians as well as reports of results. The de-identification process removed protected health information (PHI), e.g., age numbers were converted to a range.

The corpus contained 17,265 unique patient encounters. Most (~70%) included five or fewer reports; virtually all (~97%) included less than 20. The maximum

[19] http://www.informatics.jax.org/

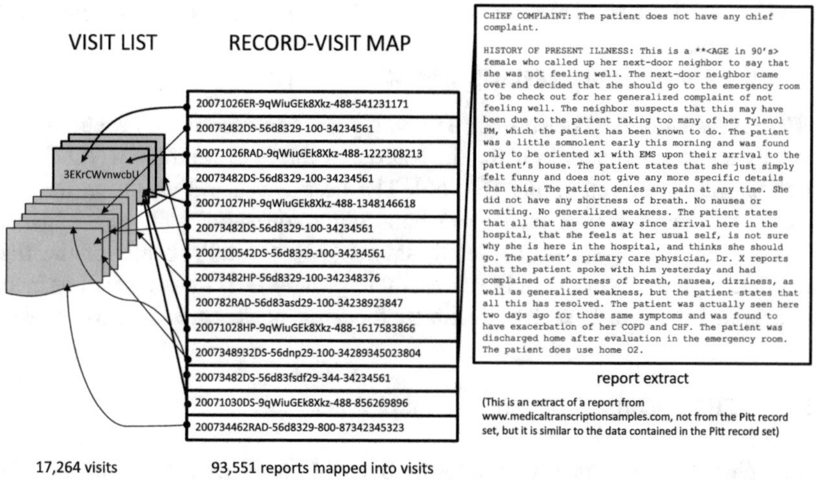
VISIT LIST
RECORD-VISIT MAP
3EKrCWvnwcbU
20071026ER-9qWiuGEk8Xkz-488-541231171
20073482DS-56d8329-100-34234561
20071026RAD-9qWiuGEk8Xkz-488-1222308213
20073482DS-56d8329-100-34234561
20071027HP-9qWiuGEk8Xkz-488-1348146618
20073482DS-56d8329-100-34234561
2007100542DS-56d8329-100-34234561
20073482HP-56d8329-100-342348376
200782RAD-56d83asd29-100-34238923847
20071028HP-9qWiuGEk8Xkz-488-1617583866
2007348932DS-56dnp29-100-34289345023804
20073482DS-56d83fsdf29-344-34234561
20071030DS-9qWiuGEk8Xkz-488-856269896
200734462RAD-56d8329-800-87342345323
CHIEF COMPLAINT: The patient does not have any chief complaint.
HISTORY OF PRESENT ILLNESS: This is a **<AGE in 90’s> female who called up her next-door neighbor to say that she was not feeling well. The next-door neighbor came over and decided that she should go to the emergency room to be check out for her generalized complaint of not feeling well. The neighbor suspects that this may have been due to the patient taking too many of her Tylenol PM, which the patient has been known to do. The patient was a little somnolent early this morning and was found only to be oriented x1 with EMS upon their arrival to the patient’s house. The patient states that she just simply felt funny and does not give any more specific details than this. The patient denies any pain at any time. She did not have any shortness of breath. No nausea or vomiting. No generalized weakness. The patient states that all that has gone away since arrival here in the hospital, that she feels at her usual self, is not sure why she is here in the hospital, and thinks she should go. The patient’s primary care physician, Dr. X reports that the patient spoke with him yesterday and had complained of shortness of breath, nausea, dizziness, as well as generalized weakness, but the patient states that all this has resolved. The patient was actually seen here two days ago for those same symptoms and was found to have exacerbation of her COPD and CHF. The patient was discharged home after evaluation in the emergency room. The patient does use home O2.
report extract
(This is an extract of a report from www.medicaltranscriptionsamples.com, not from the Pitt record set, but it is similar to the data contained in the Pitt record set)
17,264 visits
93,551 reports mapped into visits

Fig. 8.2 Structure of collection for TREC Medical Records Track (Courtesy, Ellen Voorhees, NIST)

number of notes comprising any encounter was 415. Each encounter had a chief complaint as well as one admission ICD-9 code and a set of discharge ICD-9 codes. The number of discharge ICD-9 codes varied widely from visit to visit; the median number of codes per visit was five, while the maximum was 25. Patients could not be linked across visits, i.e., be identified as having more than one visit, due to the de-identification process applied to the corpus. As such, for the purposes of this task, the "unit of retrieval" was the encounter rather than the patient, meaning that the participating systems were to produce a set of matching encounters for each topic.

In the first year of the task, the B-Pref measure was used to assess performance, since the resources available for relevance judging led to likely incomplete judgments. As often occurs with test collections, performance varied widely across different topics. An overall analysis found easy, hard, and highly variable topics.

- Easiest—best median B-Pref.
  - 105—Patients with dementia
  - 132—Patients admitted for surgery of the cervical spine for fusion or discectomy
- Hardest—worst best B-Pref and worst median B-Pref.
  - 108—Patients treated for vascular claudication surgically
  - 124—Patients who present to the hospital with episodes of acute loss of vision secondary to glaucoma
- Large differences between best and median B-Pref.
  - 103—Hospitalized patients treated for methicillin-resistant *Staphylococcus aureus* (MRSA) endocarditis

- 111—Patients with chronic back pain who receive an intraspinal pain-medicine pump
- 125—Patients coinfected with hepatitis C and HIV.

The consistently best performance in both years came from the development of manually constructed queries using the National Library of Medicine (NLM) Essie search engine described earlier [68, 69]. The best automated results in the 2011 track filtered queries by age, race, gender, and admission status, with terms expanded by synonyms from the UMLS Metathesaurus [70]. Overall, results of the track found that approaches commonly successful in general IR provided small or inconsistent value for this task, such as document focusing, negation, and term expansion.

8.2.2.3 TREC Clinical Decision Support Track

The Medical Records Track was followed by the Clinical Decision Support (CDS) Track,[20] which was started in 2014 [71, 72] and continued for two additional years [73, 74]. In some ways more of a traditional IR task, the track had the use case of providing documents that might answer three types of clinical questions about diagnosis, tests, and treatments. The document collection consisted of an open access subset of PubMed Central (PMC). The track used a subset containing 733,138 articles. Images and other supplementary material from PMC were also available, although not included in base release of documents. Each of the topics in the 2014 track consisted of a case narrative plus label designating to which basic clinical task the topic pertained. The topics were developed by physicians at the National Institutes of Health (NIH), who developed ten topics for each clinical task type. Each topic statement included both a description of the problem and a shorter, more focused summary. The case narratives were used as an idealized medical record since no collections of actual medical records were available.

8.2.2.4 TREC Precision Medicine Track

The CDS track was transformed into the Precision Medicine Track in 2017, which continued through 2020 (although the Web site continued from the CDS Track[21]) [75, 76]. This track implemented the so-called precision medicine paradigm, focused on genetic variants associated with different types of cancer. The document collection consisted of a snapshot of MEDLINE (26.8 million abstracts in 2017–2018 and 29.1 million abstracts in 2019–2020) as well as 241,006 clinical trials descriptions from ClinicalTrials.gov. (The 2017–2018 tracks also included about 70,000 abstracts from recent proceedings of the American Society of Clinical Oncology and the American Association for Cancer Research.) Topics contained disease names, genetic variant designation, and patient demographic information, with relevance defined as those matching the attributes in the topic.

---

[20] http://www.trec-cds.org/.

[21] http://www.trec-cds.org/.

8.2.2.5 CLEF Cross Language Image Retrieval Track (ImageCLEF)

The CLEF Cross Language Image Retrieval Track (ImageCLEF)[22] has had medical image retrieval among its tasks. The ImageCLEF Medical Track (ImageCLEFmed) began in the mid-2000s with relatively small collections consisting of images and their clinical annotations, collected into "cases" representing a typical study done in a medical image setting. The structure of the collection is shown in Fig. 8.3, while an example case is shown in Fig. 8.4. Early work focused on simple ad hoc retrieval of single images [77]. This early work found that mixing visual and textual approaches performed better than those using either approach alone. However, textual approaches were more robust, i.e., they were more resilient to difficult visually oriented topics than visual systems were to difficult textually oriented topics. Visual methods tended to work best when the topic specified an image modality or highly specific finding, e.g., a certain type of X-ray and/or a type of finding that always appears similar. On the other hand, textual methods tended to work best when a higher-level concept was sought, e.g., images of many modalities for a given disease or clinical finding. The early work was summarized in an overview paper [78] and a book describing all of ImageCLEF, not just the medical task [79].

The second task to be added to ImageCLEFmed was case-based retrieval. In this task, given a case description with patient demographics, limited symptoms, and test results including imaging studies (but not the final diagnosis), systems were required

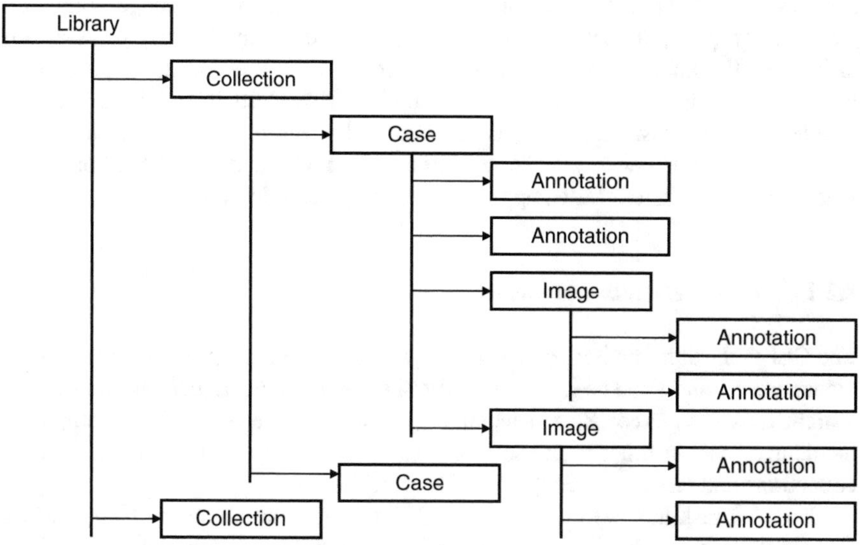

Fig. 8.3 Structure of the ImageCLEFmed test collection

[22] https://www.imageclef.org/.

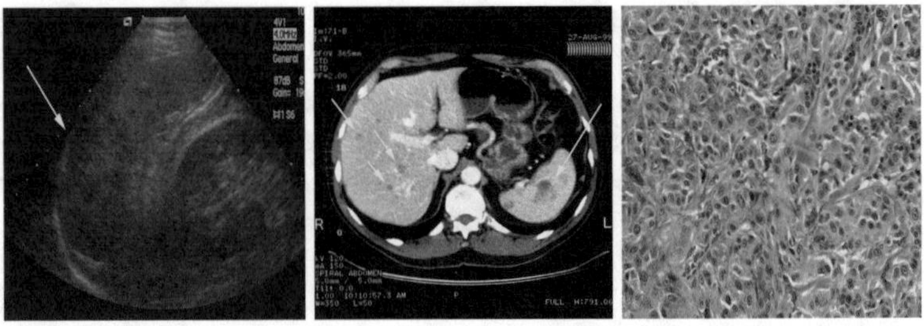

Case annotation

ID: 4272
Description: A large hypoechoic mass is seen in the spleen. CDFI reveals it to be hypovascular and distorts the intrasplenic blood vessels. This lesion is consistent with a metastatic lesion. Urinary obstruction is present on the right with pelvo-caliceal and uretreal dilatation secondary to a soft tissue lesion at the junction of the ureter and baldder. This is another secondary lesion of the malignant melanoma. Surprisingly, these lesions are not hypervascular on doppler nor on CT. Metastasis are also visible in the liver.
Diagnosis: Metastasis of spleen and ureter, malignant melanoma
Clinical Presentation: Workup in a patient with malignant melanoma. Intravenous pyelography showed no excretion of contrast on the right.

Fig. 8.4 Example case from the ImageCLEF test collection

to retrieve cases that included images that best suited the case description [80]. Similar to ad hoc retrieval, the best results came from textual and not visual queries [81, 82].

Another task to be added to ImageCLEFmed was modality classification, where systems attempted to identify the image modality (e.g., radiologic image, computerized tomography, publication figures, photographs, etc.). In the early years of this task, a small number (6–8) of modality categories were used. In 2012, however, a larger classification was developed that included over 20 items [83]. With the smaller, earlier classification set, mixed text and visual retrieval methods worked best, but with the newer and larger classification visual retrieval methods have worked better, with text-based approaches alone performing poorly [82].

8.2.2.6 CLEF eHealth Lab Series

The CLEF eHealth Lab Series[23] has focused on information extraction, information management, and IR. The latter has had tasks in patient-centered/consumer health search, cross-language IR, and technology-assisted reviews (TARs) in empirical medicine. The consumer health search tasks have run since 2013, with the specific collections and tasks for each year are listed in Table 8.4.

The TAR task has been run since 2017. They were structured by taking search statements from Cochrane systematic reviews to build a collection of PMIDs from which participants could query to retrieve. In 2017 and 2018, the TAR task focused on systematic reviews of diagnostic accuracy studies. In 2019, the task was expanded

[23] http://clef-ehealth.org/.

Table 8.4 CLEF eHealth Labs consumer health search collections and tasks

Year	Collection	Task(s)
2013	1 M documents from medical web crawl	Queries from consumers on discharge summaries
2014	Revised 1 M document medical web crawl with errors corrected	Multilingual consumer queries
2015	Same as 2014	Queries by laypeople with sign, symptom, or condition and attempt to find out more about the condition they may have
2016	ClueWeb 12 B13	Queries derived from consumer health forums, with variations and cross-language provided
2017	Same as 2016	Consumer health search with four subtasks: Ad hoc search, personalized search, query variations, and multilingual ad hoc search
2018	Extract from common Crawl[a] for about 2000 health-related domains	Consumer health search same as 2017 with addition of query intent
2019	(not run)	
2020	Same as 2018	Consumer health search with two subtasks: Ad hoc search and spoken queries

[a]https://commoncrawl.org/

to include systematic reviews of interventions as well as introduce a higher gain (score) for studies with low risk of bias (i.e., assumed to be more important to the review).

8.2.3 Ad Hoc Retrieval

Research in ad hoc retrieval in the biomedical and health domain has mostly, although not exclusively, focused on improving results over the various collections developed for TREC and CLEF. This section will focus on research in general biomedical and health ad hoc search, with subsequent sections focused on consumer, image, high-recall, and EHR search.

Follow-up research with the TREC Genomics Track ad hoc retrieval test collection has yielded a variety of findings. One study assessed word tokenization, stemming, and stop word removal, finding that varying strategies for the first resulted in substantial performance impact while changes in the latter two had minimal impact. Tokenization in genomics text can be challenging due to the use of a wide variety of symbols, including numbers, hyphens, super- and subscripts, and characters in non-English languages (e.g., Greek) [84]. Other studies found value for language modeling approaches to term weighting [85] and the related-articles feature of PubMed [86]. Additional work with TREC Genomics Track data found that language model approaches increased performance over standard TF*IDF, with further gains seen from including MeSH terms in documents and the use of blind query expansion [87].

Some researchers have used TREC CDS Track data to assess new methods to improve on this task. Most work focused on reformulating the topics, which in the original test collection were patient case descriptions, aiming to promote the most important terms for retrieving relevant articles. One approach aimed to identify important named entities in the search to re-rank search results that contain those entities [88]. Another approach also aimed to identify important terms combined with document query expansion [89]. An additional method attempted to automate the paring of the patient descriptions to more focused queries but found that human-generated queries outperformed attempts to automate querying [90].

Some research using the TREC Genomics test collection focused on improving the assignment of Medical Subject Headings (MeSH) terms by automated means. One line of work evaluated the NLM's Medical Text Indexer (MTI) introduced in Chap. 4.

The European Commission and the NLM organized a challenge evaluation to assess semantic indexing of literature called BioASQ[24] [91]. One task from this analysis found that the MTI was still useful and could possibly be augmented with machine learning approaches [92]. The study also found that assisted indexing using MTI tended to perform better with precision tasks than recall tasks. It also showed that after 12 years of use, the MTI still provided value as a tool to aid MeSH term selection by indexers [92].

Trieschnigg et al. introduced an approach called MeSH Up that uses a machine learning classification approach called k-nearest neighbor (KNN) that performed better than MetaMap, the NLM's Medical Text Indexer (MTI), and other concept-oriented approaches [93]. Aljaber et al. developed an approach that gathered MeSH terms from articles that the paper being indexed cited and ranked them based on if and where they occurred in the paper being indexed, with evaluation showing improved performance over MTI and MeSH Up [94]. Other researchers have explored this task using other test collections, with Huang et al. finding value for machine-meaning approaches [95] and Herskovic et al. showing benefit for inserting a graph-based ranking approach of MeSH terms into the MTI process [96].

Other research has focused on the development of new resources. Kim et al. developed a resource, PubMed Phrases, aiming to identify coherent groups of words that demonstrated benefit for retrieval tasks, including their use in the new relevance search methods used in PubMed [97]. The resource developed a set of 705,915 phrases, which were evaluated using PubMed user click data and manually annotation of a sample of randomly selected noun phrases.

Brown et al. developed the RElevant LIterature SearcH (RELISH) Consortium,[25] consisting of more than 1500 scientists from 84 countries who collectively annotated the relevance of over 180,000 articles indexed in PubMed with regard to their respective seed (input) article(s) [98]. The collection was found to cover over 76% of all unique Medical Subject Headings (MeSH) terms, with annotations of the same document pairs contributed by different scientists being highly concordant.

---

[24] http://www.bioasq.org/.

[25] https://relishdb.ict.griffith.edu.au/.

The authors also found that three representative baseline weighting methods used to generate recommended articles for evaluation (Okapi BM25, TF*IDF, and PubMed Related Articles) had similar overall performances, although each method tended to produce distinct collections of recommended articles, which suggested that a hybrid method may be required to completely capture all relevant articles.

Another focus of work spawned a new challenge evaluation focused on dataset retrieval using the biomedical and healthCAre Data Discovery Index Ecosystem (bioCADDIE),[26] a database of metadata about datasets available online. The bioCADDIE 2016 Dataset Retrieval Challenge used a snapshot of bioCADDIE and 30 queries to form a challenge evaluation [99, 100]. The best results came from term-based query expansion, usually employing aspects of MeSH. A number of groups used machine learning approaches, although these may have been limited by the small amount of training data that had been made available.

8.2.4 Consumer-Oriented

A good deal of consumer-oriented health search has used test collections develop from the IR portion of the CLEF eHealth Evaluation Lab. One major area of work has focused on the mismatch between the language consumers use to describe health and that use both in medical content and controlled terminologies used to index that content. Some approaches have attempted to map colloquial terms used by consumers to professional medical terms [101]. One investigation found value for a process of "query clarification," which added the most appropriate expert terms to queries submitted by users and found benefit in consumers being able to answer questions using a major search engine [102]. Additional performance was found with use of a learning-to-rank approach [103]. There may also be value to query expansion using a consumer health vocabulary [104]. Another approach assessed consumer health page readability, finding a method using machine learning worked better than traditional readability measures [105].

Somewhat related work has focused on creating automated question-answering systems for consumer health sites. As organizations like the NLM get many health-related queries for which they do not have resources to answer, automated approaches are required to handle the volume, although there is concern about the quality and correctness of answers. The NLM developed and evaluated a system, Consumer Health Information and Question Answering (CHiQA),[27] which searches over online sources known to be medically reliable [106]. A product of this research was a corpus of consumer health questions for further research[28] [107]. A related

[26] https://datamed.org/.

[27] https://chiqa.nlm.nih.gov/.

[28] https://bionlp.nlm.nih.gov/CHIQAcollections/CHQA-Corpus-1.0.zip.

approach in this area has focused on linking patient notes to consumer materials in MedlinePlus [108].

Other consumer health search work has focused on the impact of misleading or incorrect search results. This work emanates from research in the early days of the Web on efforts, manual and automated, to help searchers discern the quality of health information on the Web, e.g., [109]. Pogacar et al. assessed the influence of retrieval of correct vs. incorrect information, finding that search results biased with the latter led individuals to more frequently answer health-related questions incorrectly [110]. This led Lioma et al. to develop metrics designed to measure the effectiveness of relevance and credibility of retrieval results, with evaluation finding the measures both expressive and intuitive in their interpretation by humans [111]. This work resulted in development of a new TREC Health Misinformation Track (initially called the Decision Track) [112].

Another line of work has focused on analysis of user search logs to understand aspects of health-related searching. Early work focused on processing search logs, mostly from Microsoft Bing, to understand users' characteristics and intentions [113, 114]. This approach has uncovered "cyberchondria," defined as unnecessary escalation of health-related concern when searching [115], and "Web-scale pharmacovigilance," the uncovering of drug interactions from search logs [116, 117]. This approach has also been used to identify patients who have a higher likelihood to develop pancreatic carcinoma [118] and lung carcinoma [119]. Some limitations of these approaches are the retrospective nature of the data and the inferring of user actions and intent solely from the search logs.

8.2.5 Image Retrieval

ImageCLEFmed has continued within CLEF and branched out into other tasks, such as [120]:

- Classification.
- Compound figure separation.
- Compound figure detection.
- Multilabel classification.
- Liver CT annotation.
- Caption prediction.
- Tuberculosis.

An overview of lessons learned from ImageCLEFmed concluded [121]:

- Text retrieval worked better overall than visual retrieval.
- Visual retrieval could be effective for highly precise tasks, such as modality detection and others with small numbers of classes.
- Visual retrieval could also give high early precision, whereas text retrieval sometimes did not.

- Fusion of text and visual approaches was only occasionally helpful and had to be done with care.
- Mapping free text queries to controlled terminologies could be helpful.

Other work in image retrieval has used other image collections. Some work has focused on mapping across the "semantic gap" of what is in the image and its textual annotation [122]. This is especially so for queries that tend to be textually oriented [123]. Some research has shown value for use of relevance feedback from textual and image features [124, 125].

Other work has focused on retrieval of journal images based on captions [126, 127] and on their annotation with the goal of improving retrieval [128]. An additional analysis of journal article images, focused on figures included in PubMed, categorized images into five figure types and analyzed them related to scholarly impact. Although the distribution of figures and figure types in the literature remained constant over time, it was found to vary by field and topic. A significant correlation was noted between scientific impact and use of visual information, with higher impact papers tending to include more diagrams and plots [129].

8.2.6 High-Recall Retrieval

Some biomedical and health search tasks require high recall, i.e., attempting to find every possible relevant item. One of the best-known use cases for this type of retrieval is identifying studies for inclusion in systematic reviews. Early work in this area used a dataset for systematic reviews of drug class efficacy [130, 131]. Various machine learning approaches were found to reduce systematic review workload by prioritizing articles likely to qualify for inclusion in the reviews [132, 133]. Others have also used machine learning to recognize from the stream of new literature high-quality evidence in clinical studies [134–136].

Subsequently, challenge evaluations were developed in the technology-assisted reviews (TARs) in empirical medicine task of the CLEF eHealth Lab Series [137–139]. Another test collection[29] was developed by Scells et al. [140]. A number of methods have shown value based on the CLEF eHealth TAR collections. One challenge is that while modifications to the original Boolean queries used in the Cochrane reviews could result in better performance, predicting which one would be best for a given review was difficult to determine [141, 142]. One approach using a known relevant "seed" document to retrieve others improved performance, which was further enhanced using word embedding approaches [143].

[29] https://github.com/ielab/SIGIR2017-PICO-Collection.

8.2.7 EHR Retrieval

As evidenced by the formation of the TREC Medical Records Track, search over EHR data is an area of growing interest. The most prominent use case has been the identifying of patients who might be candidates for clinical studies. In the TREC track, a number of research groups used a variety of techniques, such as synonym and query expansion, machine learning algorithms, and matching against ICD-9 codes, but still had results that did not improve upon manually constructed queries. A failure analysis over the data from the 2011 track demonstrated why there are still challenges to overcome [144]. The first part of this analysis found reasons why visits frequently retrieved were not relevant to the topic:

- Notes contain very similar term confused with topic.
- Topic symptom/condition/procedure done in the past.
- Most, but not all, criteria present.
- All criteria present but not in the time/sequence specified by the topic description.
- Topic terms mentioned as future possibility.
- Topic terms not present—can't determine why record was captured.
- Irrelevant reference in record to topic terms.
- Topic terms denied or ruled out.

A second analysis found reasons why visits rarely retrieved were actually relevant:

- Topic terms present in record but overlooked in search.
- Visit notes used a synonym for topic terms.
- Topic terms not named and must be derived.
- Topic terms present in diagnosis list but not visit notes.

Koopman et al. further explored the "semantic gap" in medical IR and the inference required for overcoming it [145]:

- Vocabulary mismatch—synonyms including acronyms.
- Granularity mismatch—class vs. individual names.
- Conceptual implication—organisms or treatments imply diseases.
- Inferences of similarity—symptoms or diseases that commonly occur.
- Context-specific semantic gaps—negation, temporality, age and gender, and different levels of evidence (e.g., location in the history, physical exam, assessment, or plan).

Identification of these problems led Koopman et al. to carry out new experiments, which identified a substantial number of previously unjudged encounters and were subsequently judged.[30] They implemented a graph inference network approach using SNOMED CT to address the first four issues that led to improved performance for some topics but not others.

[30] https://github.com/ielab/MedIR2014-RelanceAssessment.

Other follow-on studies using the test collection reported benefit from various approaches to query expansion:

- Addition of ICD-9 codes to queries [146].
- Adding terms from other resources [147].
- Adding additional nonsynonym terms from the UMLS Metathesaurus [148].
- Using negation [149] and specialized term and concept representations [150–152].
- Learning relevance models [153].

There are some unique challenges for IR research with medical records. One of these, not limited to IR (e.g., also including NLP, machine learning, etc.), is the privacy of the patients whose records are being searched [154]. Given the growing concern over privacy and confidentiality, how can informatics (including IR) researchers carry out this work while assuring no information about patients is revealed? Some have suggested de-identification, although examples of the ability to reidentify data have kept healthcare institutions from releasing their data in this manner [155, 156]. Others have proposed use of encrypted data, although this too had allowed identification of individuals [157].

It turns out that this problem is not limited to medical records. There are many private collections of information over which we might like to search, such as email or corporate repositories. One proposal to address this problem has been dubbed, Evaluation as a Service (EaaS), based on the notion that data resides on a secure server and systems are sent to the server to run on the data [158]. Those who send systems to run on the data only see their evaluation results and not any of the actual data that their systems use. One comparison of EaaS and regular retrieval approaches found results obtained by IR research groups to be comparable [159]. This approach was used by the TREC Total Recall Track for confidential email messages [160]. Hanbury et al. proposed for sensitive medical documents [161, 162]. A major limitation to this approach is that researchers run their systems on the data (securely somewhere else), so they do not see the data and only get results of their runs.

One consequence of the privacy problem has been the inhibition of public datasets for EHR retrieval research. The UPMC test collection used for TREC has been publicly withdrawn (although many researchers still have usage agreements allowing them to continue using it), leaving the Medical Information Mart for Intensive Care (MIMIC)-III collection[31] as the only large-scale publicly available de-identified collection of medical records [163]. While many organizations have continued research on the patient cohort retrieval use case, none have been able to share their data. Researchers from Oregon Health & Science University [164] and Mayo Clinic [165] have been conducting research in parallel with a shared set of retrieval topics [166].

[31] https://mimic.physionet.org/.

8.3 General IR Research

Similar to the above section on biomedical and health IR, this section provides an overview of some important early IR research. As noted previously, the monograph by Harman describes early research in IR [5]. The major thrust of computational IR research has been to develop methods for matching relevant content items to user needs. While users have a diversity of information needs [167], and relevance is a complex notion [168], a great deal of research has focused on this notion. Although guarded by trade secrets, it is likely that commercial search engines prioritize this as well. This section begins with an overview of early research and then focuses on more recent directions, especially those involving the use of machine learning.

8.3.1 Overview of Early Research

As noted in several places already in this book, the major early leader in the IR research was Gerard Salton, who passed away in 1995 before he could see his work achieve widespread uptake in modern search systems [169, 170]. Salton focused on so-called automated retrieval, aiming to develop computer algorithms requiring minimal human involvement in indexing or retrieval. This approach was also called partial-match retrieval, because it relied on incomplete matching between query and document terms. It was also described as lexical-statistical, i.e., *lexical* because the unit of indexing was the individual word in the document and *statistical* because indexing and retrieval involved operations like weighting of terms and documents. Salton argued that these systems offered many appealing features, especially to novice end users who were less skilled in the use of controlled vocabularies, Boolean operators, and other advanced features of traditional retrieval systems. A basic approach for this type of indexing and retrieval was introduced in Chaps. 4 and 5, respectively, because some of these methods are now used in state-of-the-art systems.

Salton named his initial approach to IR as the *vector-space model*, where documents were represented as N-dimensional vectors, where N was the number of indexing terms in the database [169]. Vectors could be binary or weighted, with term weighting represented by the length of the vector in a given dimension. Queries were also represented as vectors, so that the retrieval process consisted of measuring the similarity between a query vector and all the document vectors in the database. The simplest method of doing this was to take the dot or inner product of the query and each document vector. When used with term frequency (TF) and inverse document frequency (IDF) weighting, this reduced to the partial-match indexing and retrieval approaches described in Chaps. 4 and 5. We also saw in Chap. 5 that this basic approach could be extended to include document length normalization to control for the length of documents in relevance ranking and relevance feedback to allow retrieval of more documents similar to ones already retrieved that were relevant.

The TREC era saw the development of some measures that gave somewhat better results than simple TF*IDF weighing [171]. The most prominent of these was based on a statistical model known as Poisson distributions and has been more commonly called *Okapi* or *BM25 weighting* [172]. This weighting scheme improved document normalization, yielding up to 50% improvement in mean average precision (MAP) in various TREC collections [173]. A common version of Okapi TF often used is:

$$\text{Okapi TF} = \frac{\text{frequency of term in document}}{0.5 + 1.5\dfrac{\text{length of document}}{\text{average document length}} + \text{frequency of term in document}} \tag{8.2}$$

Okapi weighting has its theoretical foundations in probabilistic IR, with its TF*IDF weighting using a "probabilistic" variant of IDF:

$$\text{Okapi IDF} = \log \frac{\text{total number of documents} - \text{number of documents with term} + 0.5}{\text{number of documents with term} + 0.5} \tag{8.3}$$

The probabilistic model has also led to a newer theoretical approach to term weighting, known as *language modeling*, which is described below.

Another approach to term weighting was to employ probability theory. This approach was not necessarily at odds with the vector-space model, and in fact its weighting approaches could be incorporated into the vector-space model. The theory underlying probabilistic IR was a model to give more weight to terms likely to occur in relevant documents and unlikely to occur in nonrelevant documents. It was based on Bayes' theorem, a common probability measure that indicates likelihood of an event based on a prior situation and new data. Probabilistic IR was predominantly a relevance feedback technique, since some relevance information about the terms in documents was required. Early attempts at probabilistic IR did not improve search results, but some success was seen with the *inference model* of Turtle and Croft [174], where documents were ranked based on how likely they are to infer belief they are relevant to the user's query.

A subsequent application of probabilistic IR was the use of *language modeling* [175]. This approach was adapted from other computer tasks, such as speech recognition and machine translation, where probabilistic principles were used to convert acoustic signals into words and words from one language to another, respectively. A key aspect of the language modeling approach was "smoothing" of the probabilities away from a purely deterministic approach of a term being present or absent in a document in a binary fashion. Theoretically, the language modeling approach measured the probability of a query term given a relevant document. Language modeling was introduced to the IR community by Ponte and Croft, who showed modest performance gains with TREC collections [176]. A variety of enhancements were subsequently found to improve retrieval performance further [177]. Zhai and

Lafferty investigated smoothing models and derived a number of new conclusions about this approach to IR [178]. Subsequent work processing text into topic signatures based on mapping to Unified Medical Language System (UMLS) Metathesaurus terms and using those instead of words found 10–20% performance gains with ad hoc retrieval data from the TREC Genomics Track [85].

Language models also allowed the measurement of query "clarity," which was defined as a measure of the deviation between the query and document language models from the general collection model [179]. Cronen-Townsend et al. found that query clarity was a good predictor of retrieval results from topics in the TREC ad hoc test collections, although application of this technique to real user queries from the TREC Interactive Track failed to uphold this association [180].

A number of other approaches were explored in the early days of IR and found to have modest benefit. One of these was stemming, which was described in Chaps. 4 and 5. Another technique explored was combining words into meaningful phrases, which aimed to enhance precision. This is especially true when broad, high-frequency terms are combined. For example, `high` and `blood` and `pressure` are relatively common words and are likely to appear in many types of medical documents. But when these terms occur adjacently, as in `high blood pressure`, they take on a very distinct meaning. Recognizing simple common phrases, however, is difficult to do algorithmically, especially without a dictionary or other linguistic resources. Furthermore, many phrases can be expressed in a variety of forms. For example, a document on high blood pressure might read, `When blood pressure is found to be high`.... In addition, a single-word synonym might be substituted, such as `elevated` for `high`. Nonetheless, consistent benefit has not been found for use of phrases.

Another approach to capturing the importance of term proximity introduced in the 1990s was *passage retrieval*, where documents were broken into smaller passages, which were used to weight the document for retrieval by the query [181]. The goal of this method was to find sections of documents that matched the query highly under the presumption that these local concentrations of query terms indicated a high likelihood of the document relevance. The main challenge to this approach was identifying appropriate passages and avoiding having highly relevant areas of documents span across passages. Callan [182] identified three types of passage in documents that could be used to subdivide documents based on content:

- Discourse passages—based on the structure of documents, such as sections and paragraphs.
- Semantic passages—based on changing conceptual content of the text.
- Window passages—based on number of words.

Salton and Buckley used discourse passages in their original experiments, which were found to work well with the highly structured text of an encyclopedia [181], but less ably with the TREC data [183]. Hearst and Plaunt utilized a vector-based approach to identifying semantic passages based on abrupt changes in document vectors between text sections, a technique that showed modest performance gains

[184]. Two groups at TREC found that overlapping text window passages of 200 words provided the best MAP performance gain of around 10–15% [185, 186]. Passages started 100 words apart and each overlaps the next to avoid the breaking up potentially relevant passages. Other groups using slightly different approaches also found benefit [173, 187, 188].

One technique that showed consistent benefit in the early years of TREC was query expansion, which was the use of relevance feedback (introduced in Chap. 5) without actual relevance information. Instead, some number of top-ranking documents were assumed to be relevant, and they were processed using the algorithm described in Chap. 5. The value of query expansion was verified by Buckley [189], who constructed a table comparing different features of TREC systems with each year's ad hoc retrieval collection (p. 311).

Can we still learn from failure analysis of early test collections? A major analysis done in 2003 but not widely published until 2009 looked at a variety of high-performing systems from TREC to determine why they failed on various topics [190]. Two "tracks" of the analysis addressed different facets and approaches to the problem. A "bottom-up" track carried out a large failure analysis, with six IR systems contributing one run each of 45 topics, with a detailed manual analysis of the results. A "top-down" track performed a number of runs using different variations of query expansion.

The "bottom-up" analysis found that systems obtained comparable performance (e.g., MAP) scores but performed differently across topics, retrieving different documents and emphasizing different aspects of the topics. However, it was concluded that all systems failed for similar reasons, usually missing some aspect of a topic that would lead to retrieval of more relevant documents. Another conclusion was that if systems could recognize the problem causing the failure, then substantially better retrieval could be obtained. In other words, emphasis on future system development should focus on what current techniques can be applied to which situations, and not on developing new retrieval techniques. The top-down analysis found that query expansion (also known as blind feedback, i.e., adding terms from highly ranked documents into a query to expand the number of terms and augment retrieval) was highly sensitive to variations in approaches. For example, the selection of the initial document set for expansion, the number of terms used, and the terms chosen greatly influenced performance.

8.3.2 Machine Learning: Uncovering Latent Meaning

A major focus of IR research has always been on the discovery of meaning, often hidden from the "surface" language in documents and other content items. One challenge for the surface approach is that the document-query matrix is sparse, in there being few overlaps between words in queries and documents. One possible approach for overcoming this problem is dimensionality reduction by trying to find the "latent" meaning across different terms and how they can be discovered computationally. Salton's original vector-space approaches aimed for this through the use of cosine similarity and term weighting [169]. Other early work focused on more explicitly reducing the dimensions of the semantic space through a technique called *latent semantic indexing* [191]. Unfortunately, this early approach was computationally expensive for the time and did not show improved retrieval effectiveness.

Like many computational tasks, IR researchers have applied machine learning techniques to search-related problems. Unlike some other areas where machine learning made rapid gains, its value took more time to be established in IR. Recent results, however, show that it has important roles to play.

The notion of machine learning has been attributed to Arthur Samuel in 1959, who described it as the "field of study that gives computers the ability to learn without being explicitly programmed" [192]. The field has come to prominence in the last decade based on both the growing amounts of digital data to be used and algorithm breakthroughs, mainly through the use of neural networks and deep learning [193, 194]. Machine learning uses two basic approaches to learning:

- *Supervised learning*—predict a known output, with learning based on training data and evaluated on test data to avoid "over-fitting".
- *Unsupervised learning*—find naturally occurring patterns or groupings within data.

In reality, these approaches are ends of the spectrum, and many approaches make use of semi-supervised learning, with a combination of labeled and unlabeled inputs and algorithms that find structure and patterns partially on their own but also with help from labeled inputs. Machine learning approaches also take advantage of *reinforcement learning*, where learning is incrementally improved from new labeled data, and *transfer learning*, where learning based on one dataset is used for another dataset.

One challenge for machine learning and IR is that different searches are often unique, based on different topics and query terms having different contexts of use. As such, there was somewhat of a lag in identifying value, unlike, for example, the success that it had with image classification or healthcare outcome prediction [195]. As the major tasks of machine learning are regression (measuring a value from a series of features) and classification (categorizing a series of features to a category), the role of machine learning for selecting documents relevant to a query is somewhat more complex. There has, however, been a great deal of recent success, mainly in the use of semi-supervised and transfer learning applied to the re-ranking of documents and passages [196]. Like other applications of machine learning, these successes have been enabled by neural networks and deep learning, particularly the latter with hidden layers that can represent the nonlinearity of relationships between terms and both their meaning and context.

Early application of machine learning in IR began with learning-to-rank (LETOR) approaches [197, 198]. As with most early approaches to machine learning, researchers aimed to identify features from which learning could occur. The challenge, however, was that obvious features, such as the content of words in queries or aspects of documents retrieved, were not readily transferrable across information needs.

More substantial advances have come from approaches that reduce that dimensionality of features, both the meaning and the context of words, in some ways similar to the latent semantic indexing approach described above. Words from documents and queries are typically mapped into these reduced dimensions, whose meaning to humans may not always be clear. One early successful approach was to build so-called word embeddings, based on the Word2vec algorithm of Mikolov et al. [198]. Additional refinements to Word2vec included global vectors for word representation (GloVe) [199] and Paragraph2vec [200]. Additional value was found from the addition of word context in the Embeddings from Language Models (ELMo) approach [201].

The most success has been achieved using deep neural networks for *autoencoding*, consisting of mapping words through their embeddings to appropriate output, and *transforming* to the word representations that are dynamically informed by other words around them, e.g., the difference of `The man was accused of robbing a bank` versus `The man went fishing by the bank of the river`. The most successful approach to this has been Bidirectional Encoder Representations from Transformers (BERT), developed by researchers at Google [202]. BERT has achieved success in many language-related tasks, in part due to the open-source availability of code libraries for its use.[32] A number of illustrative overviews of BERT have been written [203–205].

A number of early approaches to using machine learning for IR research were criticized by the methods being compared to baselines that did not represent the state of the art of other methods [206]. However, recent improvement over the highest baselines has been found, especially for approaches using semi-supervised methods, such as the application of large-scale BERT models trained on very large quantities of general language followed by finer tuning with smaller amounts of labeled data on specific IR tasks. This approach has worked particularly well as a query expansion task, although proper initial document ranking using nonneural approaches is still critical [207]. Nonetheless, different researchers have achieved improved performance over high baselines with a number of common test collections, including Robust04 and ClubWeb collections [208], early TREC newswire data [209], various LETOR datasets [210], Robust04 and ClueWeb09 [211], newswire and Web collections [212], Robust04 and various Web collections [213], several passage retrieval tasks [214, 215], Robust04 and the TREC microblog tasks [216], news tasks [217], passage re-ranking in the TREC CAR, and MS-MARCO datasets [218].

Google [219] and Microsoft Bing [220] have incorporated BERT into their live search engines. Research into these methods will likely continue based on the widespread availability of open-source code bases, e.g., the addition of BERT libraries to Anserini[33] [217] as well as the TREC Deep Learning Track making use of the MS-MARCO test collection for document and passage retrieval [221]. Of note, runs

[32] https://github.com/google-research/bert.

[33] https://github.com/amyxie361/BERTserini.

with neural networks, especially those making use of language models, consistently performed best in the TREC 2019 Deep Learning Track.[34]

The use of these approaches in biomedical and health IR is modest, although Del Fiol et al. found improvement in search filters for evidence-based medicine (EBM) categories (i.e., treatment, diagnosis, harm, and prognosis) [222]. Wei et al. focused on query term expansion, training a skip-gram model using word2vec, and found it outperformed the PubMed Related Citations (PRC) algorithm using data from the TREC 2005 Genomics and TREC 2014 Clinical Decision Support Tracks [223]. Mohan et al. developed a low-overhead, deep-learning approach targeted at IR, which requires fast run-time response [224]. A number of investigations have developed word embedding models from medically specific collections [225–228].

8.3.3 Natural Language Processing

A more explicit approach for uncovering meaning in IR is to use linguistic methods that aim to transform the "surface" language of content to a more structured and unambiguous representation. While the machine learning methods described in the previous section use mathematical methods to uncover latent semantics, the field of Natural Language Processing (NLP) aims to map from language into explicit semantics. NLP is sometimes called *computational linguistics*, since it applies computational processes to human language, i.e., linguistics.

Of course, the NLP field has also been impacted by the adoption of machine learning techniques [229]. Early work in NLP followed the general approaches of early research in artificial intelligence, with a focus on symbolic processing using handcrafted knowledge structures, which in the case of NLP were lexicons and grammars. This approach could never account for all the variation and ambiguity in human language, giving rise to a second generation of NLP that began to apply machine learning to human-derived categories. More recent successes have been achieved by use of deep learning to automate the entire process [230].

There is much rationale for use of linguistic approaches in IR. Although considerable success in indexing and retrieval can be obtained with the use of matching word stems in queries and documents, individual words do not contain all the information encoded in language. One cannot, for example, arbitrarily change the order of words in a sentence and fully understand the original meaning of that sentence (i.e., `He has high blood pressure` has a clear meaning, whereas `Blood has pressure he high` does not).

The problem of single words begins with words themselves. Many words have one or more synonyms, which are different words representing the same thing. Some common examples in healthcare include the synonyms high and elevated as well as `cancer` and `carcinoma`. Another frequent type of synonym, especially

[34] https://microsoft.github.io/TREC-2019-Deep-Learning/.

prevalent in healthcare, is the acronym, such as `AIDS` (which stands for `Acquired Immunodeficiency Syndrome`). Sometimes acronyms are embedded in multi-word terms (`AIDS-related complex`) or other acronyms (`ARC`, which stands for `AIDS-related complex`).

Conversely, many words also exhibit polysemy, which describes a word that has more than one meaning. Consider the word lead, which can represent a chemical, a component of an electrocardiogram, or a verb indicating movement. In discussing polysemy, words are noted to have different senses or meanings. Common words often have many senses. In the *Brown Corpus*, the 20 most commonly used nouns in English had an average of 7.3 senses, while the 20 most common verbs had 12.4 senses [231].

There are also problems beyond the synonymy and polysemy of single words. Words combine together to form phrases, which take on meaning beyond the sum of individual words themselves. For example, the words `high`, `blood`, and `pressure` combine in a phrase to take on a highly specific meaning. Furthermore, phrases exhibit synonymy and polysemy as well. For example, another way of describing the disease `high blood pressure` is `hypertension`. But the phrase `high blood pressure` also exhibits polysemy, inasmuch as it can indicate the disease (which is diagnosed by three consecutive elevated blood pressure readings) or a single measurement of elevated blood pressure.

These problems continue up to the most complex levels of language. Thus, certain large phrases have identical words with completely different meaning, such as `clinical decision support systems used to improve medical diagnosis` and `medical diagnosis used to improve clinical decision support systems`, as well as those that have the same meaning but share no common words, such as `post-prandial abdominal discomfort` and `epigastric pain after eating`.

These problems highlight that the biggest obstacle to computer-based understanding of text is the ambiguity of human language. As such, the major challenge of computational linguistics has been to devise algorithms that disambiguate language as well as possible to allow useful computer applications, such as IR. What are the biggest challenges in IR that motivate use of linguistic methods? Mothe and Tanguy evaluated TREC test collections and noted that the linguistic features of query statements associated with the most difficulty (i.e., lowest MAP) were syntactic link span (i.e., concepts with the longest span of words) and polysemy of query words [232].

A number of efforts to leverage NLP for IR have been tried over the years, but in general the impact has been small. One early approach aimed to apply syntactic analysis, with the goal of identifying noun phrases, the most likely location for the content words for which users would be likely to search.

Fagan modified the SMART system by adding a parser that derived NPs from the text, which were used along with words to index documents [233]. The same procedure was used for queries. This approach was shown to improve slightly on single-word indexing alone (1.2–8.7%), but performed less well than statistically generated phrases (2.2–22.7%). Salton et al. subsequently investigated the parser used in

Fagan's experiments to determine its effectiveness [234]. They concluded that the benefit for syntactic phrases was small and, since statistical methods were far more efficient with resources, both in terms of computer algorithm complexity and the human effort required to build parsers and lexicons, deemed them preferable to syntactic methods.

Another approach was the CLARIT system, which was designed to recognize noun phrases, identifying their boundaries rather than completely parsing the entire sentence [235]. CLARIT had additional features to enhance retrieval after parsing was completed [236]. Most simply, it could combine the phrases plus individual words into a vector-space approach, matching them against phrases and words in the user's query for retrieval. Another feature was thesaurus discovery, which could be based on the top-ranking documents (query expansion) or ones denoted by the user to be relevant (relevance feedback). CLARIT also had a comprehensive user interface that allowed the user to generate thesaurus discovery terms, add or delete them from the query, and vary their weighting in the query [237].

Another approach to partial parsing was used by Strzalkowski et al. [238]. Similar to CLARIT, their system aimed to recognize simple and complex NPs in concert with other lexical-statistical IR techniques, such as term weighting and query expansion. The architecture of their system separated each technique into "streams" so that each could be relatively weighted to optimize system performance and isolated for analysis in experimentation.

Similar to the concept-matching approaches described for biomedical and health IR above, none of these NLP techniques applied to general IR have performed better than statistical word-weighting approaches. While NLP appears to have benefits in other biomedical and health informatics applications, the role for comprehensive NLP in IR is still not well-determined [239].

8.3.4 Question-Answering

One of the most common uses of an IR system is to answer questions, and such users may be more interested in finding answers rather than documents. The earliest work in computer-based question-answering (QA) can be traced to the LUNAR system to answer questions in a database about lunar rocks from space missions [240]. Interest in this problem in the IR community led to formation of the TREC Question-Answering (QA) Track starting in TREC-8 and continuing ever since [19].

8.3.4.1 TREC Question-Answering Track

A variety of tasks were specified in the QA Track over the years. The original types of questions in the topics were *closed-class questions*, which assumed a definite answer in something like a noun phrase, i.e., a fact, as opposed to a procedural answer. Sample examples of questions included `Who was the first American in Space?` and `Where is the Taj Mahal?` Correct answers had to provide not only the document that answered the question but also a span of text that contained the answer, with NIST assessors judging the submitted strings for correctness. Performance was measured by the mean reciprocal rank (MRR):

$$\text{MRR} = \frac{1}{\text{Rank of answer passage}} \tag{8.4}$$

Some of the wrong answers to the sample questions above demonstrated the challenge of the task. In looking for answers to where the Taj Mahal was located, many of the newswire stories in the collection referred to the Taj Mahal Casino in Atlantic City, New Jersey, not the tomb in Agra, India. Likewise, for the other question, one document referred to former California Governor Jerry Brown as someone "who has been called the first American in space," and some searches returned that answer accordingly.

In 2000, a 5-year plan for QA under the auspices of several US government research agencies was developed [241]. This led in TREC 2001 for a new type of question to be added, list questions. In these questions, systems had to provide multiple instances, i.e., a list of answers. An example of this type of question was `What are nine countries that have imported Cuban sugar?` The list task run was scored by a measure of accuracy (i.e., the proportion of instances correct), with the range of the top ten performing systems varying from 15 to 76%.

Another change after the release of the plan, implemented in TREC 2002, was a modification in closed-class questions to become "factoid" questions. These questions required return of a single exact answer, with questions ranked by the system's confidence in its answers. Answers for questions were assigned one of the following judgments: incorrect, not supported (answer correct but document does not support answer), not exact (returned string contains more than just answer or is missing bits of it), and correct. The latter was modified later into categories of locally correct (answer correct but later document contradicts it) and globally correct (answer correct and no later document contradicts it). A third type of question was added in TREC 2003, the definition question. In this type of question, several aspects of the definition were designated as "nuggets," with a subset of nuggets classified as "vital" to adequately provide the definition.

Performance was assessed via modification of recall and precision and their aggregation into an F-score. Recall was calculated as the proportion of vital nuggets retrieved, i.e., vital nuggets retrieved/total vital nuggets. Precision was calculated as the number of correct vital nuggets provided, with a penalty for answers exceeding an allowable length, in this case 100 bytes. To encourage groups to pursue all three question types in TREC 2003, a combined score was derived for closed-class, list, and definition questions.

The most consistent performing group over the years in the QA Track was the Language Computer Corp. (LCC).[35] A summary of their approach documents many components required for accurate question-answering [242]. These include:

[35] http://www.languagecomputer.com/.

- Keyword pre-processing—spelling correction and splitting or binding of words.
- Construction of question representation—parsing of question to capture concepts and their dependencies.
- Derivation of expected answer type—disambiguating semantic category of expected answers.
- Selection of key words for searching.
- Expansion of key words for searching based on morphological, lexical, or semantic alternations.
- Retrieval of documents and passages—based on a Boolean query derived from previous steps.
- Passage post-filtering—precision is enhanced by removing passages that do not satisfy semantic constraints of questions.
- Identification of candidate answers—search within passages for answers based on expected types.
- Answer ranking—based on relevance score calculated from lexical and proximity features.
- Answer formulation—system selects candidate answers with highest relevance scores.

8.3.4.2 Recent Question-Answering

A more recent QA test collection is the Stanford Question Answering Dataset (SQuAD),[36] consisting of over 100,000 questions posed to a set of Wikipedia articles [243]. There has also been a new TREC Complex Answer Retrieval Track[37] that also makes use of a dataset of questions to Wikipedia articles [244].

8.3.4.3 Biomedical Question-Answering

Early work in biomedical QA assessed its feasibility. For example, Zweigenbaum explored the task and resources for medical QA, noting that it had a number of different attributes than general QA [245]. For example, biomedical language is highly specialized, some sources are considered trustworthy and others are not, and the availability of sources is modest, at least relative to the types of content for general QA. Rinaldi et al. explored the steps necessary to convert a general QA system to answering questions about genomics [246]. They found that the key challenges were selecting the appropriate part of the document for extracting information, handling the technical language of genomics and its synonymy and polysemy, and being able to accurately parse text.

[36] https://rajpurkar.github.io/SQuAD-explorer/.

[37] http://trec-car.cs.unh.edu/.

Other research focused in the clinical domain, with a particular emphasis on answering questions in EBM. These types of questions may have been more amenable to QA techniques because they tended to fit a semantic pattern, i.e., the patient-intervention-comparison-outcome (PICO) format, and they often had an answer. There were, however, a number of challenges. For example, while named-entity recognition was shown to be essential for general QA [242], there were several aspects of clinical questions that are not named entities, such as some outcomes of clinical studies [247]. The latter may be nouns (e.g., `death`), verbs (e.g., `improve`), or adjectives (e.g., `adverse`), and sometimes the outcome is even something that did not occur (e.g., `no difference in death rates`). This placed importance on the proper identification of semantic classes in medical texts based on the PICO framework [248] and the ability to detect the correct clinical outcome and its direction [249].

This foundational work led to systems being developed and evaluated to perform QA of EBM questions. Demner-Fushman and Lin developed a system that aimed to answer EBM questions [250]. They implemented a system based on a suite of "knowledge extractors" aiming to process the text of MEDLINE abstracts into the PICO framework, determine the strength of evidence of the article, and determine the EBM task, i.e., treatment, diagnosis, prognosis, or harm. These attributes are then matched up against EBM questions that come from users. An evaluation found the system improved substantially over the PubMed baseline in terms of ranking documents overall as well as putting answers to the questions into the top five documents retrieved.

Sneiderman et al. compared a variety of research and operational systems available at NLM for finding answers to EBM questions [251], including PubMed, Essie [252], SemRep [253], and a prototype called CQA-1.0 that used elements of the PICO approach described in the previous paragraph. In addition, the authors explored fusion of results from combinations of these systems. They developed three sets of five questions each, which they called general questions (similar to definition questions in the TREC QA Track), specific questions (requiring yes/no or factoid answers), and intermediate questions (requiring more than an overview but are not focused enough for an exact answer). Based on a variety of measures (e.g., mean average precision, precision @ N documents, and others), the fusion approaches performed best. However, Essie performed best individually for general questions, while CQA-1.0 performed best individually for intermediate and specific questions. The authors concluded that both the structuring based on the PICO format and robust concept detection are required for robust clinical QA.

As noted above, the TREC Genomics Track implemented a task of *entity-based question-answering* [50, 51]. After the ad hoc retrieval and categorization tasks of the first 2 years, the track developed a new task that focused on retrieval of short passages (from phrase to sentence to paragraph in length) that specifically addressed an information need, along with linkage to the location in the original source document. Figure 8.5 shows the relationship among passages, the entities they contained, and the documents in which they occurred.

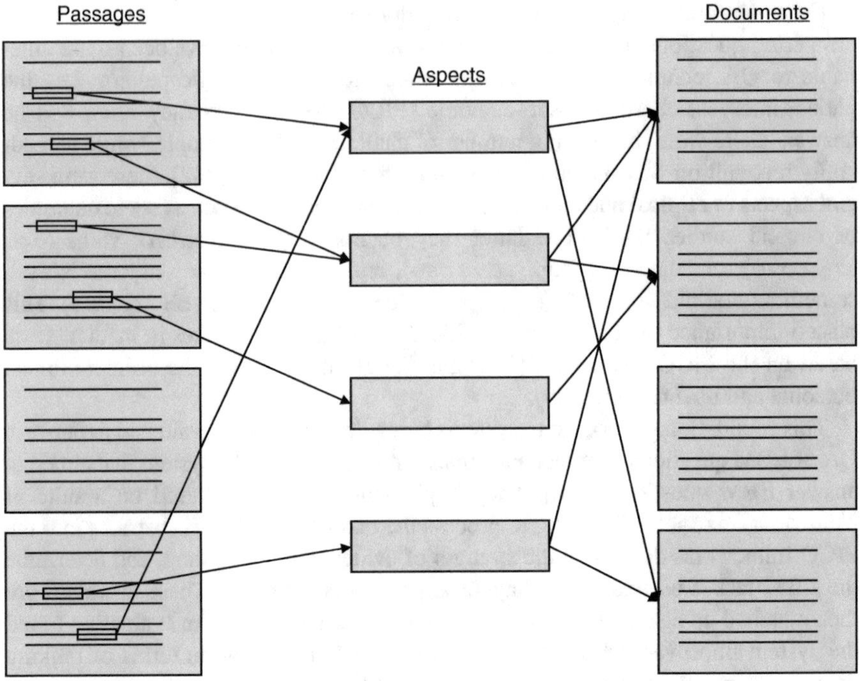

Fig. 8.5 Relationship among passages, the entities they contained, and the documents in which they occurred in the TREC Genomics entity-based question-answering task

Topics were expressed as questions and systems were measured on how well they retrieved relevant information at the passage, aspect, and document levels. Systems were required to return passages linked to source documents, while relevance judges not only rated the passages but also grouped them by aspect. For this task, aspect was defined similar to its definition in the TREC Interactive Track aspectual recall task [22], representing answers that covered a similar portion of a full answer to the topic question. The documents for this task came from a new full-text biomedical corpus, as track members had also advocated a move from bibliographic (MEDLINE) to full-text documents (journal articles). The document collection was derived from 49 journals and contained 162,259 documents, along with corresponding MEDLINE records.

The first running of the task took place in 2006, with the topics expressed as questions [50]. They were derived from the set of biologically relevant questions based on a set of Generic Topic Types (GTTs). The questions (and GTTs) all had the general format of containing one or more biological objects and processes and some explicit relationship between them. The biological objects might be genes, proteins, gene mutations, etc. The biological process could be physiological processes or diseases. The relationships could be anything but were typically verbs such as *causes*, *contributes to*, *affects*, *associated with*, or *regulates*. The GTTs, questions patterns for them, and examples are shown in Table 8.5.

Table 8.5 Generic Topic Types used in the TREC 2006 Genomics Track

GTT	Question pattern	Example
Find articles describing the role of a gene involved in a given disease	What is the role of gene in disease?	What is the role of DRD4 in alcoholism?
Find articles describing the role of a gene in a specific biological process	What effect does gene have on biological process?	What effect does the insulin receptor gene have on tumorigenesis?
Find articles describing interactions (e.g., promote, suppress, inhibit, etc.) between two or more genes in the function of an organ or in a disease	How do genes interact in organ function?	How do HMG and HMGB1 interact in hepatitis?
Find articles describing one or more mutations of a given gene and its biological impact	How does a mutation in gene influence biological process?	How does a mutation in ret influence thyroid function?

The relevance assessments were done by the usual TREC method of pooling the top-ranking passages from different groups that submitted official runs. In general, a passage was definitely relevant if it contained all required elements of the question and it answered the question. A passage was possibly relevant if it contained the majority of required elements, missing elements were within the realm of possibility (i.e., more general terms are mentioned that probably include the missing elements), and it possibly answered the question.

After determining the "best" answer passages, judges were instructed to group them into related concepts and then assign one or more Medical Subject Headings (MeSH) terms (possibly with subheadings) to capture similarities and differences among retrieved passage aspects. They were told to use the most specific MeSH term, with the option of adding subheadings, similar to the NLM literature indexing process. If one term was insufficient to denote all aspects of the gold standard passage, judges assigned additional MeSH terms. All passages judged as definitely or possibly relevant were required to have a gold standard passage and at least one MeSH term.

For this entity-based, QA task, there were three levels of retrieval performance measured: passage retrieval, aspect retrieval, and document retrieval. Each of these provided insight into the overall performance for a user trying to answer the given topic questions. Each was measured by some variant of MAP:

- Passage-level MAP—for each nominated passage, the number of characters that overlapped with those deemed relevant by the judges in the gold standard were computed.
- Aspect-level MAP—aspect retrieval was measured using the average precision for the aspects of a topic, averaged across all topics.
- Document-level MAP—for the purposes of this measure, any PMID that had a passage associated with a topic ID in the set of gold standard passages was considered a relevant document for that topic, with all other documents considered not relevant for that topic.

Table 8.6 Overall results from TREC 2006–2007 Genomics Track task

	Passage2 MAP	Passage MAP	Aspect MAP	Document MAP
TREC 2006				
Min	0.0007	0.0019	0.0110	0.0198
Median	0.0345	0.0316	0.1581	0.3083
Mean	0.0392	0.0347	0.1643	0.2887
Max	0.1486	0.1012	0.4411	0.5439
TREC 2007				
Min	0.0008	0.0029	0.0197	0.0329
Median	0.0377	0.0565	0.1311	0.1897
Mean	0.0398	0.0560	0.1326	0.1862
Max	0.1148	0.0976	0.2631	0.3286

As shown in Table 8.6, document MAP scores were highest, followed by aspect, and then passage, although these scores were not directly comparable since they measured precision at recall of different things. An analysis showed that four factors were and associated with the best performance in passage MAP [254]:

- Normalization of keywords in the query into root forms.
- Use of the Entrez Gene thesaurus for synonym terms expansion.
- Unit of text retrieved using respective IR algorithms at sentence level.
- Passage "trimming" to best sentence.

The TREC 2007 Genomics Track continued with the same task and document collection, but some modifications to the topics and relevance judging, along with adoption of a new official measure passage retrieval performance [51]. There were 36 topics for the track in 2007, which were in the form of questions asking for lists of specific entities. As in the past, information needs were gathered from working biologists. In addition to asking about information needs, there biologists were asked if their desired answer was a list of a certain type of entity, such as genes, proteins, diseases, mutations, etc., and if so, to designate that entity type. An example topic was `What [GENES] are genetically linked to alcoholism?`

Answers to this question were passages that related one or more entities of type GENE to alcoholism. For example, a valid and relevant answer to this topic would be "The DRD4 VNTR polymorphism moderates craving after alcohol consumption" (from PMID 11950104). And the GENE entity supported by this statement would be DRD4. Table 8.7 shows the entities, their definitions, potential sources of terms, and topics with each entity type.

Relevance judging was once again by pooling of top-ranking passages retrieved by participating groups. Judges were given the following instructions:

1. Review the topic question and identify key concepts.
2. Identify relevant paragraphs and select minimum complete and correct excerpts.
3. Develop controlled vocabulary for entities based on the relevant passages and code entities for each relevant passage based on this vocabulary.

Table 8.7 TREC 2007 Genomics Track entities, their definitions, potential sources of terms, and topics with each entity type

Entity type	Definition	Potential source of terms	Topics with entity type
ANTIBODIES	Immunoglobulin molecules having a specific amino acid sequence by virtue of which they interact only with the antigen (or a very similar shape) that induced their synthesis in cells of the lymphoid series (especially plasma cells)	MeSH	1
BIOLOGICAL SUBSTANCES	Chemical compounds that are produced by a living organism	MeSH	3
CELL OR TISSUE TYPES	A distinct morphological or functional form of cell, or the name of a collection of interconnected cells that perform a similar function within an organism	MeSH	2
DISEASES	A definite pathologic process with a characteristic set of signs and symptoms. It may affect the whole body or any of its parts, and its etiology, pathology, and prognosis may be known or unknown	MeSH	1
DRUGS	A pharmaceutical preparation intended for human or veterinary use	MEDLIN-EPlus	2
GENES	Specific sequences of nucleotides along a molecule of DNA (or, in the case of some viruses, RNA) which represent functional units of heredity	iHoP, harvester	11
MOLECULAR FUNCTIONS	Elemental activities, such as catalysis or binding, describing the actions of a gene product or bioactive substance at the molecular level	GO	2
MUTATIONS	Any detectable and heritable change in the genetic material that causes a change in the genotype and which is transmitted to daughter cells and to succeeding generations	MeSH	1
PATHWAYS	A series of biochemical reactions occurring within a cell to modify a chemical substance or transduce an extracellular signal	BioCarta, KEGG	2
PROTEINS	Linear polypeptides that are synthesized on ribosomes and may be further modified, cross-linked, cleaved, or assembled into complex proteins with several subunits	MeSH	5
STRAINS	A genetic subtype or variant of a virus or bacterium	Ad hoc	2
SIGNS OR SYMPTOMS	A sensation or subjective change in health function experienced by a patient, or an objective indication of some medical fact or quality that is detected by a physician during a physical examination of a patient	MeSH	1
TOXICITIES	A measure of the degree and the manner in which something is toxic or poisonous to a living organism	MeSH	2
TUMOR TYPES	An abnormal growth of tissue, originating from a specific tissue of origin or cell type, and having defined characteristic properties, such as a recognized histology	MeSH	1

The level of performance of the top systems for 2007 was somewhat lower than for 2006. This may have been due to list-entity type questions being more difficult to answer than the GTT questions. This would not be unexpected since list-entity questions were more open-ended, involved more different entity types, and were closer to natural language than the GTT question used in 2006. The top systems did consistently well on all measures, and the measures were highly correlated.

Additional work from the NLM evaluated Essie, a concept-based IR system whose main feature is to expand user queries by mapping them into concepts in the UMLS Metathesaurus [252]. Evaluation with the TREC 2006 Genomics Track test collection showed results comparable to the best-performing systems from the challenge evaluation. Another NLM research group compared a variety of document ranking strategies for TREC Genomics Track data, finding that TF*IDF ranking outperformed sentence-level co-occurrence of words and other approaches [255].

Additional follow-on work using the TREC 2006–2007 collections aimed to expand queries with the goal of optimizing diversity of query terms that could lead to improvement in aspect-oriented retrieval results [256]. Through a supervised query expansion process for term refinement, the most relevant and diversified terms were selected to expand the original query, which was then fed into a second retrieval to improve the relevance and diversity of search results. Goodwin and Harabagiu extended the TREC 2015 CDS Track into a QA format, with re-ranking of articles that resulted in an improvement over previous state-of-the-art approaches [257].

Other QA systems for biomedicine have been developed, one that attempted to parse and map questions into facts determined from journal articles [258] and another that aimed to find sentences that likely have the answer [259]. QA was also part of the BioASQ initiative, from which publicly available QA datasets have been developed[38] [91]. Some QA has focused on data from the EHR. Papari et al. explored clinical QA over i2b2 data [260], while Wen et al. developed an approach using BERT to answer "why" questions over Mayo Clinic EHR data [261].

A final system that started as a QA system and received a great deal of attention in its use for healthcare was the IBM Watson system.[39] Watson was actually developed out of IBM's participating in the TREC Question-Answering Track [19]. Watson is built around a system called DeepQA, which uses massively parallel computing to acquire knowledge from resources of a given domain [262, 263]. Watson achieved fame by defeating humans at the *Jeopardy!* television game show [264], which motivated its being applied to medicine [265].

To apply Watson to a new domain, such as medicine, three areas of adaptation were required [266]:

- Content adaptation—acquiring and modeling new content.
- Training adaptation—adding and learning from new question types.
- Functional adaptation—adapting question analysis, hypothesis scoring, and new functionality specific to the domain.

[38] http://www.bioasq.org/.

[39] https://www.ibm.com/watson-health.

In Watson's first foray into the medical domain, it was trained using several resources from internal medicine (discussed in earlier chapters), such as *ACP Medicine*, *PIER*, *Merck Manual*, and *MKSAP*. Watson was trained with 5000 questions from *Doctor's Dilemma*, a competition somewhat like *Jeopardy!*, which was run by American College of Physicians and in which medical trainees participated each year. A sample question is `Familial adenomatous polyposis is caused by mutations of this gene`, with the answer being `APC Gene`. (Googling the text of the question gave the correct answer at the top of its ranking to this and two other sample questions provided as well.)

Watson was evaluated on an additional 188 unseen questions. The primary outcome measure was recall at 10 answers, and the results varied from 0.49 for the core system to 0.77 for the fully adapted and trained system [266]. The evaluation did not compare Watson against other systems, such as Google or PubMed, or assess it using other measures, such as MRR. A subsequent use case for Watson was to apply the system to data in EHR systems, ultimately aiming to serve as a clinical decision support system. A couple of other studies found Watson able to perform comparably to humans in EHR problem list formulation [267] and in breast cancer tumor board recommendations [268]. Others have been critical of the hype around Watson and the quality of its scientific evaluation studies [269–271].

8.3.5 Text Categorization

The goal of *text categorization* is to assign documents into specific categories, usually based on their subject matter or document type [272, 273]. In the former type of category, a news producer or scientific journal may aim to assign documents to specific subject headings. In the latter type of category, documents may be classified as having certain attributes. Related to text categorization is *document routing or filtering*, which differs in that the goal is to identify relevant documents from a new stream based on queries modified by those already retrieved and determined to be relevant. The document routing task can be viewed as a form of relevance feedback, since all documents are returned to the user in a ranked order. With filtering, however, a categorization decision is made, which is whether or not to return a document to the user.

Text categorization and document filtering are usually evaluated with some sort of *utility score* that includes a penalty for nonrelevant documents that are retrieved:

$$\begin{aligned}\text{Utility} = &\left(u_r \times \text{relevant documents retrieved}\right)\\ &+ \left(u_{nr} \times \text{nonrelevant documents retrieved}\right)\end{aligned} \tag{8.5}$$

where u_r and u_{nr} are relative utilities of the value of retrieving relevant and nonrelevant documents, respectively. In the TREC Filtering Track, the values of u_r and u_{nr} were usually set at 2 and −1 [274].

The early test collections for routing and filtering came from Reuters news service data. As such, the task motivating initial text categorization research was the classification of news stories by topic, people, places, and so forth. An early widely used resource was the Reuters-21,578 collection, which was later superseded by a new collection of more recent documents and categories [275]. Other document collections have been used for text categorization research in TREC and other settings, including MEDLINE records from the OHSUMED test collection [276].

The TREC Filtering Track simulated two types of filtering, adaptive and batch [276]. In *adaptive filtering*, the documents are "released" to the system one at a time, and only documents chosen for retrieval can be used to modify the filtering query. In *batch filtering*, all documents and their relevance judgments can be used at once. Similar to other TREC tasks and tracks, participants in the Filtering Track have used a variety of methods, which yield a wide spectrum of performance [276]. In general, most approaches have aimed to optimize document weighting and then identify a threshold that maximizes inclusion of relevant document and discards nonrelevant ones. Some have used machine learning techniques, such as neural networks or logistic regression, although their results have not exceeded simpler term-weighting approaches.

A major biomedical text categorization effort was the categorization task of the TREC Genomics Track, run in 2004 and 2005 [49, 52]. The mail goal of the task was to "triage" articles for human annotators in the MGI resource described above. One of the activities of MGI is to provide structured, coded annotation of gene function from the biological literature. Human curators identify genes and assign Gene Ontology (GO)[40] and other codes about gene function with another code describing the type of experimental evidence supporting assignment of the code. In the categorization task, systems were required to classify full-text documents from a 2-year span (2002–2003) of three journals, *Journal of Biological Chemistry* (JBC), *Journal of Cell Biology* (JCB), and *Proceedings of the National Academy of Science* (PNAS). The first year's (2002) documents comprised the training data, and the second year's (2003) documents made up the test data.

The TREC Genomics text categorization tasks focused on triage of articles since this function was believed by MGI to have the most value in automating. The triage task basically considered designating whether or not an article should be designated for sending to a curator for annotation. Performance was assessed by the utility measure in Eq. 8.1 above, with the parameters u_r and u_{nr} tuned for each specific triage subtask. In TREC 2004, the triage task was to assign articles for GO annotation, whereas in 2005, the task was expanded to include triage for inclusion in databases about tumor biology [277], embryologic gene expression [278], and alleles of mutant phenotypes [279].

---

[40] http://geneontology.org/.

Table 8.8 Best and median utility scores for each subtask of the TREC Genomics text categorization task, adapted from [49]

Subtask	Best utility	Median utility
A (allele)	0.871	0.7773
E (expression)	0.8711	0.6413
G (GO annotation)	0.587	0.4575
T (tumor)	0.9433	0.761

The results from different groups are summarized in Table 8.8 and papers describing the task [49, 280]. These groups used a variety of NLP and machine learning tasks, with a wide range of results. One notable finding across all groups was the GO triage task was substantially more difficult than the tumor biology, embryologic gene expression, or alleles of mutant phenotypes tasks. Very little could be done to improve triage of articles for GO annotation beyond the presence of the MeSH term Mice. Some additional work has used a subset of the TREC Categorization data to assess the detection of figures and their types for use as features [281].

Besides the TREC Genomics Track categorization task, there has only been a small amount of other work in text categorization that has focused on biomedical topics. One exception is the high-recall IR described above that aims to categorize studies for inclusion in systematic review. Another effort focused on the identification of high-quality articles for use in EBM. Aphinyanaphongs et al. have shown that machine learning approaches can improve on the identification of such articles (as determined by their inclusion in EBM publications such as *ACP Journal Club*) [45, 282] over the techniques used by the MEDLINE Clinical Queries algorithms of Haynes et al. [31]. These authors also found ways to express these queries using Boolean operators so they could be used in exact-match retrieval systems [283]. The work of these authors was also extended to identifying unproven cancer treatments on the Web [284].

Another line of work that can be viewed as a text categorization task is the use of search engine input for *syndromic surveillance*. A great deal of press was generated by the development of a system by Google called *Flu Trends* [285]. Early work found the system to perform well retroactively in predicting H1N1 influenza in the United States [286] as well as rates of influenza and patient utilization in emergency departments [287]. However, the system performed less well in subsequent flu seasons [288], leading Lazer et al. to issue a warning against "big data hubris" [289]. Subsequent research found, however, that other approaches to flu prediction were able to outperform Google and its approach based on search queries. Additional data used includes flu data itself [290], selection of specific queries [291], and EHR data [292]. More recently, search engine input has been used for predicting healthcare utilization [293], various other health-related events [294], and emergency department utilization [295].

Additional research has looked at *literature-based discovery*, with a focus on disconnected threads in the literature [296]. For example, there might be studies that

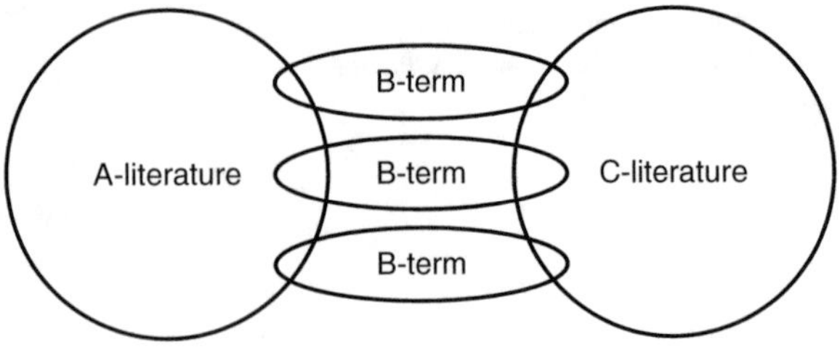

Fig. 8.6 The components of literature-based discovery, adapted from [305]

identify diseases or syndromes that result in certain manifestations and others that identify treatments that improve such manifestations, yet the treatment has never been assessed for this particular disease or syndrome. Swanson showed this (manually) to be the case in two instances:

1. Articles on `Raynaud's disease` found `blood viscosity` to be abnormally high, while others on the fish oil `eicosapentaenoic acid` found this substance to reduce `blood viscosity`, yet the latter had never been considered as a treatment for the former [297].
2. Articles on `migraine` found the disease to be implicated by spreading `depression` in the `cortex of the brain`, while others found `magnesium` to be effective in inhibiting such depression (usually in the context of treating a different condition, `epilepsy`) [298].

When first identified, the two literatures in each instance were completely disconnected, and no researchers had thought of the potential for treatment. After identification of these potential linkages, clinical trials found effectiveness for both treatments [299]. Additional disconnected complementary literatures have also been discovered in a variety of other clinical areas [300–302], and following work incorporated genomic information [303, 304]. Smalheiser et al. developed a system called ARROWSMITH[41] that was designed to facilitate further exploration [305]. ARROWSMITH combined terms common to two different literatures (the A-literature and C-literature of Fig. 8.6) with so-called B-terms that could offer conceptual explanations for linkage of the literatures. One of the challenges in using ARROWSMITH is the large number of B-terms generated, and further work has focused on methods to prune them automatically to a more manageable size [306]. Newer methods have focused on developing more complex models with the aim of acquiring additional insights from connections in the literature [307].

Additional uses of literature-based discovery have been to identify adverse drug events reported in the literature [308] as well as facilitate drug repositioning with literature [309]. There are also uses outside of medicine in the automated detection of fake news [310], use of knowledge graphs to support fact-checking [311], and rumor verification, especially when they incorporate multimedia [312].

[41] http://arrowsmith.psych.uic.edu/.

8.4 Research Systems and the User

Although the IR system user is implicit in all of the research described so far in this chapter, some have criticized the field for not paying enough attention to user studies. As noted in a number of biomedical and health IR user studies, differences among users overwhelm all system-related aspects [313, 314]. In 2007, veteran Microsoft IR researcher Susan Dumais famously said, "If in 10 years we are still using a rectangular box and a list of results, I should be fired" [315]. Dumais subsequently provided a vision for "thinking outside the (search) box" [316]. Another user-oriented researcher offered up a vision of what "natural" search interfaces might look like in the future, with the user speaking rather than typing, viewing video rather than reading text, and interacting socially rather than alone [317]. Borlund laid out a set of principles for interactive IR evaluation focused on the experiments employing simulated work tasks to which users could relate and have interest in performing [318]. Hofmann et al. have also described a framework for interactive IR evaluation [319].

Both CLEF and TREC have incorporated interactive retrieval evaluation among their tracks. CLEF began with a Living Labs Track that provided commonly asked queries to users in real time, with different systems and their features substituted as part of the study protocol. The CLEF track focused on product search and Web search, while the TREC Open Search Track focused on academic search. A good deal of user-focused IR research now is published in the proceedings of the ACM SIGIR Conference on Human Information Interaction and Retrieval (CHIIR).[42] The conference call for proposals gives an indication of the topics that are covered by the research listed in Table 8.9.

A couple of books about IR user interfaces state of the art and research have been published [320, 321]. A well-known leader in general human-computer interaction is Shneiderman, whose textbook is now in a sixth edition [322]. He is also known for his Eight Golden Rules of Interface Design[43]:

1. Strive for consistency.
2. Seek universal usability.
3. Offer informative feedback.
4. Design dialogs to yield closure.
5. Prevent errors.
6. Permit easy reversal of actions.
7. Keep users in control.
8. Reduce short-term memory load.

Another well-known leader in user interface design is Nielsen, who has a famous list of Top 10 Mistakes in Web Design,[44] the first of which is to "avoid bad search."

---

[42] https://www.chiir.org/.

[43] https://www.cs.umd.edu/~ben/goldenrules.html.

[44] https://www.nngroup.com/articles/top-10-mistakes-web-design/.

Table 8.9 User-focused research topics of the ACM SIGIR Conference on Human Information Interaction and Retrieval (CHIIR)[a]

Information seeking, including task-based and exploratory studies
Search interfaces, including those for specialized tasks, populations, and domains
User-centered design approaches to humans interacting with information and systems
Interaction techniques for information retrieval and discovery
Online information seeking, including log analysis of search and browsing
Modeling and simulation of information interaction
Information use, including measures of use as well as broader sense-making
Field and case studies relevant to understanding prerequisites for information searching, design, and access
User-centered evaluation methods and measures, including measures of user experience and performance, experiment and search task design, eye-tracking and neurophysiological approaches, data analysis methods, and usability
Human interaction and experience with conversational information systems
Context-aware and personalized search, including design, contextual features, and analysis of information interaction
Information visualization and visual analytics, including search result presentation
Collaborative information seeking and social search, including social utility and network analysis for information interaction
Conversational search and other types of stateful and multi-turn interactions between users and search applications
Insights and analyses related to human experiences and usage trends with recommendation technologies
Information interaction and seeking with mobile devices and services

[a]http://sigir.org/chiir2020/cfp.pdf

8.4.1 Early Research

A number of early systems attempted to assist the user with constructing queries. CANSEARCH was one of the first such systems in medicine. It was designed to assist novice physician searchers in retrieving documents related to cancer therapy [323]. The user did no typing and used only a touch screen to navigate menus related to cancer sites and therapies. (Recall that MEDLINE has a particularly obtuse method of representing cancers, making the newer system all the more valuable.) Once the proper menu items were chosen, a MEDLINE search statement was formed based on rules in the program. The CANSEARCH main menu had the user select the specific cancer, while submenus allowed the designation of more detail, such as the treatment. For instance, if the user chose the site as `breast cancer` and the therapy as `cisplatinum`, then the resulting search statement passed to MEDLINE would be `Breast Neoplasms/Drug Therapy AND Cisplatinum/Therapeutic Use AND Human`.

One of the most comprehensive efforts to provide expert search assistance in the medical domain came from the COACH project at the NLM [324]. COACH was added as an expert assistant to the now-defunct Internet Grateful Med. The rules used by COACH were based on an analysis of failed searches done by end users on the NLM system, as described in Chap. 7. Recall that the biggest problem found was searches with null retrieval (no documents returned). The most common reason for null retrieval was excessive ANDs, such that no documents had all the terms intersected together. Other mistakes commonly made included inappropriate use of specialty headings, improper use of subheadings, and failure to use related terms.

COACH was activated from within Internet Grateful Med after a poor search was obtained. It offered two main modes of operation: assisted increase and assisted focus. The former was invoked when the search yielded no or only a few references. In that instance, COACH may have recommended reducing the number of search terms (or at least those connected by AND), using proper specialty headings where appropriate, or adding related terms or synonyms. The assisted focus mode was called on when an excessive number of references were retrieved. It may have recommended adding a subheading to or designating as a central concept one or more of the search terms.

8.4.2 User Evaluation of Research Systems

The efficacy of many of the system-oriented approaches described in this chapter has been assessed by a general approach to evaluation that is detailed in this section. Except for some recent studies with real users to be described at the end of the chapter, virtually all evaluation of lexical-statistical systems has been based on "batch-mode" studies using test collections, which were introduced in Chap. 1. These collections typically contain a set of documents, a set of queries, and a binary determination of which documents are relevant to which query. The usual mode of comparing system performance, introduced in Chap. 1, is to generate an aggregate statistic of recall and precision, with the most commonly used metric being MAP.

Some of the test collections have been created with queries captured in the process of real interaction with a system, but others have been built by experimenters for the purpose of doing batch-style evaluation. Likewise, while some relevance judgments have been performed by domain experts, others have not. Nonetheless, these collections have achieved high usage in the research community, and evaluations of IR system performance are typically not considered meaningful to be without their use. However, there are a number of problems with batch-mode studies and the test collections on which they are based:

1. Lack of real users—simulating the behavior of users with batch-style studies does not guarantee that real users will perform identically in front of a computer.
2. Lack of meaningful measures—recall-precision tables do not capture how meaningful the information being retrieved is to the user. Furthermore, research reports often do not provide analyses of statistical significance.

3. Unrealistic databases—until TREC, most test collections were very small, on the order of a few thousand documents. There were concerns not only that such databases might have properties different from those of the large databases used in commercial systems but also that retrieval algorithms themselves might not be scalable to large databases.
4. Unrealistic queries—most queries in test collections are short statements, which in isolation do not represent the original user's (or anyone else's) information need. Also, recall from Chap. 7 that Saracevic et al. found a twofold difference in recall when an intermediary searcher had access to a taped transcript of the user's interaction with a librarian, showing that different results can occur when a searcher has access to multiple statements of the same information need [325].
5. Unrealistic relevance judgments—as seen in Chap. 7, topical relevance judgments can be inconsistent.

8.4.3 TREC Interactive Track

As noted in Sect. 8.1, the TREC experiments have for the most part used batch-style searching evaluation with no human involvement in the query process. While some manual modifications of queries have been allowed in various TREC tracks, the emphasis has always been on building automated systems. An overview of user evaluation activities at TREC, including the Interactive Track, was provided by Dumais [21]. The TREC Interactive Track shifted into full gear in TREC-5, when it adopted an *instance recall* task [22]. Recognizing that the number of relevant documents retrieved was not a good indicator of a user's performance with an IR system, the track moved toward a task-oriented approach. The approach chosen was to measure how well users could define instances (called "aspects" in TRECs 5–6 but "instances" subsequently) of a topic. Example questions included `How many stars have been discovered by the Hubble Telescope?` and `How many countries import Cuban sugar?` The database for searching was the 1991–1994 *Financial Times* database, consisting of 210,158 news articles. In the searching experiments, users were asked to save the documents that contained instances and record the specific instances identified. As with the development of document relevance judgments, assessors at NIST devised a set of "correct" instances and the documents they occurred in based on the results submitted from participating sites. This allowed instance recall to be measured:

$$\text{Instance recall} = \frac{\text{number of relevance instances in saved documents}}{\text{number of relevant instances for topic}} \tag{8.6}$$

One of the challenges for the Interactive Track was to define the degree of standardization of experiments across sites. Certainly one of the values of TREC in general was the standardization of tasks, queries, and test collections. Counter to this, however, were not only the varying research interests of different participating groups but also the diversity of users, settings, and available systems. As such, attempts to have a common control system to be matched with the different groups' experimental systems were not successful. There were, however, a number of standardized procedures undertaken. In particular, common data were collected about each user and each of their searches. The data elements were collected from common questionnaires used by all sites or extracted from search logs. Searchers were also given an explicit amount of time for searching: 20 minutes in TREC-6 and TREC-8 and 15 minutes in TREC-7. Sites were also asked to provide a narrative of one user's search on one topic each year.

With TREC-9, a QA task was adopted [326]. The TREC-9 Interactive Track continued many of the other standard approaches adopted for TREC-6 through TREC-8, although one change was an expansion of the collection used to include more documents from several additional news sources.

Most participating research groups assessed specific research questions in their experiments over the years in the Interactive Track. Hersh and colleagues, for example, compared Boolean and natural language searching interfaces in TREC-7 and compared weighted schemes shown to be more effective in batch studies with real users in TREC-8 and TREC-9. This group also attempted to determine the factors associated with successful searching, similar to the experiments they performed using MEDLINE described in Sect. 7.4.2 [313, 327, 328].

The TREC-7 study of Hersh et al. [329] compared these two approaches with the instance recall task. A group of highly experienced information professionals (mostly librarians) was recruited to take part. The Web-based interfaces used are shown in Figs. 8.7 and 8.8, respectively. Users performed virtually identical on both systems, similar to most earlier studies comparing these two types of interface. However, there were other differences between the systems. Topics using the natural language interface resulted in more documents being shown to the user (viewed). However, fewer documents were actually selected for viewing (seen) when that interface was used, probably because users had to spend more time scrolling through the document titles shown. This group of highly experienced searchers also clearly preferred the Boolean interface, no doubt in part owing to their familiarity with it.

In TREC-8 and TREC-9, Hersh and colleagues addressed the question of whether results from batch searching experiments are comparable to those obtained by real users. That is, are the results found when batch-style experiments and measures like MAP are used congruent with those obtained by real users with retrieval tasks using the same systems? To test this question, three-part experiments were performed. First, previous TREC Interactive Track data were used to determine the "best-performing" system under batch experiments. This was done by creating a test collection that designated documents with instances as relevant and running traditional batch experiments to generate MAP results. These experiments found that Okapi weighting (TREC-8) and Okapi plus PN weighting (TREC-9) performed much better than "baseline" TF*IDF weighting. Next, the interactive user experiments were carried out, with the best-performing system serving as the "experimental" intervention and the TF*IDF system as the "control." In the final step, the batch experiments were repeated with the data generated from the new interactive experiments, to verify the results held with the topics employed in the user experiments.

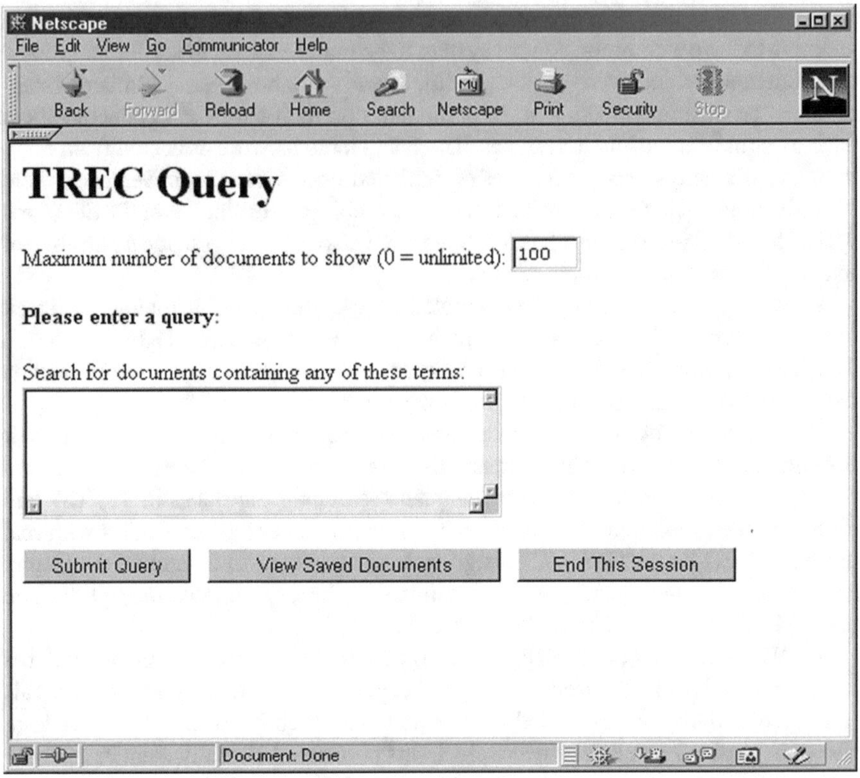

Fig. 8.7 Natural language interface for TREC Interactive Track experiments of Hersh et al. [329]

In the TREC-8 instance recall task, Hersh et al. found in the first batch experiment that Okapi weighting performed best, achieving an 81% better MAP than TF*IDF weighting [330]. For the user experiments that followed, Okapi weighting served as the experimental system and TF*IDF weighting as the control. All subjects used the natural language interface (see Fig. 8.8) to the MG system. Highly experienced searchers were again employed. The results showed a trend to better average instance recall for Okapi over TF*IDF weighting, but the results were not statistically significant. In the final batch experiments, the Okapi weighting achieved a 17.6% benefit with the data that had actually been used by the interactive searchers. These experiments also found a positive and statistically significant linear relationship for instance recall with the following variables:

- The number of documents saved as having instances by users.
- Document recall (defining a relevant document has one having one instance or more).
- The number of documents selected for viewing by the user (seen).

The same experiment was repeated in TREC-9 by Hersh et al. [331], using the question-answering task. In the initial batch experiments here, however, a combination of Okapi plus PN weighting achieved the highest MAP over the

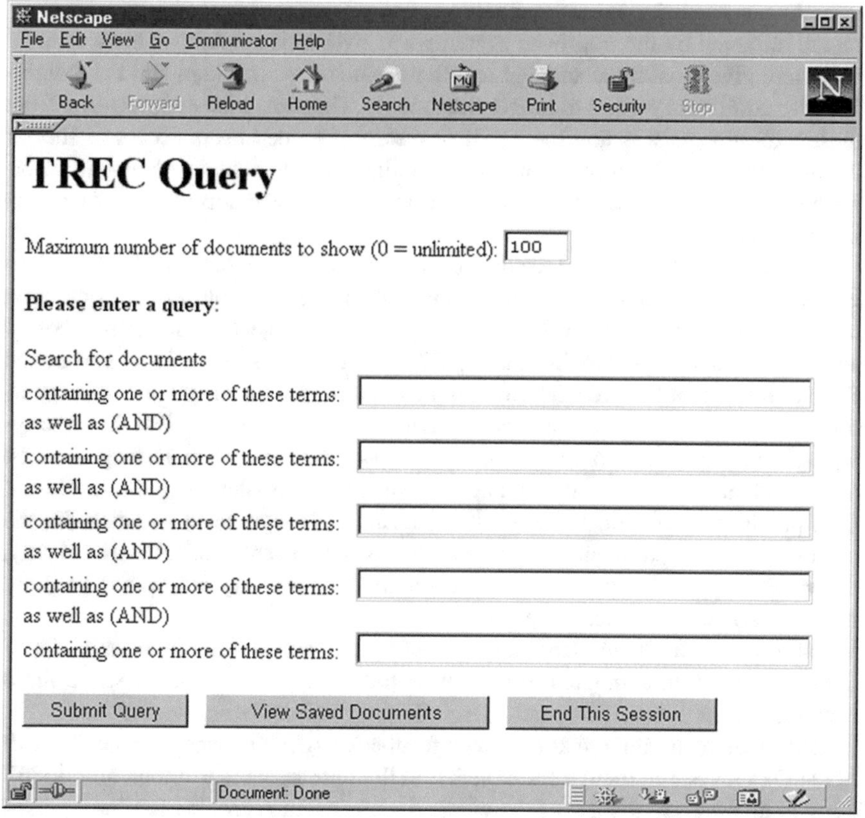

Fig. 8.8 Boolean interface for TREC Interactive Track experiments of Hersh et al. [329]

TF*IDF baseline, 58%. The user experiments thus employed Okapi plus PN weighting as the experimental system. The same user types of as well as the same natural language interface to the MG system were used. In the user experiments, the proportion of questions answered correctly was virtually identical between systems, 43.0% for TF*IDF weighting and 41.0% for Okapi plus PN weighting. In both the TREC-8 and TREC-9 experiments, use of the same user interface precluded measuring user satisfaction differences between systems. The results of the final batch experiments were comparable to those of the TREC-8 experiment: Okapi plus PN weighting achieved a 31.5% MAP improvement over the TF*IDF weighting.

A follow-up experiment attempted to determine why the "improved" (Okapi weighting in TREC-8 and Okapi plus PN weighting in TREC-9) systems failed to lead to better performance over the TF*IDF system in the hands of real users [332]. Analysis of the search output found that the users retrieved more relevant documents as well as more instances in the top ten documents with the improved systems. However, the overall number of relevant documents retrieved was comparable for both systems, although the improved system retrieved fewer nonrelevant documents. Further analysis showed that the average length of documents retrieved by the improved systems was over twice as long. This was to be expected, given that the document length normalization in Okapi and PN weighting give additional weight to longer documents. The most likely explanation from these experiments was that the TF*IDF system provided users access to shorter documents, albeit fewer relevant ones, enabling users to achieve comparable performance with the outcomes measures: instance recall and correctness of answering questions.

Further work has explored the discordant results between batch and user searching. Allan et al. found that as "system accuracy" (as measures by clusters containing increasing amounts of relevant content) increased, subject time and number of answers found to a question increased [333]. However, another study by Turpin and Scholer found that time required to find the first relevant document and the proportion of queries with no relevant answer had no association with MAP of the underlying system [334]. The only measure that was associated with finding the first relevant document was whether the first document in the system output was relevant (i.e., precision at one document). These results have significant meaning for the myriad of batch experiments performed in TREC and other IR evaluations. Namely, the MAP of systems without human users in the loop is a very limited and possibly misleading measure of performance.

Other groups used the TREC Interactive Track to assess different research questions. Belkin et al. attempted to determine the utility to users of relevance feedback [335].

Robertson et al. found that relevance feedback slightly enhanced instance recall in the Okapi system, though a simple TF*IDF approach outperformed both [336]. Yang et al. assessed the use of the whole document for relevance feedback versus selection by the user of specific passages in documents [337]. They hypothesized that the user would do better with the latter, more focused approach. Their results showed no significant difference, but a definite trend in favor of the whole-document approach.

Additional research in the TREC Interactive Track looked at the presentation of search results. Wu et al. used the instance recall tasks to assess the value of users' clustering of documents (TREC-7) or classifications of terms (TREC-8) [338]. In the TREC-9 QA interactive task, Wu et al. compared two systems that differed in how they displayed their document output (or "surrogates") [339]. One system displayed "answer-indicative sentences" that showed three sentences containing the highest number of words from the query. The other displayed the title and first 20 words of the document. Users had a higher rate of answering questions correctly with the former system (65% vs. 47%).

Other researchers investigated presentation of search results. In the TREC-7 instance recall task, Allan et al. found that separate "aspect windows" allowing a user to maintain different queries and result sets did not improve performance over a baseline TF*IDF system, but a 3D interface highlighting documents belonging to the different instances produced an improvement that was statistically significant [340].

8.5 Looking Forward

The early and middle chapters of this book show that IR systems are ubiquitous for searching for information within and outside of biomedical and health. The last few chapters show, however, that some challenges remain, both from within IR applications and external to them in those having information needs being able to access content. As the editions of this book have shown, the way we access IR systems and what we retrieve from them have evolved over several decades, from text-only information accessed using command-line interfaces on time-share networks to the multimedia content we now access on devices from watches to phones to tablets to computers. The quantity and variety of information continue to grow, as do new machine learning and artificial intelligence methods to process it. Will the methods currently used at the time of this edition being published be seen as outdated as those that represented the state of the art when the first edition was published? Will new technologies change the way we search for and otherwise interact with information? Only time will tell.

References

1. Callan J, Moffat A. Panel on use of proprietary data. SIGIR Forum. 2012;46(2):10–8.
2. Voorhees E, Harman D, editors. TREC: experiment and evaluation in information retrieval. Cambridge, MA: MIT Press; 2005.
3. Ferro N, Peters C, editors. Information retrieval evaluation in a changing world – lessons learned from 20 years of CLEF. Cham: Springer; 2019.
4. Harman D. Information retrieval evaluation. San Rafael, CA: Morgan and Claypool; 2011.
5. Harman D. Information retrieval: the early years. Foundations and trends in information retrieval, vol. 5. Hanover, MA: Now Publishers; 2019.
6. Carterette B., editor. System effectiveness, user models, and user utility: a conceptual framework for investigation. In: The 34th annual ACM SIGIR conference. Beijing: ACM; 2011.
7. Sanderson M, Croft W. The history of information retrieval research. Proc IEEE. 2012; 100:1444–51.
8. Talmon J, Ammenwerth E, Brender J, de Keizer N, Nykänen P, Rigby M. STARE-HI – statement on reporting of evaluation studies in health informatics. Int J Med Inform. 2009;78:1–9.
9. Brender J, Talmon J, de Keizer N, Nykanen P, Rigby M, Ammenwerth E. STARE-HI – statement on reporting of evaluation studies in health informatics: explanation and elaboration. Appl Clin Inform. 2013;4:331–58.
10. Culpepper J, Diaz F, Smucker M. Research Frontiers in information retrieval: report from the third strategic workshop on information retrieval in Lorne (SWIRL 2018). SIGIR Forum. 2018;52(1):34–90.
11. Voorhees E. The TREC 2005 robust track. SIGIR Forum. 2006;40(1):41–8.
12. Carterette B., editor. Robust test collections for retrieval evaluation. In: Proceedings of the 30th annual international ACM SIGIR conference on research and development in information retrieval. New York: ACM; 2007.
13. Nguyen T, Rosenberg M, Song X, Gao J, Tiwary S, Majumder R, et al., editors. MS MARCO: a human generated machine reading comprehension dataset. In: Proceedings of the workshop on cognitive computation: integrating neural and symbolic approaches 2016. Barcelona, Spain; 2016.

14. Bajaj P, Campos D, Craswell N, Deng L, Gao J, Liu X, et al. MS MARCO: a human generated machine reading comprehension dataset. arXivorg. 2016:arXiv:1611.09268.
15. Robertson S, Callan J. Routing and filtering. In: Voorhees E, Harman D, editors. TREC: experiment and evaluation in information retrieval. Cambridge, MA: MIT Press; 2005. p. 99–121.
16. Harman D. Beyond English. In: Voorhees E, Harman D, editors. TREC: experiment and evaluation in information retrieval. Cambridge, MA: MIT Press; 2005. p. 153–82.
17. Kantor P, Voorhees E. The TREC-5 confusion track: comparing retrieval methods for scanned text. Inf Retr. 2000;2:165–76.
18. Voorhees E, Garofolo J. Retrieving Noisy text. In: Voorhees E, Harman D, editors. TREC – experiment and evaluation in information retrieval. Cambridge, MA: MIT Press; 2005. p. 183–97.
19. Voorhees E. Question answering in TREC. In: Voorhees E, Harman D, editors. TREC – experiment and evaluation in information retrieval. Cambridge, MA: MIT Press; 2005. p. 233–57.
20. Hersh W, Voorhees E. TREC genomics special issue overview. Inf Retr. 2009;12:1–15.
21. Dumais S, Belkin N. The TREC interactive tracks: putting the user into search. In: Voorhees E, Harman D, editors. TREC – experiment and evaluation in information retrieval. Cambridge, MA: MIT Press; 2005. p. 123–52.
22. Hersh W. Interactivity at the text retrieval conference (TREC). Inf Process Manag. 2001;37:365–6.
23. Allan J, editor. HARD track overview in TREC 2005 – high accuracy retrieval from documents. The fourteenth text retrieval conference (TREC 2005). Gaithersburg, MD: National Institute of Standards and Technology; 2005.
24. Hawking D, Craswell N. The very large collection and web tracks. In: Voorhees E, Harman D, editors. TREC: experiment and evaluation in information retrieval. Cambridge, MA: MIT Press; 2005. p. 199–232.
25. Clarke C, Scholer F, Soboroff I, editors. The TREC 2005 terabyte track. The fourteenth text REtrieval conference (TREC 2005) proceedings. Gaithersburg, MD: National Institute of Standards and Technology; 2005.
26. Cormack G, Smucker M, Clarke C. Efficient and effective spam filtering and re-ranking for large web datasets. Inf Retr. 2011;14:441–65.
27. Macdonald C, Santos R, Ounis I, Soboroff I. Blog track research at TREC. SIGIR Forum. 2010;44(1):58–75.
28. Frisse M. Searching for information in a hypertext medical handbook. Commun ACM. 1988;31:880–6.
29. Evans D, Hersh W, Monarch I, Lefferts R, Handerson S. Automatic indexing of abstracts via natural language processing using a simple thesaurus. Med Decis Mak. 1991;11:S108–S15.
30. Hersh W, Hickam D. Information retrieval in medicine: the SAPHIRE experience. J Am Soc Inf Sci. 1995;46:743–7.
31. Haynes R, Wilczynski N, McKibbon K, Walker C, Sinclair J. Developing optimal search strategies for detecting clinically sound studies in MEDLINE. J Am Med Inform Assoc. 1994;1:447–58.
32. Salton G. A new comparison between conventional indexing (MEDLARS) and automatic text processing (SMART). J Am Soc Inf Sci. 1972;23(2):75–84.
33. Schuyler P, McCray A, Schoolman H, editors. A test collection for experimentation in bibliographic retrieval. MEDINFO 89 – proceedings of the sixth congress on medical informatics. Singapore: North-Holland; 1989.
34. Hersh W, Buckley C, Leone T, Hickam D, editors. OHSUMED: an interactive retrieval evaluation and new large test collection for research. In: Proceedings of the 17th annual international ACM SIGIR conference on research and development in information retrieval. Dublin: Springer; 1994.
35. Hersh W. Evaluation of Meta-1 for a concept-based approach to the automated indexing and retrieval of bibliographic and full-text databases. Med Decis Mak. 1991;11:S120–S4.
36. Hersh W, Hickam D. A comparison of retrieval effectiveness for three methods of indexing medical literature. Am J Med Sci. 1992;303:292–300.

37. Hersh W, Hickam D, Haynes R, McKibbon K. A performance and failure analysis of SAPHIRE with a MEDLINE test collection. J Am Med Inform Assoc. 1994;1:51–60.
38. Hersh W, Hickam D. A comparison of two methods for indexing and retrieval from a full-text medical database. Med Decis Mak. 1993;13:220–6.
39. Hersh W, Hickam D, Leone T, editors. Word, concepts, or both: optimal indexing units for automated information retrieval. In: Proceedings of the 16th annual symposium on computer applications in medical care. Baltimore, MD: McGraw-Hill; 1992.
40. Hersh W, Hickam D. An evaluation of interactive Boolean and natural language searching with an on-line medical textbook. J Am Soc Inf Sci. 1995;46:478–89.
41. Srinivasan P. Query expansion and MEDLINE. Inf Process Manag. 1996;32:431–44.
42. Srinivasan P. Optimal document-indexing vocabulary for MEDLINE. Inf Process Manag. 1996;32:503–14.
43. Aronson A, Rindflesch T, editors. Query expansion using the UMLS Metathesaurus. In: Proceedings of the 1997 AMIA annual fall symposium; Nashville, TN: Hanley and Belfus; 1997.
44. Bernstam E, Herskovic J, Aphinyanaphongs Y, Aliferis C, Sriram M, Hersh W. Using citation data to improve retrieval from MEDLINE. J Am Med Inform Assoc. 2006;13:96–105.
45. Aphinyanaphongs Y, Statnikov A, Aliferis C. A comparison of citation metrics to machine learning filters for the identification of high quality MEDLINE documents. J Am Med Inform Assoc. 2006;13:446–55.
46. Hersh W, Bhupatiraju R, editors. TREC genomics track overview. The twelfth text retrieval conference (TREC 2003). Gaithersburg, MD: NIST; 2003.
47. Mitchell J, Aronson A, Mork J, Folk L, Humphrey S, Ward J, editors. Gene indexing: characterization and analysis of NLM's GeneRIFs. Proceedings of the AMIA 2003 annual symposium. Washington, DC: Hanley and Belfus; 2003.
48. Hersh W, Bhuptiraju R, Ross L, Johnson P, Cohen A, Kraemer D, editors. TREC 2004 genomics track overview. The thirteenth text retrieval conference (TREC 2004). Gaithersburg, MD: National Institute for Standards and Technology; 2004.
49. Hersh W, Cohen A, Yang J, Bhupatiraju R, Roberts P, Hearst M, editors. TREC 2005 genomics track overview. The fourteenth text retrieval conference – TREC 2005. Gaithersburg, MD: National Institute for Standards and Technology; 2005.
50. Hersh W, Cohen A, Roberts P, Rekapalli H, editors. TREC 2006 genomics track overview. The fifteenth text retrieval conference (TREC 2006). Gaithersburg, MD: National Institute for Standards and Technology; 2006.
51. Hersh W, Cohen A, Ruslen L, Roberts P, editors. TREC 2007 genomics track overview. The sixteenth text retrieval conference (TREC 2007) proceedings. Gaithersburg, MD: National Institute for Standards and Technology; 2007.
52. Hersh W, Bhupatiraju R, Ross L, Johnson P, Cohen A, Kraemer D. Enhancing access to the bibliome: the TREC 2004 genomics track. J Biomed Discov Collab. 2006;1:3.
53. Fujita S, editor. Revisiting again document length hypotheses – TREC 2004 genomics track experiments at Patolis. The thirteenth text retrieval conference: TREC 2004. Gaithersburg, MD: National Institute of Standards and Technology; 2004.
54. Buttcher S, Clarke C, Cormack G, editors. Domain-specific synonym expansion and validation for biomedical information retrieval (MultiText experiments for TREC 2004). The thirteenth text retrieval conference: TREC 2004. Gaithersburg, MD: National Institute of Standards and Technology; 2004.
55. Seki K, Costello J, Singan V, Mostafa J, editors. TREC 2004 genomics track experiments at IUB. The thirteenth text retrieval conference: TREC 2004. Gaithersburg, MD: National Institute of Standards and Technology; 2004.
56. Nakov P, Schwartz A, Stoica E, Hearst M, editors. BioText team experiments for the TREC 2004 genomics track. The thirteenth text retrieval conference: TREC 2004. Gaithersburg, MD: National Institute of Standards and Technology; 2004.
57. Aronson A, Demmer D, Humphrey S, Ide N, Kim W, Loane R, et al., editors. Knowledge-intensive and statistical approaches to the retrieval and annotation of genomics MEDLINE

citations. The thirteenth text retrieval conference: TREC 2004. Gaithersburg, MD: National Institute of Standards and Technology; 2004.
58. Huang X, Zhong M, Si L, editors. York University at TREC 2005: genomics track. The fourteenth text REtrieval conference proceedings (TREC 2005). Gaithersburg, MD: National Institute for Standards and Technology; 2005.
59. Ando R, Dredze M, Zhang T, editors. TREC 2005 genomics track experiments at IBM Watson. The fourteenth text REtrieval conference proceedings (TREC 2005). Gaithersburg, MD: National Institute for Standards and Technology; 2005.
60. Aronson A, Demner-Fushman D, Humphrey S, Lin J, Ruch P, Ruiz M, et al., editors. Fusion of knowledge-intensive and statistical approaches for retrieving and annotating textual genomics documents. The fourteenth text REtrieval conference proceedings (TREC 2005). Gaithersburg, MD: National Institute for Standards and Technology; 2005.
61. Zheng Z, Brady S, Garg A, Shatkay H, editors. Applying probabilistic thematic clustering for classification in the TREC 2005 genomics track. The fourteenth text REtrieval conference proceedings (TREC 2005). Gaithersburg, MD: National Institute for Standards and Technology; 2005.
62. Voorhees E, Tong R, editors. Overview of the TREC 2011 medical records track. The twentieth text REtrieval conference proceedings (TREC 2011). Gaithersburg, MD: National Institute of Standards and Technology; 2011.
63. Voorhees E, Hersh W, editors. Overview of the TREC 2012 medical records track. The twenty-first text REtrieval conference proceedings (TREC 2012). Gaithersburg, MD: National Institute of Standards and Technology; 2012.
64. Voorhees E, editor. The TREC medical records track. In: Proceedings of the international conference on bioinformatics, computational biology and biomedical informatics. ACM, Washington, DC; 2013.
65. Safran C, Bloomrosen M, Hammond W, Labkoff S, Markel-Fox S, Tang P, et al. Toward a national framework for the secondary use of health data: an American medical informatics association white paper. J Am Med Inform Assoc. 2007;14:1–9.
66. Friedman C, Wong A, Blumenthal D. Achieving a nationwide learning health system. Sci Transl Med. 2010;2(57):57cm29.
67. Meystre S, Lovis C, Bürkle T, Tognola G, Budrionis A, Lehmann C. Clinical data reuse or secondary use: current status and potential future progress. Yearb Med Inform. 2017;26(1):38–52.
68. Demner-Fushman D, Abhyankar S, Jimeno-Yepes A, Loane R, Rance B, Lang F, et al., editors. A knowledge-based approach to medical records retrieval. In: The twentieth text REtrieval conference proceedings (TREC 2011). Gaithersburg, MD: National Institute for Standards and Technology; 2011.
69. Demner-Fushman D, Abhyankar S, Jimeno-Yepes A, Loane R, Lang F, Mork J, et al., editors. NLM at TREC 2012 medical records track. In: The twenty-first text REtrieval conference proceedings (TREC 2012). Gaithersburg, MD: National Institute for Standards and Technology; 2012.
70. King B, Wang L, Provalov I, editors. Cengage learning at TREC 2011 medical track. In: The twentieth text REtrieval conference proceedings (TREC 2011). Gaithersburg, MD: National Institute for Standards and Technology; 2011.
71. Simpson M, Voorhees E, Hersh W, editors. Overview of the TREC 2014 clinical decision support track. In: The twenty-third text REtrieval conference proceedings (TREC 2014). Gaithersburg, MD: National Institute of Standards and Technology; 2014.
72. Roberts K, Simpson M, Demner-Fushman D, Voorhees E, Hersh W. State-of-the-art in biomedical literature retrieval for clinical cases: a survey of the TREC 2014 CDS track. Inform Retrieval J. 2016;19:113–48.
73. Roberts K, Simpson M, Voorhees E, Hersh W, editors. Overview of the TREC 2015 clinical decision support track. In: The twenty-fourth text REtrieval conference (TREC 2015) proceedings. TREC, Gaithersburg, MD; 2015.
74. Roberts K, Demner-Fushman D, Voorhees E, Hersh W, editors. Overview of the TREC 2016 clinical decision support track. In: The twenty-fifth text REtrieval conference (TREC 2016) proceedings. Gaithersburg, MD, TREC; 2016.

75. Roberts K, Demner-Fushman D, Voorhees E, Hersh W, Bedrick S, editors. Overview of the TREC 2017 precision medicine track. In: The twenty-sixth text REtrieval conference (TREC 2017) proceedings. TREC, Gaithersburg, MD; 2017.
76. Roberts K, Demner-Fushman D, Voorhees E, Hersh W, Bedrick S, Lazar A, editors. Overview of the TREC 2018 precision medicine track. In: The twenty-seventh text REtrieval conference (TREC 2018) proceedings. TREC, Gaithersburg, MD; 2018.
77. Hersh W, Müller H, Jensen J, Yang J, Gorman P, Ruch P. Advancing biomedical image retrieval: development and analysis of a test collection. J Am Med Inform Assoc. 2006;13:488–96.
78. Hersh W, Müller H, Kalpathy-Cramer J. The ImageCLEFmed medical image retrieval task test collection. J Digit Imaging. 2009;22:648–55.
79. Müller H, Clough P, Deselaers T, Caputo B, editors. ImageCLEF: experimental evaluation in visual information retrieval. Heidelberg: Springer; 2010.
80. Kalpathy-Cramer J, Bedrick S, Radhouani S, Hersh W, Eggel I, Kahn C, et al. Retrieving similar cases from the medical literature – the ImageCLEF experience. In: MEDINFO 2010. ISO Press: Cape Town; 2010.
81. Kalpathy-Cramer J, Müller H, Bedrick S, Eggel I, Alba G, de Herrera S, et al., editors. Overview of the CLEF 2011 medical image classification and retrieval tasks. In: CLEF 2011 Labs and Workshops Notebook Papers. Amsterdam, Netherlands; 2011.
82. Müller H, Seco De Herrera A, Kalpathy-Cramer J, Demmer-Fushman D, Antani S, Eggel I, editors. Overview of the ImageCLEF 2012 medical image retrieval and classification tasks. In: CLEF 2012 working notes, Rome; 2012.
83. Müller H, Kalpathy-Cramer J, Demner-Fushman D, Antani S, editors. Creating a classification of image types in the medical literature for visual categorization. Medical imaging 2012: Advanced PACS-based imaging informatics and therapeutic applications. San Diego, CA: SPIE; 2012.
84. Jiang J, Zhai C. An empirical study of tokenization strategies for biomedical information retrieval. Inf Retr. 2007;10:341–63.
85. Zhou X, Hu X, Zhang X. Topic signature language models for ad hoc retrieval. IEEE Trans Knowl Data Eng. 2007;19:1276–87.
86. Lin J, Wilbur W. PubMed related articles: a probabilistic topic-based model for content similarity. BMC Bioinform. 2007;8:423.
87. Abdou S, Savoy J. Searching in MEDLINE: query expansion and manual indexing evaluation. Inf Process Manag. 2008;44:781–99.
88. Fafalios P, Tzitzikas Y. Stochastic reranking of biomedical search results based on extracted entities. J Am Soc Inform Sci Technol. 2017;68:2572–86.
89. Soldaini L, Yates A, Goharian N. Learning to reformulate long queries for clinical decision support. J Am Soc Inform Sci Technol. 2017;68:2602–19.
90. Koopman B, Cripwell L, Zuccon G, editors. Generating clinical queries from patient narratives: a comparison between machines and humans. In: Proceedings of the 40th international ACM SIGIR conference on Research and Development in information retrieval. ACM, Tokyo; 2017.
91. Tsatsaronis G, Balikas G, Malakasiotis P, Partalas I, Zschunke M, Alvers M, et al. An overview of the BIOASQ large-scale biomedical semantic indexing and question answering competition. BMC Bioinform. 2015;16:138.
92. Mork J, Aronson A, Demner-Fushman D. 12 years on – is the NLM medical text indexer still useful and relevant? J Biomed Semant. 2017;2017(8):8.
93. Trieschnigg D, Pezik P, Lee V, de Jong F, Kraaij W, Rebholz-Schuhmann D. MeSH Up: effective MeSH text classification for improved document retrieval. Bioinformatics. 2009;25:1412–8.
94. Aljaber B, Martinez D, Stokes N, Bailey J. Improving MeSH classification of biomedical articles using citation contexts. J Biomed Inform. 2011;44:881–96.
95. Huang M, Neveol A, Lu Z. Recommending MeSH terms for annotating biomedical articles. J Am Med Inform Assoc. 2011;18:660–7.
96. Herskovic J, Cohen T, Subramanian D, Iyengar M, Smith J, Bernstam E. MEDRank: using graph-based concept ranking to index biomedical texts. Int J Med Inform. 2011;80:431–41.

97. Kim S, Yeganova L, Comeau D, Wilbur W, Lu Z. PubMed phrases, an open set of coherent phrases for searching biomedical literature. Sci Data. 2018;5:180104.
98. Brown P, Zhou Y. Large expert-curated database for benchmarking document similarity detection in biomedical literature search. Database. 2019;2019:baz085.
99. Cohen T, Roberts K, Gururaj A, Chen X, Pournejati S, Hersh W, et al. A publicly available benchmark for biomedical dataset retrieval: the reference standard for the 2016 bioCADDIE dataset retrieval challenge. Database. 2017;27:bax061.
100. Roberts K, Gururaj A, Chen X, Pournejati S, Hersh W, Demner-Fushman D, et al. Information retrieval for biomedical datasets: the 2016 bioCADDIE dataset retrieval challenge. Database. 2017;2017:bax068.
101. Stanton I, Leong S, Mishra N, editors. Circumlocution in diagnostic medical queries. In: Proceedings of the 37th international ACM SIGIR conference on research and development in information retrieval. Gold Coast: ACM; 2014.
102. Soldaini L, Yates A, Yom-Tov E, Frieder O, Goharian N. Enhancing web search in the medical domain via query. Inform Retrieval J. 2016;19:149–73.
103. Soldaini L, Goharian N, editors. Learning to rank for consumer health search: a semantic approach. In: Proceedings of the ACM SIGIR international conference on theory of information retrieval. Amsterdam: ACM; 2017.
104. Jimmy, Zuccon G, Koopman B. Payoffs and pitfalls in using knowledge-bases for consumer health search. Inform Retrieval J. 2018;22:350–94.
105. Palotti J, Zuccon G, Hanbury A. Consumer health search on the web: study of web page understandability and its integration in ranking algorithms. J Med Internet Res. 2018;21(1):e10986.
106. Demner-Fushman D, Mrabet Y, Abacha A. Consumer health information and question answering: helping consumers find answers to their health-related information needs. J Am Med Inform Assoc. 2019;27:194–201.
107. Kilicoglu H, Abacha A, Mrabet Y, Shooshan S, Rodriguez L, Masterton K, et al. Semantic annotation of consumer health questions. BMC Bioinform. 2018;19:34.
108. Zheng J, Yu H. Methods for linking EHR notes to education materials. Inform Retrieval J. 2016;19:174–88.
109. Silberg W, Lundberg G, Musacchio R. Assessing, controlling, and assuring the quality of medical information on the internet: caveat lector et viewor – let the reader and viewer beware. J Am Med Assoc. 1997;277:1244–5.
110. Pogacar F, Ghenai A, Smucker M, Clarke C, editors. The positive and negative influence of search results on people's decisions about the efficacy of medical treatments. In: 2017 ACM SIGIR international conference on the theory of information retrieval. Amsterdam, ACM; 2017.
111. Lioma C, Simonsen J, Larsen B, editors. Evaluation measures for relevance and credibility in ranked lists. In: Proceedings of the ACM SIGIR international conference on theory of information retrieval. ACM, Amsterdam; 2017.
112. Lioma C, Maistro M, Smucker M, Zuccon G, editors. Overview of the TREC 2019 decision track. In: The twenty-eighth text REtrieval conference (TREC 2019) proceedings. Gaithersburg, MD: TREC; 2019.
113. Cartright M, White R, Horvitz E, editors. Intentions and attention in exploratory health search. In: Proceedings of the 34th annual international ACM SIGIR conference on research and development in information retrieval (SIGIR 2011). Beijing: ACM; 2011.
114. White R, Horvitz E, Editors. Studies of the onset and persistence of medical concerns in search logs. In: Proceedings of the 35th annual international ACM SIGIR conference on research and development in information retrieval (SIGIR 2012). Portland, OR: ACM; 2012.
115. White R, Horvitz E. Cyberchondria: studies of the escalation of medical concerns in web search. ACM Trans Inf Syst. 2009;4:23–37.
116. White R, Tatonetti N, Shah N, Altman R, Horvitz E. Web-scale pharmacovigilance: listening to signals from the crowd. J Am Med Inform Assoc. 2013;20:404–8.
117. Nguyen T, Larsen M, O'Dea B, Phung D, Venkatesh S, Christensen H. Estimation of the prevalence of adverse drug reactions from social media. J Biomed Inform. 2017;102:130–7.

118. Paparrizos J, White R, Horvitz E. Screening for pancreatic adenocarcinoma using signals from web search logs: feasibility study and results. J Oncol Pract. 2016;12:737–44.
119. White R, Horvitz E. Evaluation of the feasibility of screening patients for early signs of lung carcinoma in web search logs. JAMA Oncol. 2017;3:398–401.
120. Müller H, Kalpathy-Cramer J, García A, de Herrera A. Experiences from the ImageCLEF medical retrieval and annotation tasks. In: Ferro N, Peters C, editors. Information retrieval evaluation in a changing world – lessons learned from 20 years of CLEF. Cham: Springer; 2019.
121. Kalpathy-Cramer J, SecodeHerrera A, Demner-Fushman D, Antani S, Bedrick S, Müller H. Evaluating performance of biomedical image retrieval systems – an overview of the medical image retrieval task at ImageCLEF 2004–2013. Comput Med Imaging Graph. 2015;39:55–61.
122. Kurtz C, Beaulieu C, Napel S, Rubin D. A hierarchical knowledge-based approach for retrieving similar medical images described with semantic annotations. J Biomed Inform. 2014;49:227–44.
123. de Herrera A, Schaer R, Müller H. Shangri–La: a medical case–based retrieval tool. J Am Soc Inform Sci Technol. 2017;68:2587–2601.
124. Markonis D, Schaer R, Müller H. Evaluating multimodal relevance feedback techniques for medical image retrieval. Inform Retrieval J. 2016;19:100–12.
125. Ayadi H, Torjmen-Khemakhem M, Daoud M, Huang J, Jemaa M. MF-re-rank: a modality feature-based re-ranking model for medical image retrieval. J Am Soc Inform Sci Technol. 2018;69:1095–108.
126. Yu H, Agarwal S, Johnston M, Cohen A. Are figure legends sufficient? Evaluating the contribution of associated text to biomedical figure comprehension. J Biomed Discov Collab. 2009;4:1.
127. Kahn C, Rubin D. Automated semantic indexing of figure captions to improve radiology image retrieval. J Am Med Inform Assoc. 2009;16:380–6.
128. Demner-Fushman D, Antani S, Simpson M, Thoma G. Annotation and retrieval of clinically relevant images. Int J Med Inform. 2009;78:e59–67.
129. Lee P, West J, Howe B. Viziometrics: analyzing visual information in the scientific literature. IEEE Trans Big Data. 2017;4:117–29.
130. Cohen A, Hersh W, Peterson K, Yen P. Reducing workload in systematic review preparation using automated citation classification. J Am Med Inform Assoc. 2006;13:206–19.
131. Cohen A, Ambert K, McDonagh M. Cross-topic learning for work prioritization in systematic review creation and update. J Am Med Inform Assoc. 2009;16:690–704.
132. Cohen A, Ambert K, McDonagh M. Studying the potential impact of automated document classification on scheduling a systematic review update. BMC Med Inform Decis Mak. 2012;12:33.
133. Cohen A, Smalheiser N, McDonagh M, Yu C, Adams C, Davis J, et al. Automated confidence ranked classification of randomized controlled trial articles: an aid to evidence-based medicine. J Am Med Inform Assoc. 2015;22:707–17.
134. Kilicoglu H, Demner-Fushman D, Rindflesch T, Wilczynski N, Haynes R. Towards automatic recognition of scientifically rigorous clinical research evidence. J Am Med Inform Assoc. 2009;16:25–31.
135. Paynter R, Bañez L, Berliner E, Erinoff E, Lege-Matsuura J, Potter S, et al. EPC methods: an exploration of the use of text-mining software in systematic reviews. Rockville, MD: Agency for Healthcare Research and Quality; 2016. Contract No.: Report No.: 16-EHC023-EF.
136. Shekelle P, Shetty K, Newberry S, Maglione M, Motala A. Machine learning versus standard techniques for updating searches for systematic reviews: a diagnostic accuracy study. Ann Intern Med. 2017;167:213–5.
137. Kanoulas E, Li D, Azzopardi L, Spijker R, editors. CLEF 2017 technologically assisted reviews in empirical medicine overview. In: Working notes of CLEF 2017 – conference and labs of the evaluation forum. Dublin: CLEF; 2017.
138. Kanoulas E, Li D, Azzopardi L, Spijker R, editors. CLEF 2018 technologically assisted reviews in empirical medicine overview. In: Working notes of CLEF 2018 – conference and labs of the evaluation forum. Avignon: CLEF; 2018.

139. Kanoulas E, Li D, Azzopardi L, Spijker R, editors. CLEF 2019 technology assisted reviews in empirical medicine overview. In: Working notes of CLEF 2019 – conference and labs of the evaluation forum. Lugano: CLEF; 2019.
140. Scells H, Zuccon G, Koopman B, Deacon A, Azzopardi L, Geva S, editors. A test collection for evaluating retrieval of studies for inclusion in systematic reviews. In: Proceedings of the 40th international ACM SIGIR conference on research and development in information retrieval. Tokyo: ACM; 2017.
141. Scells H, Azzopardi L, Zuccon G, Koopman B, editors. Query variation performance prediction for systematic reviews. In: 41st international ACM SIGIR conference on research and development in information retrieval. Ann Arbor, MI: ACM; 2018.
142. Scells H, Zuccon G, editors. Generating better queries for systematic reviews. In: Proceedings of the 41st international ACM SIGIR conference on research and development in information retrieval. Ann Arbor, MI: ACM; 2018.
143. Lee G, Sun A, editors. Seed-driven document ranking for systematic reviews in evidence-based medicine. In: Proceedings of the 41st international ACM SIGIR conference on research and development in information retrieval. Ann Arbor, MI: ACM; 2018.
144. Edinger T, Cohen A, Bedrick S, Ambert K, Hersh W, editors. Barriers to retrieving patient information from electronic health record data: failure analysis from the TREC medical records track. In: AMIA 2012 annual symposium. Chicago, IL: AMIA; 2012.
145. Koopman B, Zuccon G, Bruza P, Sitbon L, Lawley M. Information retrieval as semantic inference: a graph inference model applied to medical search. Inform Retrieval J. 2016;19:6–37.
146. Amini I, Martinez D, Li X, Sanderson M. Improving patient record search: a meta-data based approach. Inf Process Manag. 2016;52:258–72.
147. Zhu D, Wu S, Carterette B, Liu H. Using large clinical corpora for query expansion in text-based cohort identification. J Biomed Inform. 2014;49:275–81.
148. Martinez D, Otegi A, Soroa A, Agirre E. Improving search over electronic health records using UMLS-based query expansion through random walks. J Biomed Inform. 2014;51:100–6.
149. Limsopatham N, Macdonald C, Ounis I, editors. Learning to handle negated language in medical records search. In: CIKM 13: proceedings of the 22nd ACM international conference on information and knowledge management. San Francisco, CA: ACM; 2013.
150. Limsopatham N, Macdonald C, Ounis I, editors. Learning to combine representations for medical records search. In: Proceedings of the 35th annual international ACM SIGIR conference on research and development in information retrieval (SIGIR 2012). Dublin: Association for Computing Machinery; 2013.
151. Limsopatham N, Macdonald C, Ounis I, editors. Inferring conceptual relationships to improve medical records search. In: OAIR 13: proceedings of the 10th conference on open research areas in information retrieval. Lisbon: ACM; 2013.
152. Limsopatham N, Macdonald C, Ounis I. Aggregating evidence from hospital departments to improve medical records search. Adv Inf Retrieval, Lect Notes Comput Sci. 2013;7814:279–91.
153. Goodwin T, Harabagiu S. Learning relevance models for patient cohort retrieval. JAMIA Open. 2018;1:265–74.
154. Friedman C, Rindflesch T, Corn M. Natural language processing: state of the art and prospects for significant progress, a workshop sponsored by the National Library of medicine. J Biomed Inform. 2013;46:765–73.
155. Sweeney L, editor. Replacing personally-identifying information in medical records, the Scrub system. In: Proceedings of the 1996 AMIA annual fall symposium. Washington, DC: Hanley and Belfus; 1996.
156. Sweeney L. Matching known patients to health records in Washington State data. arXivorg. 2013;arXiv:1307.70.
157. Naveed M, Kamara S, Wright C. Inference attacks on property-preserving encrypted databases. In: Proceedings of the 22nd ACM SIGSAC conference on computer and communications security. Denver, CO: ACM; 2015.

158. Lin J, Efron M. Evaluation as a service for information retrieval. SIGIR Forum. 2013;47(2):8–14.
159. Paik J, Lin J, editors. Retrievability in API-based "evaluation as a service". In: Proceedings of the 2016 ACM international conference on the theory of information retrieval. Newark, DE: ACM; 2016.
160. Roegiest A, Cormack G, editors. An architecture for privacy-preserving and replicable high-recall retrieval experiments. In: Proceedings of the 39th international ACM SIGIR conference on research and development in information retrieval. Pisa: ACM; 2016.
161. Hanbury A, Müller H, Balog K, Brodt T, Cormack G, Eggel I, et al. Evaluation-as-a-service: overview and outlook. arXivorg. 2015;arXiv:1512.07454.
162. Hopfgartner F, Hanbury A, Müller H, Kando N, Mercer S, Kalpathy-Cramer J, et al. Report on the evaluation-as-a-service (EaaS) expert workshop. SIGIR Forum. 2015;49(1):57–65.
163. Johnson A, Pollard T, Shen L, Lehman L, Feng M, Ghassemi M, et al. MIMIC-III, a freely accessible critical care database. Sci Data. 2016;3:160035.
164. Chamberlin S, Bedrick S, Cohen A, Wang Y, Wen A, Liu S, Liu H, Hersh W. Evaluation of patient-level retrieval from electronic health record data for a cohort discovery task. JAMIA Open, 2020;ooaa026.
165. Wang Y, Wen A, Liu S, Hersh W, Bedrick S, Liu H. Test collections for electronic health record-based clinical information retrieval. JAMIA Open. 2019;2:360–8.
166. Wu S, Liu S, Wang Y, Timmons T, Uppili H, Bedrick S, et al. Intra-institutional EHR collections for patient-level information retrieval. J Am Soc Inf Sci Tec. 2017;68:2636–48.
167. Marchionini G. Information concepts: from books to cyberspace identities. San Rafael, CA: Morgan and Claypool; 2010.
168. Saracevic T. The notion of relevance in information science: everybody knows what relevance is. But, what is it really? San Rafael, CA: Morgan and Claypool; 2016.
169. Salton G, McGill M. Introduction to modern information retrieval. New York: McGraw-Hill; 1983.
170. Salton G. Developments in automatic text retrieval. Science. 1991;253:974–80.
171. Zobel J, Moffat A. Exploring the similarity space. SIGIR Forum. 1998;32:18–34.
172. Robertson S, Walker S, editors. Some simple effective approximations to the 2-Poisson model for probabilistic weighted retrieval. In: Proceedings of the 17th annual international ACM SIGIR conference on research and development in information retrieval. Dublin: Springer; 1994.
173. Robertson S, Walker S, Jones S, Hancock-Beaulieu M, Gatford M, editors. Okapi at TREC-3. In: Overview of the third text REtrieval conference (TREC-3). Gaithersburg, MD: National Institute of Standards and Technology; 1994.
174. Turtle H, Croft W. Evaluation of an inference network-based retrieval model. ACM Trans Inf Syst. 1991;9:187–222.
175. Hiemstra D, Kraaij W. A language-modeling approach to TREC. In: Voorhees E, Harman D, editors. TREC: experiment and evaluation in information retrieval, vol. 373–396. Cambridge, MA: MIT Press; 2005.
176. Ponte J, Croft W, editors. A language modeling approach to information retrieval. In: Proceedings of the 21st annual international ACM SIGIR conference on research and development in information retrieval. Melbourne: ACM; 1998.
177. Berger A, Lafferty J, editors. Information retrieval as statistical translation. In: Proceedings of the 22nd annual international ACM SIGIR conference on research and development in information retrieval. Berkeley, CA: ACM; 1999.
178. Zhai C, Lafferty J. A study of smoothing methods for language models applied to information retrieval. ACM Trans Inf Syst. 2004;22:179–214.
179. Cronen-Townsend S, Zhou Y, Croft W, editors. Predicting query performance. In: Proceedings of the 25th annual international ACM SIGIR conference on research and development in information retrieval. Tampere: ACM; 2002.
180. Turpin A, Hersh W, editors. Do clarity scores for queries correlate with user performance? In: Proceedings of the fifteenth Australasian database conference (ADC2004). Dunedin: Australian Computer Society; 2004.

181. Salton G, Buckley C. Global text matching for information retrieval. Science. 1991;253:1012–5.
182. Callan J, editor. Passage level evidence in document retrieval. In: Proceedings of the 17th annual international ACM SIGIR conference on research and development in information retrieval. Dublin: Springer; 1994.
183. Buckley C, Allan J, Salton G, editors. Automatic routing and ad-hoc retrieval using SMART: TREC-2. In: The second text REtrieval conference (TREC-2). Gaithersburg, MD: National Institute of Standards and Technology; 1993.
184. Hearst M, Plaunt C, editors. Subtopic structuring for full-length document access. In: Proceedings of the 16th annual international ACM SIGIR conference on research and development in information retrieval. Pittsburgh, PA: ACM; 1993.
185. Broglio J, Callan J, Croft W, Nachbar D, editors. Document retrieval and routing using the INQUERY system. In: Overview of the third text REtrieval conference (TREC-3). Gaithersburg, MD: National Institute of Standards and Technology; 1994.
186. Buckley C, Salton G, Allan J, Singhal A, editors. Automatic query expansion using SMART: TREC 3. In: Overview of the third text REtrieval conference (TREC-3). Gaithersburg, MD: National Institute of Standards and Technology; 1994.
187. Knaus D, Mittendorf E, Schauble P, editors. Improving a basic retrieval method by links and passage level evidence. In: Overview of the third text REtrieval conference (TREC-3). Gaithersburg, MD: National Institute of Standards and Technology; 1994.
188. Kwok K, Grunfeld L, Lewis D, editors. TREC-3 ad-hoc, routing retrieval, and thresholding experiments using PIRCS. In: Overview of the third text REtrieval conference (TREC-3). Gaithersburg, MD: National Institute of Standards and Technology; 1994.
189. Buckley C. The SMART project at TREC. In: Voorhees E, Harman D, editors. TREC: experiment and evaluation in information retrieval. Cambridge, MA: MIT Press; 2005. p. 301–20.
190. Buckley C. Why current IR engines fail. Inf Retr. 2009;12:652–65.
191. Deerwester S, Dumais S, Furnas G, Landauer T, Harshman R. Indexing by latent semantic analysis. J Am Soc Inf Sci. 1990;41:391–407.
192. McCarthy J, Feigenbaum E. In memoriam Arthur Samuel: Pioneer in machine learning. AI Mag. 1990;11(3):10–1.
193. Alpaydin E. Machine learning: The new AI. Cambridge, MA: MIT Press; 2016.
194. Goodfellow I, Bengio Y, Courville A. Deep learning. Cambridge, MA: MIT Press; 2016.
195. Esteva A, Robicquet A, Ramsundar B, Kuleshov V, DePristo M, Chou K, et al. A guide to deep learning in healthcare. Nat Med. 2019;25:24–9.
196. Mitra B, Craswell N. An introduction to neural information retrieval. Foundations and trends in information retrieval. Delft: Now Publishers; 2018.
197. Liu T. Learning to rank for information retrieval. Foundations and trends in information retrieval. Delft: Now Publishers; 2009.
198. Qin T, Liu T, Xu J, Li H. LETOR: a benchmark collection for research on learning to rank for information retrieval. Inf Retr. 2010;13:346–74.
199. Pennington J, Socher R, Manning C, editors. GloVe: global vectors for word representation. In: Proceedings of the 2014 conference on empirical methods in natural language processing (EMNLP). Doha: Association for Computational Linguistics; 2014.
200. Le Q, Mikolov T, editors. Distributed representations of sentences and documents. In: Proceedings of the 31st international conference on machine learning. Bejing: PMLR; 2014.
201. Peters M, Neumann M, Iyyer M, Gardner M, Clark C, Lee K, et al. Deep contextualized word representations. arXivorg. 2018;arXiv:1802.05365.
202. Devlin J, Chang M, Lee K, Toutanova K, editors. BERT: pre-training of deep bidirectional transformers for language understanding. In: Proceedings of the 2019 Conference of the north American chapter of the association for computational linguistics: human language technologies. MinneapolisMN: Association for Computational Linguistics; 2019.
203. Alammar J. The Illustrated BERT, ELMo, and Co. (How NLP cracked transfer learning). Visualizing machine learning one concept at a time 2018
204. Latysheva N. The year of BERT – The boom in deeper transfer learning in NLP. Toward data science, 2019

205. Ruder S. NLP's ImageNet moment has arrived. The gradient, 2018
206. Yang W, Lu K, Yang P, Lin J, editors. Critically examining the "neural hype": weak baselines and the additivity of effectiveness gains from neural ranking. In: Proceedings of the 42nd international ACM SIGIR conference on Research and Development in information retrieval. Paris: ACM; 2019.
207. Mitra B, Diaz F, Craswell N, editors. Learning to match using local and distributed representations of text for web search. In: Proceedings of the 26th international conference on the world wide web. Geneva: International World Wide Web Conferences Steering Committee; 2017.
208. Dehghani M, Zamani H, Severyn A, Kamps J, Croft W, editors. Neural ranking models with weak supervision. In: Proceedings of the 40th international ACM SIGIR conference on research and development in information retrieval (SIGIR2017). Tokyo: ACM; 2017.
209. Van Gysel C, de Rijke M, Kanoulas E. Neural vector spaces for unsupervised information retrieval. ACM Trans Inf Sys. 2018;36(3):38.
210. Ai Q, Bi K, Guo J, Croft W, editors. Learning a deep listwise context model for ranking refinement. In: Proceedings of the 41st international ACM SIGIR conference on research and development in information retrieval, Ann Arbor, MI; 2018.
211. Dai Z, Callan J, editors. Deeper text understanding for IR with contextual neural language modeling. In: Proceedings of the 42nd international ACM SIGIR conference on Research and Development in information retrieval. Paris, France; 2019.
212. Imani A, Vakili A, Montazer A, Shakery A. Deep neural networks for query expansion using word embeddings. arXivorg. 2018;arXiv:1811.03514.
213. MacAvaney S, Yates A, Cohan A, Goharian N, editors. CEDR: contextualized embeddings for document ranking. In: Proceedings of the 42nd international ACM SIGIR conference on Research and Development in information retrieval, Paris, France; 2019.
214. Qiao Y, Xiong C, Liu Z, Liu Z. Understanding the behaviors of BERT in ranking. arXivorg. 2019;arXiv:1904.07531.
215. Padigela H, Zamani H, Croft W. Investigating the successes and failures of BERT for passage re-ranking. arXivorg. 2019;arXiv:1905.01758.
216. Yang W, Zhang H, Lin J. Simple applications of BERT for ad hoc document retrieval. arXivorg. 2019;arXiv:1903.10972.
217. Yilmaz Z, Yang W, Zhang H, Lin J, editors. Cross-domain modeling of sentence-level evidence for document retrieval. In: Proceedings of the 2019 Conference on empirical methods in natural language processing and the 9th international joint conference on natural language processing (EMNLP-IJCNLP). Hong Kong: EMNLP; 2019.
218. Nogueira R, Cho K. Passage re-ranking with BERT. arXivorg. 2019;arXiv:1901.04085.
219. Lardinois F. Google brings in BERT to improve its search results. Tech Crunch; 2019. https://techcrunch.com/2019/10/25/google-brings-in-bert-to-improve-its-search-results/
220. Nguyen G. Bing says it has been applying BERT since April. Search Engine Land; 2019. https://searchengineland.com/bing-says-it-has-been-applying-bert-since-april-325371
221. Yang W, Xie Y, Lin A, Li X, Tan L, Xiong K et al., editors. End-to-end open-domain question answering with BERTserini. In: Proceedings of the 2019 conference of the North American chapter of the association for computational linguistics; Minneapolis: Association for Computational Linguistics; 2019.
222. DelFiol G, Michelson M, Iorio A, Cotoi C, Haynes R. A deep learning method to automatically identify reports of scientifically rigorous clinical research from the biomedical literature: comparative analytic study. J Med Internet Res. 2018;20(6):e10281.
223. Wei W, Marmor R, Singh S, Wang S, Demner-Fushman D, Kuo T et al., editors. Finding related publications: extending the set of terms used to assess article similarity. AMIA joint summits on translational science, San Francisco, CA; 2016.
224. Mohan S, Fiorini N, Kim S, Lu Z, editors. A fast deep learning model for textual relevance in biomedical information retrieval. In: Proceedings of the 2018 World wide web conference, Lyon, France; 2018.
225. Choi E, Bahadori T, Searles E, Coffey C, Thompson M, Bost J et al., editors. Multi-layer representation learning for medical concepts. In: Proceedings of the 22nd ACM SIGKDD international conference on knowledge discovery and data mining. San Francisco: ACM; 2016.

226. Wang Y, Liu S, Afzal N, Rastegar-Mojarad M, Wang L, Shen F, et al. A comparison of word embeddings for the biomedical natural language processing. J Biomed Inform. 2018;87:12–20.
227. Beam A, Kompa B, Schmaltz A, Fried I, Weber G, Palmer N, et al. Clinical concept embeddings learned from massive sources of multimodal medical data. arXivorg. 2018;arXiv:1804.01486.
228. Agarwal K, Eftimov T, Addanki R, Choudhury S, Tamang S, Rallo R. Snomed2Vec: random walk and poincaré embeddings of a clinical knowledge base for healthcare analytics. arXivorg. 2019;arXiv:1907.08650.
229. Deng L, Liu Y, editors. Deep learning in natural language processing. New York, NY: Springer; 2018.
230. Tenney I, Das D, Pavlick E, editors. BERT rediscovers the classical NLP pipeline. In: Proceedings of the 57th annual meeting of the Association for Computational Linguistics, Florence, Italy; 2019.
231. Kucera H, Francis W. Computational analysis of present-day American English. Providence, RI: Brown University Press; 1967.
232. Mothe J, Tanguy L, editors. Linguistic features to predict query difficulty. Workshop on predicting query difficulty – methods and applications, Salvador, Brazil; 2005.
233. Fagan J. Experiments in automatic phrase indexing document retrieval: a comparison of syntactic and non-syntactic methods [Ph.D.]. Ithaca, NY: Cornell University; 1987.
234. Salton G, Buckley C, Smith M. On the application of syntactic methodologies in automatic text analysis. Inf Process Manag. 1990;26:73–92.
235. Evans D, Lefferts R, Greffenstette G, Handerson S, Hersh W, Archbold A, editors. CLARIT TREC design, experiments, and results. The first text REtrieval conference (TREC-1). Gaithersburg, MD: National Institute of Standards and Technology; 1992.
236. Evans D, Zhai C, editors. Noun-phrase analysis in unrestricted text for information retrieval. In: Proceedings of the 34th annual meeting on association for computational linguistics. Santa Cruz, CA: Association for Computational Linguistics; 1994.
237. Hersh W, Campbell E, Evans D, Brownlow N, editors. Empirical, automated vocabulary discovery using large text corpora and advanced natural language processing tools. In: Proceedings of the 1996 AMIA annual fall symposium. Washington, DC: Hanley and Belfus; 1996.
238. Strzalkowski T, Lin F, Wang J, Perez-Carballo J. Evaluating natural language processing techniques in information retrieval. In: Strzalkowski T, editor. Natural language information retrieval. Dordrecht: Kluwer; 1999. p. 113–46.
239. Demner-Fushman D, Elhadad N, Friedman C. Natural language processing for health-related texts. In: Shortliffe E, Cimino J, Elhadad N, Chiang M, editors. Biomedical informatics: computer applications in health care and biomedicine. 5th ed. London: Springer; 2020.
240. Woods W. Transition network grammars for natural language analysis. Commun ACM. 1970;13:591–602.
241. Burger J, Cardie C, Chaudhri V, Gaizauskas R, Harabagiu S, Israel D et al. Issues, tasks and program structures to roadmap research in Question and Answering (Q&A); 2000. http://www-nlpir.nist.gov/projects/duc/papers/qa.Roadmap-paper_v2.doc. Accessed July 1, 2002.
242. Moldovan D, Pasca M, Harabagiu S, Surdeanu M. Performance issues and error analysis in an open-domain question answering system. ACM Trans Inf Syst. 2003;21(2):133–54.
243. Rajpurkar P, Zhang J, Lopyrev K, Liang P, editors. SQuAD: 100,000+ questions for machine comprehension of text. Proceedings of the 2016 conference on empirical methods in natural language processing. Austin, TX: Association for Computational Linguistics; 2016.
244. Nanni F, Mitra B, Magnusson M, Dietz L, editors. Benchmark for complex answer retrieval. In: Proceedings of the ACM SIGIR international conference on theory of information retrieval. New York: ACM; 2017.

245. Zweigenbaum P, editor. Question answering in biomedicine. European chapter of the association for computational linguistics workshop on natural language processing for question answering. Budapest: Association for Computational Linguistics; 2003.
246. Rinaldi F, Dowdall J, Schneider G, Persidis A, editors. Answering questions in the genomics domain. ACL 2004 workshop on question answering in restricted domains. Barcelona: Association for Computational Linguistics; 2004.
247. Niu Y, Hirst G, Mc Arthur G, Rodriguez-Gianolli P, editors. Answering clinical questions with role identification. In: Proceedings, workshop on natural language processing in biomedicine, 41st annual meeting of the Association for Computational Linguistics. Sapporo: Association for Computational Linguistics; 2003.
248. Niu Y, Hirst G, editors. Analysis of semantic classes in medical text for question answering. Workshop on question answering in restricted domains, 42nd annual meeting of the Association For Computational Linguistics. Barcelona: Association for Computational Linguistics; 2004.
249. Niu Y, Zhu X, Hirst G, editors. Using outcome polarity in sentence extraction for medical question-answering. Proceedings of the AMIA 2006 annual symposium. Washington, DC: American Medical Informatics Association; 2006.
250. Demner-Fushman D, Lin J. Answering clinical questions with knowledge-based and statistical techniques. Comput Linguist. 2007;33:63–103.
251. Sneiderman C, Demner-Fushman D, Fiszman M, Ide N, Rindflesch T. Knowledge-based methods to help clinicians find answers in MEDLINE. J Am Med Inform Assoc. 2007;14:772–80.
252. Ide N, Loane R, Demner-Fushman D. Essie: a concept-based search engine for structured biomedical text. J Am Med Inform Assoc. 2007;14:253–63.
253. Fiszman M, Rindflesch T, Kilicoglu H, editors. Abstraction summarization for managing the biomedical research literature. Proceedings of the HLT-NAACL workshop on computational lexical semantics. Boston, MA: North American Association for Computational Linguistics; 2004.
254. Rekapalli H, Cohen A, Hersh W, editors. A comparative analysis of retrieval features used in the TREC 2006 genomics track passage retrieval task. Proceedings of the AMIA 2007 annual symposium. Chicago, IL: American Medical Informatics Association; 2007.
255. Lu Z, Kim W, Wilbur W. Evaluating relevance ranking strategies for MEDLINE retrieval. J Am Med Inform Assoc. 2009;16:32–6.
256. Xu B, Lin H, Yang L, Xu K, Zhang Y, Zhang D, et al. A supervised term ranking model for diversity enhanced biomedical information retrieval. BMC Bioinform. 2019;20:590.
257. Goodwin T, Harabagiu S. Knowledge representations and inference techniques for medical question answering. ACM Trans Intell Syst Technol. 2017;9, 14(2)
258. Neves M, Leser U. Question answering for biology. Methods. 2015;74:36–46.
259. Hristovski D, Dinevski D, Kastrin A, Rindflesch T. Biomedical question answering using semantic relations. BMC Bioinform. 2015;16:6.
260. Pampari A, Raghavan P, Liang J, Peng J, editors. emrQA: a large corpus for question answering on electronic medical records. Proceedings of the 2018 Conference on empirical methods in natural language processing. Brussels: University of Illinois at Urbana-Champaign; 2018.
261. Wen A, Elwazir M, Moon S, Fan J. Adapting and evaluating a deep learning language model for clinical why-question answering. JAMIA Open; 2020. Epub ahead of print.
262. Ferrucci D, Brown E, Chu-Carroll J, Fan J, Gondek D, Kalyanpur A, et al. Building Watson: an overview of the DeepQA project. AI Mag. 2010;31(3):59–79.
263. Ferrucci D. Introduction to "this is Watson". IBM J Res Dev. 2012;56(3/4):1–15.
264. Markoff J. Computer wins on 'jeopardy!': trivial, it's not New York Times, New York 2011 February 16
265. Lohr S. The future of high-tech health care — and the challenge. New York Times, New York; 2012 February, 13.
266. Ferrucci D, Levas A, Bagchi S, Gondek D, Mueller E. Watson: beyond Jeopardy! Artif Intell. 2012;199–200:93–105.

267. Devarakonda M, Mehta N, Tsou C, Liang J, Nowacki A, Jelovsek J. Automated problem list generation and physicians perspective from a pilot study. J Biomed Inform. 2017;105:121–9.
268. Somashekhar S, Sepúlveda M, Puglielli S, Norden A, Shortliffe E, RohitKumar C, et al. Watson for oncology and breast cancer treatment recommendations: agreement with an expert multidisciplinary tumor board. Ann Oncol. 2018;29:418–23.
269. Schank R. The fraudulent claims made by IBM about Watson and AI. They are not doing "cognitive computing" no matter how many times they say they are; 2016.
270. Ross C, Swetlit I. IBM pitched its Watson supercomputer as a revolution in cancer care. It's nowhere close STAT; 2017 September 5.
271. Coiera E. Journal review: Watson for oncology in breast cancer. The guide to health informatics 3rd edn.; 2018.
272. Lewis D, editor. Evaluating and optimizing autonomous text classification systems. In: Proceedings of the 18th annual international ACM SIGIR conference on research and development in information retrieval. Seattle, WA: ACM; 1995.
273. Sebastiani F. Text categorization. In: Zanasi A, editor. Text mining and its applications. Southampton: WIT Press; 2005. p. 109–29.
274. Robertson S, Soboroff I, editors. The TREC 2001 filtering track report. The tenth text REtrieval conference (TREC 2001). Gaithersburg, MD: National Institute of Standards and Technology; 2001.
275. Lewis D, Yang Y, Rose T, Li F. RCV1: a new benchmark collection for text categorization research. J Mach Learn Res. 2004;5:361–97.
276. Robertson S, Hull D, editors. The TREC-9 filtering track final report. The ninth text REtrieval conference (TREC-9). Gaithersburg, MD: National Institute of Standards and Technology; 2000.
277. Krupke D, Naf D, Vincent M, Allio T, Mikaelian I, Sundberg J, et al. The mouse tumor biology database: integrated access to mouse cancer biology data. Exp Lung Res. 2005;31:259–70.
278. Hill D, Begley D, Finger J, Hayamizu T, McCright I, Smith C, et al. The mouse gene expression database (GXD): updates and enhancements. Nucleic Acids Res. 2004;32:D568–D71.
279. Strivens M, Eppig J. Visualizing the laboratory mouse: capturing phenotype information. Genetica. 2004;122:89–97.
280. Cohen A, Hersh W. The TREC 2004 genomics track categorization task: classifying full-text biomedical documents. J Biomed Discov Collab. 2006;1:4.
281. Shatkay H, Chen N, Blostein D. Integrating image data into biomedical text categorization. Bioinformatics. 2006;22:e446–e53.
282. Aphinyanaphongs Y, Tsamardinos I, Statnikov A, Hardin D, Aliferis C. Text categorization models for high-quality article retrieval in internal medicine. J Am Med Inform Assoc. 2005;12:207–16.
283. Aphinyanaphongs Y, Aliferis C, editors. Learning Boolean queries for article quality filtering. MEDINFO 2004 – proceedings of the eleventh world congress on medical informatics. San Francisco, CA: IOS Press; 2004.
284. Aphinyanaphongs Y, Aliferis C, editors. Text categorization models for identifying unproven cancer treatments on the web. MEDINFO 2007 – proceedings of the twelfth world congress on health (medical) informatics. Brisbane: IOS Press; 2007.
285. Carneiro H, Mylonakis E. Google trends: a web-based tool for real-time surveillance of disease outbreaks. Clin Infect Dis. 2009;49:1557–64.
286. Cook S, Conrad C, Fowlkes A, Mohebbi M. Assessing Google flu trends performance in the United States during the 2009 influenza virus A (H1N1) pandemic. PLoS One. 2011;6(8):e23610.
287. Dugas A, Hsieh Y, Levin S, Pines J, Mareiniss D, Mohareb A, et al. Google flu trends: correlation with emergency department influenza rates and crowding metrics. Clin Infect Dis. 2012;54:463–9.
288. Butler D. When Google got flu wrong. Nature. 2013;494:155–6.

289. Lazer D, Kennedy R, King G, Vespignani A. Big data. The parable of Google flu: traps in big data analysis. Science. 2014;343:1203–5.
290. Martin L, Xu B, Yasui Y. Improving Google flu trends estimates for the United States through transformation. PLoS One. 2014;10(4):e0122939.
291. Santillana M, Zhang D, Althouse B, Ayers J. What can digital disease detection learn from (an external revision to) Google flu trends? Am J Prev Med. 2014;47:341–7.
292. Yang S, Santillana M, Brownstein J, Gray J, Richardson S, Kou S. Using electronic health records and internet search information for accurate influenza forecasting. BMC Infect Dis. 2017;17:332.
293. Agarwal V, Zhang L, Zhu J, Fang S, Cheng T, Hong C, et al. Impact of predicting health care utilization via web search behavior: a data-driven analysis. J Med Internet Res. 2016;9:e251.
294. Yom-Tov E, Borsa D, Hayward A, McKendry R, Cox I. Automatic identification of web-based risk markers for health events. J Med Internet Res. 2016;17(1):e29.
295. Tideman S, Santillana M, Bickel J, Reis B. Internet search query data improve forecasts of daily emergency department volume. J Am Med Inform Assoc. 2019;26:1574–83.
296. Henry S, McInnes B. Literature based discovery: models, methods, and trends. J Biomed Inform. 2017;74:20–32.
297. Swanson D. Two medical literatures that are logically but not bibliographically connected. Perspect Biol Med. 1986;30:7–18.
298. Swanson D. Migraine and magnesium: eleven neglected connections. Perspect Biol Med. 1988;31:526–57.
299. Swanson D, Smalheiser N. An interactive system for finding complementary literatures: a stimulus to scientific discovery. Artif Intell. 1997;91:183–203.
300. Weeber M, Vos R, Klein H, DeJong-VanDenBerg L, Aronson A, Molema G. Generating hypotheses by discovering implicit associations in the literature: a case report of a search for new potential therapeutic uses for thalidomide. J Am Med Inform Assoc. 2003;10:252–9.
301. Srinivasan P. Text mining: generating hypotheses from MEDLINE. J Am Soc Inf Sci Tec. 2004;55:396–413.
302. Srinivasan P, Libbus B. Mining MEDLINE for implicit links between dietary substances and diseases. Bioinformatics. 2004;20:i290–i6.
303. Seki K, Mostafa J, editors. Discovering implicit associations between genes and hereditary diseases. Pacific symposium on biocomputing. Maui, Hawaii: World Scientific; 2007.
304. Hettne K, Weeber M, Laine M, tenCate H, Boyer S, Kors J, et al. Automatic mining of the literature to generate new hypotheses for the possible link between periodontitis and atherosclerosis: lipopolysaccharide as a case study. J Clin Peridontol. 2007;34:1016–24.
305. Smalheiser N, Swanson D. Using ARROWSMITH: a computer-assisted approach to formulating and assessing scientific hypotheses. Comput Methods Prog Biomed. 1998;57:149–53.
306. Torvik V, Smalheiser N. A quantitative model for linking two disparate sets of articles in MEDLINE. Bioinformatics. 2007;23:1658–65.
307. Smalheiser N. Literature-based discovery: beyond the ABCs. J Am Soc Inf Sci Tec. 2012;63:218–24.
308. Tafti A, Badger J, LaRose E, Shirzadi E, Mahnke A, Mayer J, et al. Adverse drug event discovery using biomedical literature: a big data neural network adventure. JMIR Med Inform. 2017;4:e51.
309. Brown A, Patel C. MeSHDD: literature-based drug-drug similarity for drug repositioning. J Am Med Inform Assoc. 2017;24:614–8.
310. Pérez-Rosas V, Kleinberg B, Lefevre A, Mihalcea R. Automatic detection of fake news. arXivorg. 2017;arXiv:1708.07104.
311. Shiralkar P, Flammini A, Menczer F, Ciampaglia G. Finding streams in knowledge graphs to support fact checking. arXivorg. 2017;arXiv:1708.07239.
312. Wen W, Su S, Yu Z. Cross-lingual cross-platform rumor verification pivoting on multimedia content. arXivorg. 2018;arXiv:1808.04911.

313. Hersh W, Crabtree M, Hickam D, Sacherek L, Friedman C, Tidmarsh P, et al. Factors associated with success for searching MEDLINE and applying evidence to answer clinical questions. J Am Med Inform Assoc. 2002;9:283–93.
314. Koopman B, Zuccon G, Bruza P. What makes an effective clinical query and querier? J Am Soc Inf Sci Tec. 2017;68:2557–71.
315. Markoff J. Searching for Michael Jordan? Microsoft wants a better way. New York: New York Times; 2007 March 7.
316. Dumais S, editor. Thinking outside the (search) box. User modeling, adaptation, and personalization, 17th international conference, UMAP 2009 proceedings, Trento, Italy. Berlin: Springer; 2009.
317. Hearst M. 'Natural' search user interfaces. Commun ACM. 2011;54(11):60–7.
318. Borlund P. Interactive information retrieval: an introduction. J Inf Sci Theory Pract. 2013;1:12–32.
319. Hofmann K, Li L, Radlinski F. Online evaluation for information retrieval. Foundations and trends in information retrieval. Delft: Now Publishers; 2016.
320. Hearst M. Search user interfaces. Cambridge: Cambridge University Press; 2009.
321. Wilson M. Search user interface design. Synthesis lectures on information concepts, retrieval, and services. San Rafael: Morgan and Claypool; 2012.
322. Shneiderman B, Plaisant C, Cohen M, Jacobs S, Elmqvist N, Diakopoulos N. Designing the user Interface: strategies for effective human-computer interaction. 6th ed. London: Pearson; 2016.
323. Pollitt A. CANSEARCH: an expert systems approach to document retrieval. Inf Process Manag. 1987;23:119–36.
324. Kingsland L, Harbourt A, Syed E, Schuyler P. COACH: applying UMLS knowledge sources in an expert searcher environment. Bull Med Libr Assoc. 1993;81:178–83.
325. Saracevic T, Kantor P. A study of information seeking and retrieving. III. Searchers, searches, and overlap. J Am Soc Inf Sci. 1988;39:197–216.
326. Hersh W, Over P, editors. TREC-9 interactive track report. The ninth text REtrieval conference (TREC-9). Gaithersburg, MD: National Institute of Standards and Technology; 2000.
327. Rose L, Crabtree K, Hersh W, editors. Factors influencing successful use of information retrieval systems by nurse practitioner students. In: Proceedings of the AMIA 1998 annual symposium. Orlando, FL: Hanley and Belfus; 1998.
328. Hersh W, Crabtree M, Hickam D, Sacherek L, Rose L, Friedman C. Factors associated with successful answering of clinical questions using an information retrieval system. Bull Med Libr Assoc. 2000;88:323–31.
329. Hersh W, Turpin A, Price S, Kraemer D, Olson D, Chan B, et al. Challenging conventional assumptions of automated information retrieval with real users: Boolean searching and batch retrieval evaluations. Inf Process Manag. 2001;37:383–402.
330. Hersh W, Turpin A, Price S, Kraemer D, Chan B, Sacherek L, et al., editors. Do batch and user evaluations give the same results? In: Proceedings of the 23rd annual international ACM SIGIR conference on research and development in information retrieval. Athens, Greece: ACM; 2000.
331. Hersh W, Turpin A, Sacherek L, Olson D, Price S, editors. Further analysis of whether batch and user evaluations give the same results with a question-answering task. The ninth text REtrieval conference (TREC-9). Gaithersburg, MD: National Institute of Standards and Technology; 2000.
332. Turpin A, Hersh W, editors. Why batch and user evaluations do not give the same results. In: Proceedings of the 24th annual international ACM SIGIR conference on research and development in information retrieval. New Orleans, LA: ACM; 2001.
333. Allan J, Carterette B, Lewis J, editors. When will information retrieval be "good enough?": user effectiveness as a function of retrieval accuracy. In: Proceedings of the 28th international ACM SIGIR conference on research and development in information retrieval. Salvador: ACM;2005.

334. Turpin A, Scholer F, editors. User performance versus precision measures for simple search tasks. In: Proceedings of the 29th annual international ACM SIGIR conference on research and development in information retrieval. Seattle, WA: ACM; 2006.
335. Belkin N, Cool C, Kelly D, Lin S, Park S, Perez-Carballo J, et al. Iterative exploration, design and evaluation of support for query reformulation in interactive information retrieval. Inf Process Manag. 2000;37:403–34.
336. Robertson S, Walker S, Beaulieu M, editors. Okapi at TREC-7: automatic ad hoc, filtering, VLC, and interactive track. The seventh text REtrieval conference (TREC-7). Gaithersburg, MD: National Institute of Standards and Technology; 1998.
337. Yang K, Maglaughlin K, Newby G. Passage feedback with IRIS. Inf Process Manag. 2000;37:521–41.
338. Wu M, Fuller M, Wilkinson R. Using clustering and classification approaches in interactive retrieval. Inf Process Manag. 2000;37:459–84.
339. Wu M, Fuller M, Wilkinson R, editors. Searcher performance in question answering. In: Proceedings of the 24th annual international ACM SIGIR conference on research and development in information retrieval. New Orleans, LA: ACM; 2001.
340. Allan J. Building hypertext using information retrieval. Inf Process Manag. 1997;33:145–60.

Correction to: Retrieval

Correction to: Chapter 5 in: W. Hersh, *Information Retrieval: A Biomedical and Health Perspective*, Health Informatics, https://doi.org/10.1007/978-3-030-47686-1_5

The original version of the book was inadvertently published with wrong Equations 5.2, 5.3 and 5.4, and the revised equations were updated in the chapter as follows,

$$\text{Document weight} = \frac{\sum\limits_{\text{all query terms}} (\text{Weight of term in query} * \text{Weight of term in document})}{\sqrt{\left(\sum\limits_{\text{all query terms}} \text{Weight of term in query}^2\right) * \left(\sum\limits_{\text{all document terms}} \text{Weight of term in document}^2\right)}} \tag{5.2}$$

$$\begin{aligned} &\text{New query weight} = \\ &\alpha * \text{Original query weight} \\ &+\beta * \frac{1}{\text{number of relevant documents}} * \sum_{\text{all relevant documents}} \text{weight in document} \\ &-\gamma * \frac{1}{\text{number of nonrelevant documents}} * \sum_{\text{all nonrelevant documents}} \text{weight in document} \end{aligned} \tag{5.3}$$

$$\begin{aligned} &\text{New query weight} = \\ &\text{Original query weight} \\ &+\text{Average term weight in relevant documents} \\ &-\text{Average term weight in nonrelevant documents} \end{aligned} \tag{5.4}$$

The updated online version of this chapter can be found at https://doi.org/10.1007/978-3-030-47686-1_5

W. Hersh, *Information Retrieval: A Biomedical and Health Perspective*,
Health Informatics, https://doi.org/10.1007/978-3-030-47686-1_9

Index

W. Hersh, *Information Retrieval: A Biomedical and Health Perspective*,
Health Informatics, https://doi.org/10.1007/978-3-030-47686-1

J

K

R

S

T

U

Printed in the United States
by Baker & Taylor Publisher Services